BIOLOGICALLY
INSPIRED
ROBOTICS

T0076473

BIOLOGICALLY INSPIRED
INSPIRED
ROBOTICS

Edited by
Yunhui Liu and Dong Sun

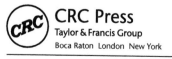

CRC Press
Taylor & Francis Group
Boca Raton London New York

CRC Press is an imprint of the
Taylor & Francis Group, an **informa** business

Cover images courtesy of Professor Hu Huosheng, University of Essex (robot fish, top), and © 2006 Lehrstuhl fürSteuerungs- und Regelungstechnik (EDDIE, bottom).

CRC Press
Taylor & Francis Group
6000 Broken Sound Parkway NW, Suite 300
Boca Raton, FL 33487-2742

First issued in paperback 2019

© 2012 by Taylor & Francis Group, LLC
CRC Press is an imprint of Taylor & Francis Group, an Informa business

No claim to original U.S. Government works

ISBN-13: 978-1-4398-5488-4 (hbk)
ISBN-13: 978-0-367-38178-3 (pbk)

Library of Congress Cataloging-in-Publication Data

Biologically inspired robotics / editors, Yunhui Liu and Dong Sun.
    p. cm.
  Includes bibliographical references and index.
  ISBN 978-1-4398-5488-4 (hardback)
    1. Robotics. 2. Bionics. 3. Biomimicry. 4. Biomechanics. I. Liu, Yunhui. II. Sun, Dong, 1967- III. Title.

TJ211.B5553 2011
629.8'92--dc22   2011008352

Visit the Taylor & Francis Web site at
http://www.taylorandfrancis.com

and the CRC Press Web site at
http://www.crcpress.com

Contents

Preface... vii

Contributors...xi

1 **Introduction to Biologically Inspired Robotics**......................... 1
   Yunhui Liu and Dong Sun

2 **CPG-Based Control of Serpentine Locomotion of a Snake-Like Robot** 13
   Xiaodong Wu and Shugen Ma

3 **Analysis and Design of a Bionic Fitness Cycle** 33
   Jun Zhang, Ying Hu, Haiyang Jin, and Zhijian Long, and Jianwei Zhang

4 **Human-Inspired Hyper Dynamic Manipulation** 55
   Aiguo Ming and Chunquan Xu

5 **A School of Robotic Fish for Pollution Detection in Port** 85
   Huosheng Hu, John Oyekan, and Dongbing Gu

6 **Development of a Low-Noise Bio-Inspired Humanoid Robot Neck**.. 105
   Bingtuan Gao, Ning Xi, Jianguo Zhao, and Jing Xu

7 **Automatic Single-Cell Transfer Module** 125
   Huseyin Uvet, Akiyuki Hasegawa, Kenichi Ohara, Tomohito Takubo, Yasushi Mae, and Tatsuo Arai

8 **Biomechanical Characterization of Human Red Blood Cells with Optical Tweezers**.. 147
   Youhua Tan, Dong Sun, and Wenhao Huang

9 **Nanorobotic Manipulation for a Single Biological Cell**................... 165
   Toshio Fukuda, Masahiro Nakajima, and Mohd Ridzuan Ahmad

10 **Measurement of Brain Activity Using Optical and Electrical Methods**... 189
   Atsushi Saito, Alexsandr Ianov, and Yoshiyuki Sankai

11 **Bowel Polyp Detection in Capsule Endoscopy Images with Color and Shape Features** 205
    Baopu Li and Max Q.-H. Meng

12 **Classification of Hand Motion Using Surface EMG Signals** 219
    Xueyan Tang, Yunhui Liu, Congyi Lu, and Weilun Poon

13 **Multifunctional Actuators Utilizing Magnetorheological Fluids for Assistive Knee Braces** 239
    H. T. Guo and W. H. Liao

14 **Mathematical Modeling of Brain Circuitry during Cerebellar Movement Control** 263
    Henrik Jörntell, Per-Ola Forsberg, Fredrik Bengtsson, and Rolf Johansson

15 **Development of Hand Rehabilitation System Using Wire-Driven Link Mechanism for Paralysis Patients** 277
    Hiroshi Yamaura, Kojiro Matsushita, Ryu Kato, and Hiroshi Yokoi

16 **A Test Environment for Studying the Human-Likeness of Robotic Eye Movements** 295
    Stefan Kohlbecher, Klaus Bartl, Erich Schneider, Jürgen Blume, Alexander Bannat, Stefan Sosnowski, Kolja Kühnlenz, Gerhard Rigoll, and Frank Wallhoff

Index 313

Preface

Biologically inspired robotics is an interdisciplinary subject between robotics and biology that mainly involves two technical areas. The first technical area concerns how to apply biological ideas and phenomena to engineering problems in robotics. In this area, robotics scientists are extensively engaging in design of new robots or robot mechanisms that mimic creatures, invention of new types of sensors that function similarly to biological sensing systems, development of control algorithms that perform as well as a biological sensory–motor control scheme does, design of new actuators that function as muscles, etc. These efforts are indeed robotic engineering inspired by biology and are also called *biomimetics*. The primary issue of the second technical area is how to apply robotics technology to understanding of biological systems and their behaviors. The topics in the second area include robotic modeling of biological systems, simulations of biological behaviors, understanding of biological recognition and motor functions, etc. The second area is also called *bio-robotic modeling/analysis* and its objective is to bring robotics technology to biology via new breakthroughs.

The research of biologically inspired engineering can be traced back to a few centuries ago. A famous example is the development of flying machines that mimic flying birds. Probably the earliest work on biologically inspired robotics is the humanoid robots developed by Ichiro Kato and his colleagues in the early 1970s. Since then, biologically inspired robotics has been one of the hottest and fastest-growing topics in robotics and many important achievements have been made. For example, humanoid robots that are similar to humans in appearance and behaviors, robotic snakes, insects, fish, and so on, have been developed in the last 20 years. Efforts in biologically inspired robotics are not only restricted to research work in laboratories; novel applications of the technology are also being extensively explored in services, education, rehabilitation, medical care, and other sectors.

The objective of this book is to introduce the latest efforts in research on biologically inspired robotics. It is edited based on the original works presented at the 2009 IEEE International Conference on Robotics and Biomimetics (ROBIO) held during December 20–23, 2009, in Guilin, China. ROBIO is an international conference particularly focused on biologically inspired robotics. More than 500 robotics researchers from around the world took part in ROBIO 2009. We selected 15 excellent works from 450 presentations at the conference and requested that the authors contribute extended versions of the papers as chapters of this book. The content covers both biomimetics and bio-robotic modeling/analysis. Chapters on biologically inspired robot design and control, bio-sensing, bio-actuation, and micro/nano bio-robotic systems address the subject of biomimetics. Works on human hand motion recognition using biological signals, modeling of human brain activities, characterization of cell properties using robotic systems, etc., deal with bio-robotic modeling/analysis. In order to provide readers with a better understanding of organization of this book, we classified the content into the following four parts: biologically inspired robot design and control, micro/nano bio-robotic systems, biological measurement and actuation, and applications of robotics technology to biological problems.

This book starts with a brief introduction to biologically inspired robotics in Chapter 1. Chapters 2–6, which form the first part of the book, are focused on biologically inspired robot design and control. Chapter 2 presents a biomimetic controller for controlling the motion of a robotic snake with a large number of degrees of freedom based on the concept of central pattern generator, which is a rhythmical motion generator existing in most animals. Chapter 3 introduces a bionic fitness cycle called the Bio-Cycle, inspired by the cheetah, for physical exercises and relaxation. By mimicking the running and walking mechanisms of a cheetah, the Bio-Cycle enables user to easily change speed of type of motion in order to fit different fitness needs. Chapter 4 addresses the realization of highly skilled manipulation/motion performed by some athletes using a smart mechanical mechanism. Chapter 5 is focused on the biologically inspired design of autonomous robotic fish and their application to pollution detection in port. Chapter 6 presents the design of a low-noise neck mechanism of a humanoid robot by mimicking the motion of a human neck.

The second part of the book consists of Chapters 7, 8, and 9 with a focus on the state of the art of micro/nano bio-robotic systems. Chapter 7 presents an automated single-cell transfer module with a vision-based nondestructive cell detection system for microfluidic applications examining or processing cells. Chapter 8 addresses biomechanical characterization of mechanical properties of human red blood cells using a microrobotic system, which is a problem in bio-robotic analysis. Chapter 9 introduces the state-of-the-art technology of nanorobotic manipulation of single biological cells.

We introduce biological measurement and actuation in the third part, consisting of Chapters 10–15. Chapter 10 proposes a noninvasive brain activity scanning method using an innovative hybrid sensor that simultaneously measures both optical and electrical signals of the brain. This hybrid sensor makes it possible to measure the brain activities of patients who cannot produce bioelectric brain signals due to severe spinal cord injury or advanced stages of amyotrophic lateral sclerosis. Chapter 11 addresses biomedical detection using capsule endoscopy (CE) and presents a novel scheme for bowel polyp detection using CE images. Chapter 12 discusses classification of hand motion using surface electromyography (EMG). A novel measure that is robust to positions of the sensors, velocity of hand motion, and grasping forces is developed for classifying human hand motion. Chapter 13 proposes a multifunctional actuator using magnetorheological fluids for assistive knee braces. The novelty of the actuator lies in that it can work with multiple functions as motor, clutch, and brake in order to meet the requirements of normal human walking.

Applications of robotics technology to biological problems are addressed in the last part, which consists of Chapters 14, 15, and 16. Chapter 14 copes with mathematical modeling of brain circuitry during cerebellar movement control by characterizing incoming and outgoing signals of individual neurons during sensory activation. This is a typical example of using an engineering model to investigate the behaviors of biological systems. Chapter 15 presents a rehabilitation system for recovery of motor function of human hands after injury. The design of the system is based on a mechanical model of human fingers. Chapter 16 studies gaze and movement behaviors of human eyes in human–robot interactions for the design of a human-likeness vision system for robots.

The editors would like to express their sincere gratitude to the authors of all of the chapters in this book. We are also grateful to Li-Ming Leong and Jocelyn Banks-Kyle of CRC Press and Taylor & Francis Asia Pacific for their invaluable comments and help in proposing and preparing this book. It was the greatest pleasure to work with the authors and the editorial staff and to learn from them while working on this exciting project.

Yunhui Liu
Dong Sun
City University of Hong Kong

Contributors

Mohd Ridzuan Ahmad
Department of Electronic Engineering
Universiti Teknologi Malaysi
Skudai Johor, Malaysia
(e-mail: ridzuan@fke.utm.my)

Tatsuo Arai
Department of Systems Innovation
Osaka University
Osaka, Japan
(e-mail: t_chayooth@arai-lab.
sys.es.osaka-u.ac.jp)

Alexander Bannat
Institute for Human–Machine
Communication
Technische Universität München
Munich, Germany
(e-mail: bannat@tum.de)

Klaus Bartl
Institute of Clinical Neurosciences
University of Munich Hospital
Munich, Germany
(e-mail: kbartl@nefo.med.
uni-muenchen.de)

Fredrik Bengtsson
Section for Neurophysiology
Department of Experimental
Medical Science
Lund University
Lund, Sweden
(e-mail: fredrik.bengtsson@med.lu.se)

Jürgen Blume
Institute for Human–Machine
Communication
Technische Universität München
Munich, Germany
(e-mail: blume@tum.de)

Per-Ola Forsberg
Section for Neurophysiology
Department of Experimental
Medical Science
Lund University
Lund, Sweden
(e-mail: perola.forsberg@gmail.com)

Toshio Fukuda
Department of Micro-Nano
Systems Engineering
Nagoya University
Nagoya, Japan
(e-mail: fukuda@mein.nagoya-u.ac.jp)
and
Center For Micro-Nano Mechatronics
Nagoya University
Nagoya, Aichi, Japan

Bingtuan Gao
School of Electrical Engineering
Southeast University
Nanjing, China
(e-mail: gaobingtuan@seu.edu.cn)
and
Department of Electrical and
Computer Engineering
Michigan State University
East Lansing, Michigan
(e-mail: xin@egr.msu.edu)

Dongbing Gu
School of Computer Science and
Electronic Engineering
University of Essex
Colchester, UK
(e-mail: dgu@essex.ac.uk)

H. T. Guo
Department of Mechanical and
  Automation Engineering
The Chinese University of Hong Kong
Hong Kong, China
(e-mail: htguo@mae.cuhk.edu.hk)

Akiyuki Hasegawa
Institute of Advanced Biomedical
  Engineering and Science
Tokyo Women's Medical University
Tokyo, Japan
(email: ahasegawa@abmes.twmu.ac.jp)

Huosheng Hu
School of Computer Science and
  Electronic Engineering
University of Essex
Colchester, UK
(e-mail: hhu@essex.ac.uk)

Ying Hu
Shenzhen Institutes of
  Advanced Technology
Chinese Academy of Sciences
Shenzhen, China
(e-mail: ying.hu@siat.ac.cn)
and
The Chinese University of Hong Kong
Hong Kong, China

Wenhao Huang
Department of Precision Machinery
  and Precision Instrumentation
University of Science and
  Technology of China
Hefei, China
(e-mail: whuang@ustc.edu.cn)

Alexsandr Ianov
Systems and Information Engineering
University of Tsukuba
Tsukuba, Japan
(e-mail: ianov@golem.kz.tsukuba.ac.jp)

Haiyang Jin
Shenzhen Institutes of
  Advanced Technology
Chinese Academy of Sciences
Shenzhen, China
(e-mail: hy.jin@sub.siat.ac.cn)
and
The Chinese University of Hong Kong
Hong Kong, China

Rolf Johansson
Department of Automatic Control
Lund University
Lund, Sweden
(e-mail: Rolf.Johansson@control.lth.se)

Henrik Jörntell
Section for Neurophysiology
Department of Experimental
  Medical Science
Lund University
Lund, Sweden
(e-mail: Henrik.Jorntell@med.lu.se)

Ryu Kato
Department of Mechanical Engineering
  and Intelligent Sytems
The University of
  Electro-Communications
Tokyo, Japan
(e-mail: kato@mce.uec.ac.jp)

Stefan Kohlbecher
Institute of Clinical Neurosciences
University of Munich Hospital
Munich, Germany
(e-mail: skohlbecher@nefo.
  med.uni-muenchen.de)

Kolja Kühnlenz
Institute for Advanced Study
  (IAS) / Institute of Automatic
  Control Engineering (LSR)
Technische Universität München
Munich, Germany
(e-mail: koku@tum.de)

Baopu Li
Department of Electronic Engineering
The Chinese University of Hong Kong
Hong Kong, China
(e-mail: bpli@ee.cuhk.edu.hk)

W. H. Liao
Department of Mechanical and
  Automation Engineering
The Chinese University of Hong Kong
Shatin, N.T., Hong Kong, China
(e-mail: whliao@mae.cuhk.edu.hk)

Yunhui Liu
Department of Precision Mechanical
  and Automation Engineering
The Chinese University of Hong Kong
Hong Kong, China
(e-mail: yhliu@mae.cuhk.edu.hk)

Zhijian Long
Shenzhen Institutes of
  Advanced Technology
Chinese Academy of Sciences
Shenzhen, China
(e-mail: zj.long@sub.siat.ac.cn)
and
The Chinese University of Hong Kong
Hong Kong, China

Congyi Lu
Department of Mechanical and
  Automation Engineering
The Chinese University of Hong Kong
Hong Kong, China
(e-mail: cylu@mae.cuhk.edu.hk)

Shugen Ma
Department of Robotics
Ritsumeikan University
Shiga, Japan
(e-mail: shugen@se.ritsumei.ac.jp)

Yasushi Mae
Department of Systems Innovation
Osaka University
Osaka, Japan
(e-mail: mae@sys.es.osaka-u.ac.jp)

Kojiro Matsushita
Osaka University Medical School
Osaka, Japan
(e-mail: matsushita@nsurg.
  med.osaka-u.ac.jp)

Max Q.-H. Meng
Department of Electronic Engineering
The Chinese University of Hong Kong
Hong Kong, China
(e-mail: max@ee.cuhk.edu.hk)

Aiguo Ming
Department of Mechanical Engineering
  and Intelligent Systems
The University of
  Electro-Communications
Tokyo, Japan
(e-mail: ming@mce.uec.ac.jp)

Masahiro Nakajima
Center For Micro-Nano Mechatronics
Nagoya University
Nagoya, Japan
(e-mail: nakajima@mein.nagoya-u.ac.jp)

Kenichi Ohara
Department of Systems Innovation
Osaka University
Osaka, Japan
(e-mail: k-oohara@ari-lab.
  sys.es.osaka-u.ac.jp)

John Oyekan
School of Computer Science and
  Electronic Engineering
University of Essex
Colchester, UK
(e-mail: jooyek@essex.ac.uk)

Weilun Poon
Department of Mechanical and
  Automation Engineering
The Chinese University of Hong Kong
Hong Kong, China
(e-mail: wlpoon@mae.cuhk.edu.hk)

Gerhard Rigoll
Institute for Human–Machine
  Communication
Technische Universität München
Munich, Germany
(e-mail: rigoll@tum.de)

Atsushi Saito
Systems and Information Engineering
University of Tsukuba
Tsukuba, Japan
(e-mail: saito@golem.kz.tsukuba.ac.jp)

Yoshiyuki Sankai
Systems and Information Engineering
University of Tsukuba
Tsukuba, Japan
(e-mail: sankai@golem.kz.tsukuba.ac.jp)

Erich Schneider
Institute of Clinical Neurosciences
University of Munich Hospital
Munich, Germany
(e-mail: eschneider@nefo.
  med.uni-muenchen.de)

Stefan Sosnowski
Institute of Automatic Control
  Engineering (LSR)
Technische Universität München
Munich, Germany
(e-mail: sosnowski@tum.de)

Dong Sun
Department of Manufacturing
  Engineering and Engineering
  Management
City University of Hong Kong
Hong Kong, China
(e-mail: medsun@cityu.edu.hk)

Tomohito Takubo
Department of Systems Innovation
Osaka University
Osaka, Japan
(e-mail: takubo@arai-lab.
  sys.es.osaka-u.ac.jp)

Youhua Tan
Department of Manufacturing
  Engineering and Engineering
  Management
City University of Hong Kong
Hong Kong, China
(e-mail: youhuatan2@cityu.edu.hk)

Xueyan Tang
Department of Mechanical and
  Automation Engineering
The Chinese University of Hong Kong
Hong Kong, China
(e-mail: xytang@mae.cuhk.edu.hk)

Huseyin Uvet
Department of Mechatronics Engineering
College of Mechanical Engineering
Yildiz Technical University
Istanbul, Turkey
(e-mail: huvet@yildiz.edu.tr)

Frank Wallhoff
Institute of Hearing Technology
  and Audiology
Jade University of Applied Sciences
Oldenburg, Germany
(e-mail: frank.wallhoff@jade-hs.de)

Xiaodong Wu
Department of Robotics
Ritsumeikan University
Shiga, Japan
(e-mail: gr041087@ed.ritsumei.ac.jp)

Ning Xi
Department of Electrical and
  Computer Engineering
Michigan State University
East Lansing, Michigan
(e-mail: xin@egr.msu.edu)

Chunquan Xu
Department of Mechanical Engineering
  and Intelligent Systems
The University of
  Electro-Communications
Tokyo, Japan
(e-mail: xu@rm.mce.uec.ac.jp)

Jing Xu
*Department of Electrical and
    Computer Engineering
Michigan State University
East Lansing, Michigan
(e-mail: xujing0829@gmail.com)*

Hiroshi Yamaura
*Panasonic Corporation
Osaka, Japan
(e-mail: yamaura.hiroshi@
    jp.panasonic.com)*

Hiroshi Yokoi
*Department of Mechanical Engineering
    and Intelligent Sytems
The University of
    Electro-Communications
Tokyo, Japan
(e-mail: yokoi@mce.uec.ac.jp)*

Jianwei Zhang
*TAMS
University of Hamburg
Hamburg, Germany
(e-mail: jw.zhang@siat.ac.cn)*

Jun Zhang
*Shenzhen Institutes of
    Advanced Technology
Chinese Academy of Sciences
Shenzhen, China
(e-mail: jun.zhang@siat.ac.cn)
and
The Chinese University of Hong Kong
Hong Kong, China*

Jianguo Zhao
*Department of Electrical and
    Computer Engineering
Michigan State University
East Lansing, Michigan
(e-mail: zhaojia1@msu.edu)*

1

Introduction to Biologically Inspired Robotics

Yunhui Liu

The Chinese University of Hong Kong
Hong Kong, China

Dong Sun

City University of Hong Kong
Hong Kong, China

CONTENTS

1.1 What Is Biologically Inspired Robotics? 1
1.2 History...2
1.3 Biologically Inspired Robot Design..5
1.4 Biologically Inspired Robot Control..5
1.5 Biologically Inspired Actuation and Sensing 9
1.6 Conclusion 11
References...11

Abstract

This chapter gives a brief introduction to biologically inspired robotics. We will discuss what biological inspired robotics is, its major topics, and brief history. Some well-known biologically inspired robots and technology will be also introduced.

1.1 What Is Biologically Inspired Robotics?

Biologically inspired robotics is an interdisciplinary subject of robotics and biology and consists of mainly two broad areas: biomimetics and bio-robotic modeling/analysis. Biomimetics draws inspiration from biology, and its primary concern is the application of biological ideas and phenomena to engineering problems in robotics. The topics cover almost every technical aspect of robotics including biologically inspired design, motion control, sensing, and

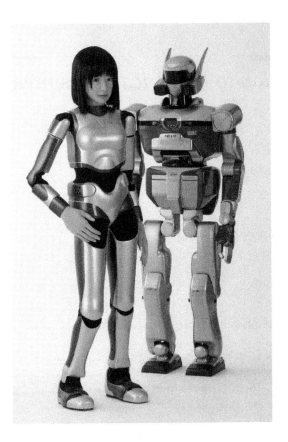

FIGURE 1.1
The humanoid robot, HRP-2 developed at AIST, Japan.

actuation of robotic systems. A typical example of biomimetic robots is the humanoid robot, which is analogous with a human being in appearance and behavior (Figure 1.1). *Bio-robotic modeling/analysis* is the application of robotic models and principles to address biological issues such as recognition processes of the human brain, behaviors of animals and insects, etc. For example, by using a model of a biomimetic robotic fish, it is possible to study the swimming dynamics of fish; it may be possible to model sensory motor control of human arms using a bionic arm.

1.2 History

Humans have tried to create mechanical systems that mimic the behaviors of animals and other living creatures for a long time. The history can be traced back to development of the mechanical drink-serving waitress and musical players by Arab scholar and craftsman Al-Jazari in the thirteenth century and mechanical puppets or dolls such as the well-known Japanese *karakuri ningyo* in the eighteenth and nineteenth centuries. Probably the most famous example is the tremendous effort made to development of flying machines in the early twentieth century.

Designing robots that mimic animals and other living creatures dates back to the 1940s and 1950s (Beer 2009). The robotic tortoises developed by W. Gray Walter (Walter 1963) are most closely related to biologically inspired robotics. The tortoises are driven by motorized wheels and equipped with a light sensor and touch sensor. They are mobile robots indeed! When talking about the history of biomimetic robotics, it is necessary to note the work of Ichiro Kato's group at Waseda University in the early 1970s on design and control of biped robots (http://www.wikipedia.org/wiki/Humanoid_robot). They developed the first biped robot, WaBOT-1, in 1973 and a musician robot that played the piano in 1984. Their work laid the foundation for the research and development of present-day humanoid robots. Since the early 1980s, inspired by motion of snakes and spiders, Hirose and his group have designed several snake robots and legged robots (Hirose and Yamda 2009). Figure 1.2 shows the latest design of a snake robot created at the Shenyang Institute of Automation (China; Z. Liu et al. 2006). In 1997, Honda presented the first humanoid robot, Asimo, that truly has a humanoid appearance and integrates computer, control, sensing systems, power, and into a single stand-alone body (Hirai 1997). Since then, several humanoid robots, such as the Sony humanoid robot QRIO (Movellan et al. 2004), the AIST humanoid robot HRP-2 (Kaneko et al. 2004; Figure 1.1), and the BIT humanoid robot

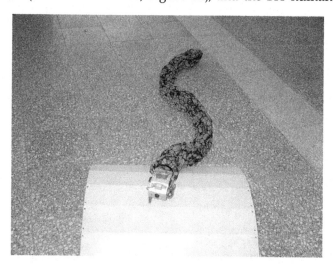

FIGURE 1.2
Robotic snake developed by Z. Liu et al. (2006) at the Shenyang Institute of Automation and Ritsumeikan University.

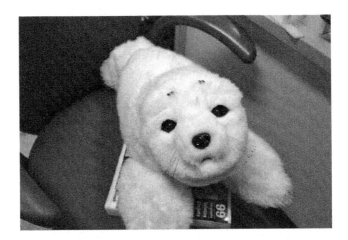

FIGURE 1.3
Seal-mimetic robot PARO developed by Shibata (2004) at AIST, Japan.

BHR-2 (Huang et al. 2005), have been developed in Japan, Europe, and China. The early biomimetic robots for entertainment include the robotic dog AIBO developed by Sony and the seal-mimetic robot PARO by Shibata (2004; Figure 1.3). With the advancement of sensing, actuation, and information technology, biologically inspired robotics is advancing rapidly with extensive study by robotics researchers and increasing investment from industries and governments worldwide. Different robots or robotic systems inspired by animals, insects, and fish have been developed. Figure 1.4 shows a robotic fish developed by Hu at the University of Essex (J. Liu, Dukes, and Hu 2005). Biomimetics has become one of the fastest growing topics in robotics in recent years.

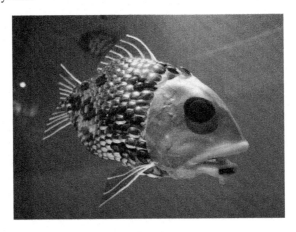

FIGURE 1.4
Robotic fish developed by J. Liu et al. (2005) at the University of Essex.

1.3 Biologically Inspired Robot Design

Designing mechanisms for robots that mimic the motion of animals and other living creatures is one of the core problems in biologically inspired robotics. The mechanisms of movement vary for different animals and other living creatures. Many mammals, such as cats, tigers, horses, etc., use four legs to move around, but humans rely on two legs to move. Spiders use legs to climb, but snakes climb without legs. The challenging issue here is how to realize biological movement using mechanical structures. Biological motion is generated by the interaction of muscles, joints, and tissues of a continuum deformable body. There are no actuators that are as sophisticated as muscles, materials that are as soft as tissues, or joints that generate the complicated yet smooth motion that human and animal joints perform. Therefore, it is crucial to develop simplified mechanisms that can generate motion similar to biological motion.

For example, a snake moves forward and backward using the frictional force between its body and the ground. Its body is a deformable continuum whose geometric shape is used to control the frictional force. The snake can change its speed by changing the shape of its body. Because it is difficult to design a mechanical structure that can deform freely and continuously by active control, existing robotic snakes employ a series of movable segments that are connected by a joint (Figure 1.5). Moreover, the snake relies on its skin to slide on the ground, and such skin cannot be made by current technologies, so wheels are attached to the segments. If the connection joint allows the rotation about one axis, the robotic snake moves in a plane. If the connection joint is a spherical joint that allows rotation about two perpendicular axes, the robotic snake can move in three-dimensional space; for example, to climb a tree.

By observing the motion of animals and insects, researchers have designed legged robots including biped or humanoid robots, four-legged robots that mimic the mechanisms of animal movement, and robots with eight, twelve, or even more legs. Legged robots move by repeatedly lifting and moving their legs backward or forward as animals do. Figure 1.6 shows a four-legged and a six-legged mobile robot. Other examples of biomimetic robots include the robotic fish developed at the University of Essex (see Figure 1.4).

1.4 Biologically Inspired Robot Control

The behaviors of animals and other living creatures inspire the development of new ideas for controlling the motion or behaviors of robots. In principle, robotic control and biological control systems are similar. They all work

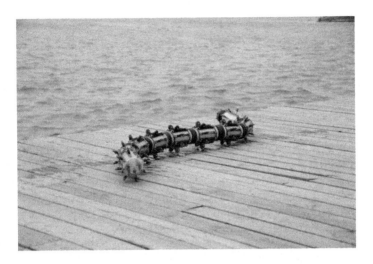

FIGURE 1.5
Design of a robotic snake by Z. Liu et al. (2006).

on the basis of sensory motor control. Biological systems are controlled by expansion and contraction of the muscles based on information collected by the biological sensors such as eyes, skin, ears, nose, etc. Robotic systems are controlled based on information feedback from robotic sensors using their actuators. The underlying principle for both robotic and biological systems is feedback control. Traditionally, researchers have designed control algorithms for robots using conventional methodologies and theories in controlling engineering. Different from traditional approaches, biologically inspired controllers are designed based on new philosophy inspired by biological systems. Typical examples of biologically inspired approaches for robot control are behavior control, proposed by Brooks at the Massachusetts Institute of Technology (Brooks 1987); iterative learning control, developed by Arimoto et al. (1985); and intelligent control methods including genetic algorithms (Parker, Khoogar, and Goldberg 1989) and swarm control (Fukuda and Kawauchi 1990).

Behavior control was originally developed to solve the problem of motion control for mobile robots. Traditionally, researchers have followed the procedure of sensing–perception–planning–control for controlling the motion of a mobile robot. In this method, the robot first uses its sensors to acquire information from the surrounding environment. Second, the acquired information is processed and interpreted. As the third step, a motion is planned for the robot based on the information interpreted. Finally, the robot executes the planned motion. It was found that this sequential approach was not very useful for navigation of mobile robots because it took a lot of time to process and interpret the information and to plan the motion. Behavior control employs the idea of *reactive control*, which is a typical behavior of biological

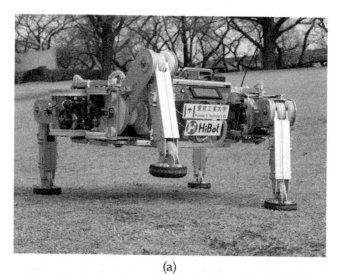

(a)

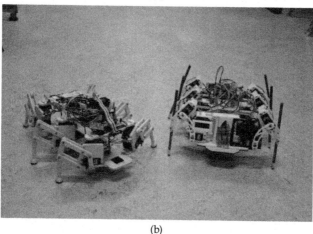

(b)

FIGURE 1.6
(a) Four-legged robot designed by Hirose and Yamada (2009) at the Tokyo Institute of Technology and (b) six-legged mobile robots.

systems. When physical stimulation is received by the human body, the body will immediately react to the stimulation. For example, when your hand gets too close to a hot stove, your hand will automatically move away from the source of heat once it feels hot. In behavior control, there are a number of primitive behaviors that are reactive responses to information collected by a sensor or a group of sensors in parallel (Figure 1.7). Primitive behaviors are arranged in a hierarchical structure so that coordination among them can be easily carried out. This approach is widely used in navigation control of mobile robots.

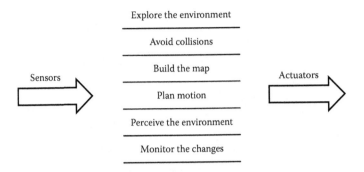

FIGURE 1.7
Concept of behavior-based control.

Iterative learning control was developed by Arimoto in 1982 based on observation of the human learning process of drawing lines, circles, and letters. When I was in primary school, whenever the teacher taught us a new Chinese character, he always asked us to write the character twenty or thirty times after class. The process of learning new characters is as follows: we first tried to write the character and then compared what we wrote (real trajectory in robotics) with the model (desired trajectory) so that we could correct our hand inputs the next time. By repeating this cycle several times, we could always write the character well. Iterative learning control actually simulates this process. Consider the case of a robot drawing a circle using iterative learning. Denote the desired trajectory of the robot in drawing the circle by $\left(\mathbf{q}_d(t), \dot{\mathbf{q}}_d(t), \ddot{\mathbf{q}}_d(t)\right)$ and the real trajectory of the robot at the kth trial by $\left(\mathbf{q}_k(t), \dot{\mathbf{q}}_k(t), \ddot{\mathbf{q}}_k(t)\right)$. Let $\mathbf{u}_k(t)$ represent the joint input of the robot manipulator at the kth trial. $\mathbf{y}_k(t)$ denotes the output of the robot at the kth trial, and $\mathbf{y}_d(t)$ is the desired output. The output could be either the velocity or the position of the robot. The input $\mathbf{u}_{k+1}(t)$ of the robot at the next trial, that is, the $(k+1)$-th trial, is given by the following P-type learning process:

$$\mathbf{u}_{k+1}(t) = \mathbf{u}_k(t) + \mathbf{K}(\mathbf{y}_d(t) - \mathbf{y}_k(t)) \tag{1.1}$$

where K is the positive-definite learning gain. The asymptotic convergence of the position error of the robot manipulator under iterative learning control has been proved using Lyapunov's theory. Figure 1.8 shows a block diagram of the iterative learning controller. Arimoto, Naniwa, and Suzuki (1990) also developed a D-type learning controller and a learning controller with a forgetting factor.

A *genetic algorithm* is a heuristic optimization method inspired by natural evolution of biological systems. It uses evolution algorithms to search for the optimal solution. Genetic algorithms have been used in robotics for optimal control, planning, etc. Swarm control is inspired by the group behaviors of ants. A single ant has very limited ability to transport food. However, a group of

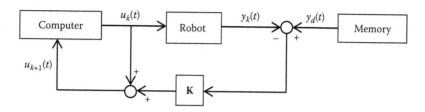

FIGURE 1.8
Block diagram of *P*-type iterative learning control.

ants can transport a large amount of food that is much heavier than the weight of a single ant. *Swarm control* is a decentralized and self-organized method for achieving collective behaviors of multiple robots, such as formation control, etc.

1.5 Biologically Inspired Actuation and Sensing

Sensors and actuators are major components of robotic systems. Development of robot actuators that function similar to muscles has long been a goal in the field of robotics. Muscles generate force by contraction of muscle fibers. The rubbertuator (Wang et al. 1992), developed by Bridgestone Corporation (Japan) in 1985, was the first commercial actuator that had similar characteristics to human muscles. The rubbertuator is made from rubber tubes covered by braided fibers. By shortening and lengthening the rubber tubes as compressed air is fed in or blended out, it is possible to rotate a joint in a robotic arm. The advantage of using rubber as the actuator is that it can control not only the position but the impedance/force of the robotic system. Unfortunately, the rubbertuator was not a successful product mainly because it was not suitable for many applications. In recent years, different artificial muscles, such as those using ionic polymer–metal composites (IPMCs; Kaneda et al. 2003; Oguro, Kawami, and Takenaka 1992), nanotubes, and polyacrylonitrile, have been developed. The IMPC-based artificial muscle uses electricity to control its deformation. The IMPC is made by coating a platinum or gold layer on an ion-exchange membrane, which is a perfluorosulfonic acid membrane. When an external voltage is applied to the metal layers, the ions of the ion-exchange membrane are attracted to the electrodes with water molecules. As a result, one side of the membrane will expand and the other side will shrink, so the IPMC bends at a high speed. The polyacrylonitrile artificial muscle uses the change of the pH value to contract. Artificial muscles have many potential applications such as in design of prosthetic limbs and in robotics, but tremendous efforts must still be made in design, modeling, analysis of characteristics, and control before the technology is mature.

Biologically inspired sensing involves two aspects: design of robot sensors based on biological sensors such as skin, eyes, ears, etc., and sensing biological signals of humans for robotic applications. Research on biologically inspired sensors includes efforts made in computer vision, in particular stereo vision, and development of tactile sensors, artificial ears and noses, etc. The work in sensing biological signals includes electromyography (EMG) and electroencephalography (EEG) measurements for robot control and human–robot interactions. Figure 1.9 shows the surface EMG signals

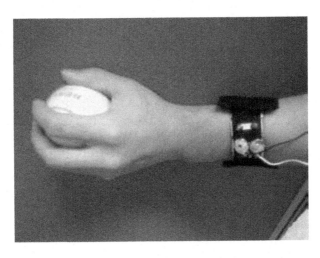

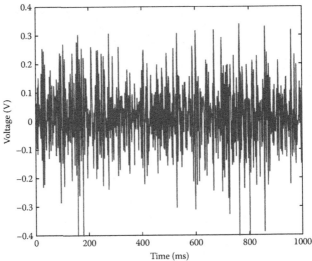

FIGURE 1.9
EMG measurement: (a) the surface EMG sensing ring developed by Liu et al. (see Chapter 12) at the Chinese University of Hong Kong and (b) measured signals.

measured when a hand grasps a ball. If it is possible to directly understand the intention of a person from his EEG/EMG signals, we can develop an EEG/EMG-based closed-loop control system for prosthetic limbs so that the artificial limbs could perform as well as the original limbs do. Similarly, by understanding the EEG signals generated by the brain when it is thinking, it will be possible to develop a mind-reading interface for robots to directly read the human mind.

1.6 Conclusion

Biologically inspired robotics is an emerging and fast growing area. It is an interdisciplinary subject that encompasses biology and engineering areas, including mechanical, electronic, control, and computer engineering. Biologically inspired robotics covers the topics of robot design, sensors, actuators, control systems/algorithms, etc. Tremendous research efforts are being made in biologically inspired robotics worldwide. This book presents a collection of works on the latest developments in related topics in this ever-growing area. The purpose is to help our readers gain insight and understanding of the technology and principles in this area.

References

http://www.wikipedia.org/wiki/Humanoid_robot. Last modified August 7, 2011.

Arimoto, S., Kawamura, S., Miyazaki, F., and Tamaki, S. 1985. Learning control theory for dynamic systems. *Proceedings of the 24th IEEE International Conference on Decision and Control*, 24(1): 1375–1380.

Arimoto, S., Naniwa, T., and Suzuki, H. 1990. Robustness of P-type learning control with a forgetting factor for robot motions. *Proceedings of the 29th IEEE Conference on Decision and Control*, Honolulu, HI, December 5–7, 1990.

Beer, R.D., 2009. Biologically inspired robotics. Scholarpedia. http://www.scholarpedia.org/article/Biologically_inspired_robotics

Brooks, R.A. 1987. A hardware retargetable distributed layered architecture for mobile robot control. Paper read at the IEEE International Conference on Robotics and Automation, Raleigh, NC, March 31–April 3, 1987.

Fukuda, T. and Kawauchi, Y. 1990. Cellular robotic system (CEBOT) as one of the realization of self-organizing intelligent universal manipulator. Paper read at the IEEE International Conference on Robotics and Automation, Cincinnati, OH, May 13–18, 1990.

Hirai, K. 1997. Current and future perpectives of Honda humanoid robot. *Proceedings of IEEE/RSJ Interntional Conference on Intelligent Robots and Systems*, 2: 500–509.

Hirose, S. and Yamda, H. 2009. Snake-like robots. *IEEE Robotics and Automation Magazine*, 167(1): 88–98.

Huang, Q. Peng, Z., Zhang, W., Zhang, L. and Li, K. 2005. Design of humanoid complicated dynamic motion based on human motion capture. *Proceedings of IEEE/ RSJ International Conference on Intelligent Robots and Systems*, pp. 3536–3541, Edmonton, Canada, August 2–5, 2005.

Kaneda, Y., Kamamichi, N., Yamakita, Y., Asaka, K., and Luo, Z.W. 2003. Control of linear artificial muscle actuator using IPMC. Paper read at the SICE Annual Conference, Fukui, Japan, August 4–6, 2003.

Kaneko, K., Kanehiro, F., Kajita, S., Hirukawa, H., Kawasaki, T., Hirata, M., Akachi, K., and Isozumi, T. 2004. Humanoid Robot HRP-2. *Proceedings of 2004 IEEE/RSJ International Conference on Robotics and Automation*, New Orleans, Louisiana, April 2004.

Liu, J., Dukes, I., and Hu, H. 2005. Novel mechatronics design for a robotic fish. Paper read at the IEEE/RSJ International Conference on Intelligent Robots and Systems, Edmonton,Canada, August 2–6, 2005.

Liu, Z., Ma, S., Li, B., and Wang, Y.C. 2006. 3D locomotion of a snake-like robot controlled by cyclic inhibitory CPG model. Paper read at the IEEE/RSJ International Conference on Intelligent Robots and Systems, Beijing, October 9–15, 2006.

Movellan, J.R., Tanaka, F., Fortenberry, B., and Aisaka, K. 2005. The RUBI-QRIO Project: Origins, principles, and first steps. *Proceedings of the 4th International Conferneces on Development and Learning*, pp. 80–86, Osaka, Japan, July 19–21, 2005.

Oguro, K., Kawami, Y., and Takenaka, H. 1992. Bending of an ion-conducting polymer film-electrode composite by an electric stimulus at low voltage. *Journal of the Micromachine Society*, 5: 27–30. (in Japanese)

Parker, J.K., Khoogar, A.R., and Goldberg, D.E. 1989. Inverse kinematics of redundant robots using genetic algorithms. Paper read at the IEEE International Conference on Robotics and Automation, Scottsdale, AZ, May 14–19, 1989.

Shibata, T. 2004. An overview of human interactive robot for psychological enrichment. *Proceedings of the IEEE*, 92(11): 1794–1758.

Walter, W.G. 1963. *The Living Brain*, 2nd ed. New York: W. W. Norton and Company.

Wang, X., Matsushita, T., Sagara, S., Katoh, R., and Yamashita, T. 1992. Two approaches to force control by rubbertuator-driven mechanism applications of IMC and SMC. Paper read at the International Conference on Industrial Electronics, Control, Instrumentation and Automation, San Diego, CA, November 9–13, 1992.

2

CPG-Based Control of Serpentine Locomotion of a Snake-Like Robot

Xiaodong Wu and Shugen Ma

Ritsumeikan University
Shiga, Japan

CONTENTS

2.1   Introduction 14
2.2   CPG Models for Generation of Rhythmic Motion 15
2.3   CPG Network for Control of a Snake-Like Robot 16
        2.3.1   CPG Network with Feedback Connection 17
        2.3.2   Analysis of a CPG Network 20
2.4   CPG-Controlled Snake-Like Robot 22
        2.4.1   Control of the Locomotion Curvature 23
        2.4.2   Control of the Locomotion Speed 24
        2.4.3   Control of the Number of S-Shapes 24
        2.4.4   Control of the Turning Motion 25
        2.4.5   Control of the Round Motion 26
2.5   Experiments 26
2.6   Summary 29
References 31

Abstract

A biomimetic approach is proposed to solve the difficulty in controlling a snake-like robot with a large number of degrees of freedom. This method is based on the central pattern generator (CPG), which is a rhythmical motion generator existing in most animals. To solve the problems in the previous CPG network, a new network with a feedback connection is presented that can generate uniform outputs without any adjustment. Furthermore, the relation characteristics between the CPG parameters and the outputs are investigated. Based on the results of the influence of each parameter, desired motion patterns can be achieved by adjusting the CPG parameters correspondingly. Both simulation of and experiments with the snake-like robot have been taken for the analysis of the locomotion control.

2.1 Introduction

With elongated and limbless bodies, as well as scales, snakes perform many kinds of nimble motions, adapting to different kinds of environments. By using such advantageous characteristics of snakes, snake-like robots are expected to be applied to perform search or rescue tasks in an unstructured environment, where traditional mobile mechanisms cannot move well. However, it is difficult to control a snake-like robot effectively due to the fact that the robot has high degrees of freedom. Some eel-like or snake-like robots present elegant mechanical designs or life-like movements (see Ma 2001; McIsaac and Ostrowski 2000; Mori and Hirose 2002). These snake-like robots were designed to imitate the shape of snakes. Most are complicated models with numerous calculations or little environmental adaptability. Furthermore, it is difficult to change gait patterns using simple commands.

Recently, researchers have turned their attention to bio-inspired locomotion control methods. Animals can spontaneously carry out walking, respiration, and flying without any careful planning. Most of these rhythmic motions are controlled by a rhythm-generating mechanism, which is called the *central pattern generator* (CPG) (Mattia, Paolo, and Luigi 2004). The CPG can generate self-induced oscillation even without a high level command. Due to the advantage of the CPG in rhythmic motion control, many researchers have placed CPG schemes into the control of robots. By implementing CPG oscillators in the mechanism of a robot arm, more adaptive movement was performed (Williamson 1998). A dynamic gait was achieved through the use of a neural system model in a quadruped robot (Fukuoka, Kimura, and Cohen 2003). Based on biomimetic CPGs and on information from distributed distance sensors, neuromuscular motion control for an undulatory robot model was presented (Sfakiotakis and Tsakiris 2008). An amphibious robotic snake realized a crawl motion by utilizing an onboard CPG (Crespi and Ijspeert 2008). The generation of rhythmic and voluntary patterns of mastication has been tested on a humanoid chewing robot by using a CPG oscillator (Xu et al. 2009).

The rhythmic creeping motion of a snake can also be generated with a CPG mechanism. Much research has been conducted on snake-like robotic locomotion controlled by a CPG (see Conradt and Varshavskaya 2003; Inoue, Ma, and Jin 2004; Matsuo, Yokoyama, and Ishii 2007). Most of these studies employed a CPG network with a unilateral open-loop connection. The output of the CPG oscillator in this network requires an additional calculation to develop more suitable rhythmic signals for robot control due to its irregular output wave. In order to achieve a better signal without any additional calculation, a network with feedback connection was proposed to generate rhythmic output with uniform amplitude and phase difference (Wu and Ma 2010). The influence of each CPG parameter on the output of CPG was also analyzed. Based on results of the analysis, the locomotion control of a snake-like robot was verified through both simulation and experiment. The relation between the locomotion patterns and the CPG parameters were additionally obtained. In addition, how to obtain a different number of loco-motive *S*-shapes was analyzed for this kind of CPG network.

2.2 CPG Models for Generation of Rhythmic Motion

Various models of a CPG neuron have been proposed (Ekeberg 1993; Matsuoka 1985). The CPG model proposed by Ekeberg (1993) is structurally complicated and difficult to analyze numerically. However, the model of a CPG neuron proposed by Matsuoka (1985) has the features of continuous-time and continuous-variable in its simple structure and can thus be easily implemented into the control of the robot. Moreover, because Matsuoka's (1985) CPG model has been proven mathematically to generate rhythmic output, this neuron model was thus adopted for the control of our snake-like robot.

Several neurons are usually included in a CPG model (Matsuoka 1985). The neurons of the CPG are affected by each other. Through the interaction of neurons, a group of rhythmic outputs is provided. The structure of the individual neuron model is shown in Figure 2.1a. The mathematical model of each neuron can be expressed as

$$\tau_1 \dot{u} + u = u_0 - \beta v - \sum_{j=1}^{m} wy_j$$

$$\tau_2 \dot{v} + v = y \tag{2.1}$$

$$y = g(u) = \max(0, u)$$

where u is the membrane potential of the neuron; v is the variable that represents the degree of adaptation; y is the output of the CPG neuron, and its value is always positive; u_0 is the tonic driving input; τ_1 and τ_2 are the parameters that specify the time constants for membrane potential and adaptation degree, respectively; β is the adaptation coefficient; w is the weight between neurons; $\sum wy_j$ represents the input from other neurons; and m is the number of all of the neurons in the CPG model.

Usually, there are several ways to construct a CPG model by connecting different numbers of neurons. For instance, a dual-neuron model and a tri-neuron CPG model are shown in Figures 2.1b and 2.1c, respectively. These two CPG models have been adopted in the control systems of many bionic robots (Kimura, Akiyama, and Sakurama 1999; Lu et al. 2005). Due to the complicated structure and numerous computations, a CPG model with four or more neurons is not often used in practical applications. Because the

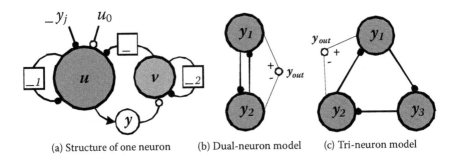

(a) Structure of one neuron   (b) Dual-neuron model   (c) Tri-neuron model

FIGURE 2.1
CPG models of neural oscillator.

output of an individual neuron always has a positive value, the output of the CPG module y_{out}, which is defined by subtracting the output of the second neuron y_2 from the first neuron y_1, is used to get a symmetrical rhythmic signal with both positive and negative values.

$$y_{out} = y_1 - y_2 \qquad (2.2)$$

For a CPG model, an initial stimulation is needed to promote the neurons to generate a group of rhythmic signals with a certain phase, like a high-level command from the cerebrum in a biological CPG.

2.3 CPG Network for Control of a Snake-Like Robot

The propelling force of the serpentine motion of a snake-like robot comes from the interaction of the robot with the ground by swinging the joints from side to side (Hirose 1993). The rhythmic signals implemented in the joint motors can be easily generated by a CPG network, as shown in Figure 2.2. Due to the fact that one joint angle corresponds to one CPG output, a series of successive rhythmic signals with a certain phase difference are required to realize snake-like locomotion control. Thus, several CPG modules are needed to construct a kind of network for mimicking the neural system of a snake.

For simplicity, an open-loop unilaterally connected CPG network has been efficiently employed for the control of s snake-like robot (Inoue, Ma, and Jin 2004; Lu et al. 2006). However, additional calculation is required to adjust the irregular output signal of this network. A CPG network with a cross-connected architecture has been used in the work of Matsuo, Yokoyama, and Ishii (2007). However, the number of connections in this network is two times more than our network and the calculations increased correspondingly. Furthermore, the phase difference in this network cannot be changed conveniently because of the strong couplings between the CPGs. To solve the

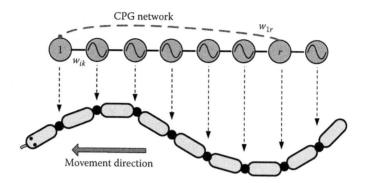

FIGURE 2.2
CPG network implemented to control a snake-like robot.

problems in these CPG networks, a closed-loop network with unidirectional couplings between the oscillators is proposed. This CPG network with a feedback connection can generate uniform outputs with the same amplitude and specific phase difference without any additional adjustment.

2.3.1 CPG Network with Feedback Connection

Based on the mathematical model of a single neuron as stated in Section 2.2, a CPG network that includes n CPG modules and has m neurons can be described in a group of basic equations. Regarding the jth neuron of the ith CPG module, the mathematical model can be described by

$$\tau_{1,i}\dot{u}_{j,i} + u_{j,i} = u_{0,i} - \beta v_{j,i} - wy_{s,i} - \sum_{k=1}^{n} w_{ik}y_{j,k}$$

$$\tau_{2,i}\dot{v}_{j,i} + v_{j,i} = y_{j,i}$$

$$y_{j,i} = g(u_{j,i}) = \max(0, u_{j,i})$$

$$y_{out,i} = y_{1,i} - y_{2,i} \qquad (2.3)$$

$$i, k = 1, 2, \ldots n, i \neq k; j = 1, 2, \ldots m;$$

$$s = \begin{cases} m, & \text{if } j = 1 \\ j-1, & \text{others} \end{cases}$$

$$w_{ik} = \begin{cases} w_0, & k = i-1 \\ w_0, & k = r, i = 1 \\ 0, & \text{others} \end{cases}$$

where n is the number of CPG modules in the network; m is the number of neurons in one CPG module; s is the serial number of neurons connected to the jth neuron; $u_{j,i}$ is the membrane potential of the jth neuron in the ith CPG module; $v_{j,i}$ is the variable that represents the degree of adaptation; $u_{0,i}$ is the tonic driving input; $\tau_{1,i}$ and $\tau_{2,i}$ are the time constants; β is the adaptation coefficient; w is the weight between neurons; w_{ik} is the connection weight of the ith module from the kth module; $y_{j,i}$ is the output of the jth neuron in the ith CPG module; $y_{out,i}$ is the output of the ith CPG module; w_0 is a constant value for connection weight; and r is the number of the CPG in the network with feedback connection.

The basic concept of this network is shown in Figure 2.2. Compared with the unilaterally connected network, this network has the same unidirectional couplings between the oscillators. The difference is that the output of the the rth CPG module is provided as feedback to the first module to form a closed loop. The connection weight between CPGs w_{ik} takes the same value from Equation (2.3). In addition, the weight of the feedback w_{1r} from the rth module to the first one should adopt a weight value, given by $w_{1r} = w_0$.

Because the rth CPG module transmits the same value to the $(r + 1)$-th and the first CPG module, the output waves of the $(r + 1)$-th and the 1st module have completely identical shapes and phases. The $(r + 1)$-th module will also transmit its output to the $(r + 2)$-th module as the first module transmits its output to the second module. Thus, the $(r + 2)$-th module will generate the same output as that of the second module. In the same way, the following output of CPG modules will take the similar process mentioned above as CPGs in the loop. Thus, the output of the CPG modules on the outside of the loop can be represented as

$$y_{out,pr+q} = y_{out,q} \quad p = 1, 2, ..., \quad q = 1, 2, ...r \quad (2.4)$$

To compare the output of a CPG network with a unilateral connection and feedback connection, a network composed of six CPG modules is constructed. For the network with feedback connection, the sixth module is selected to provide feedback to the first CPG module. The results are simulated by use of both the dual-neuron mutual inhibition model and the tri-neuron cyclic inhibitory model. Rhythmic outputs of CPG models with respect to the set of CPG parameters in Table 2.1 are shown in Figures 2.3 and 2.4.

As shown in Figure 2.3, the amplitude of the CPG outputs in the unilaterally connected network is not of uniform size and the waveforms cannot form a perfect traveling wave to suit the control of the multilink robot. Thus, it is necessary to make adjustments to obtain applicable rhythmic signals for control of the robot. The output of CPGs in Figure 2.4 has a feedback connection with the same amplitude and phase difference. Furthermore, it is obvious that all of the output waves of the CPG modules in the loop are

TABLE 2.1

Configuration of Parameters in the CPG Neuron

Driving input	u_0	2.5
Time constant	τ_1	2.0
Time constant	τ_2	6.0
Adaptation coefficient	β	2.5
Connection weight inner neurons	w	2.7
Connection weight among CPGs	w_0	0.1

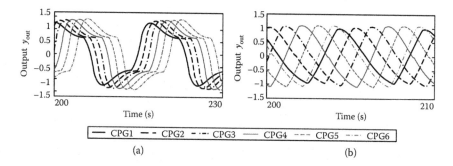

FIGURE 2.3

Rhythmic outputs of two kinds of CPG models using a unilaterally connected network: (a) mutual inhibitory model and (b) cyclic inhibitory model.

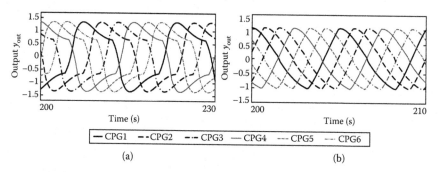

FIGURE 2.4

Rhythmic outputs of two kinds of CPG models in a closed-loop network: (a) mutual inhibitory model and (b) cyclic inhibitory model.

homogeneously distributed in one period (see Figure 2.4). Because the output of the CPG modules on the outside of the loop has the same phase as the CPGs in the loop, the phase difference between the two neighboring CPG modules in the whole network can be obtained by

$$\Phi = 2\pi / r \tag{2.5}$$

From the above discussion, we know that it is more convenient to obtain a uniform output from the CPG network by feeding one of the CPG signals back to the first module. This kind of closed-loop network can be applied to snake-like robot control without any additional modification on the output signals of the CPG. Thus, the system computation is decreased dramatically. Moreover, the characteristic of the phase difference as stated in Equation (2.5) can be used to control the number of S-shapes in snake-like robot locomotion. Therefore, this network with the feedback connection is more suitable for the control of a snake-like robot.

2.3.2 Analysis of a CPG Network

To figure out how to employ the CPG network to control locomotion of a snake-like robot, the influence of each CPG parameter on the signal output has to be investigated. In Matsuoka's early work (Matsuoka 1985, 1987), some partial and qualitative conclusions on the influence of the parameters on the oscillator behavior were indicated. But a detailed analysis of the CPG characteristics to generate the desired rhythmic signals in the network was not provided. Because there is a strong coupling relation between the parameters and the output, herein a numerical method is used to obtain the characteristics of the CPG model. To determine the influence of each parameter on the output, the output characteristic is studied with the value of one parameter varied in a certain range while the rest of the parameters remain unchanged.

From the mathematical model of the CPG model in Equation (2.1), the output is mainly determined by several parameters. The influence of these parameters on the amplitude and the period of oscillator output are primarily investigated. A cyclic inhibitory CPG model with three neurons is selected to study the influence of parameters, and the numerical results are shown in Figure 2.5. The value ranges of these parameters conform to the mathematical analysis for stable oscillation in Matsuoka (1987), where every parameter should meet the following numerical condition:

$$\begin{cases} w/(1+\beta) \le 1 \\ 1+\tau_1/\tau_2 < w \end{cases} \tag{2.6}$$

Summarizing these characteristics, a concise conclusion can be obtained from Table 2.2. Two important linear relations can be easily found: output amplitude increases linearly with the driving input u_0; time constant τ_1, τ_2 keeps a linear relation with the period of output while the value of τ_1/τ_2 is a constant. However, if τ_1/τ_2 is not a constant, the linear relation between time constant τ_1, τ_2 and the period of output will be broken. The change of parameter u_0 does not influence the period of the output, whereas the change of τ_1, τ_2 has no influence on the amplitude of the output. Furthermore, the basic

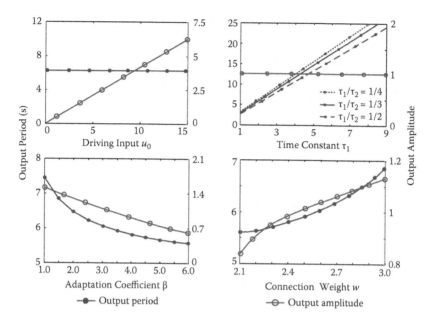

FIGURE 2.5
Results to show the relation between the CPG parameters and the CPG output.

TABLE 2.2
Change of the CPG Output with Respect to Each CPG Parameter

Parameters	Amplitude	Period	Wave Shape	Values Range
u_0	↗	—	No	$u_0 > 0$
τ_1, τ_2 with constant τ_1/τ_2	—	↗	No	$\tau_1 / \tau_2 \leq w - 1$
w	⤴	⤴	Yes	$1 + \tau_1 / \tau_2 \leq w < 1 + \beta$
β	⤵	⤵	No	$\beta > w - 1$

Linear increase: ↗ , unchanged: — , nonlinear increase: ⤴ , nonlinear decrease: ⤵

shape of the output wave is not affected by the driving input and time constant. For the parameters of the coefficient β and connection weight w, there are no such advantages. Thus, the driving input and time constant can be employed to adjust the CPG output by these two useful linear relations.

A snake-like robot performs locomotion with one S-shape when the sum of the total phase differences of the joints is 2π. The number of the locomotive S-shapes increases with respect to the increasing phase difference of joint angles. As stated in Section 2.3.1, the phase differences of CPG outputs are homogeneously distributed in one period if the network is a closed-loop type. From Equation (2.5), the sum of the total phase differences of a CPG's outputs can be derived by $(n-1)\Phi$ where n is the numbers of CPGs. Because one locomotive S-shape can be obtained by a group of rhythmic signals with total 2π, the number of the locomotive S-shapes, N, can be given by

$$N = \frac{(n-1)\Phi}{2\pi} = \frac{n-1}{r} \qquad (2.7)$$

Therefore, the number of the locomotive S-shape can be varied by changing the connection of rth CPG module to the first CPG module.

2.4 CPG-Controlled Snake-Like Robot

To verify the proposed CPG-based control method, a simulator for a snake-like robot has been developed in an open dynamics engine (ODE) environment, as shown in Figure 2.6. In the simulation, the interaction between the robot and the ground is modeled with asymmetric friction by using a larger normal friction coefficient μ_N and a smaller tangential friction coefficient μ_T. To realize this kind of friction model, a passive wheel is utilized for each link of the snake-like robot. The actuators are installed on the joints of the robot to make each joint swing from side to side, like the behavior of a snake. The physical parameters of our snake-like robot platform are given in Table 2.3. In the experiment, a closed-loop network with a feedback connection using a cyclic inhibitory CPG model was selected as the oscillation generator for the control of the snake-like robot. The output of the ith CPG was implemented

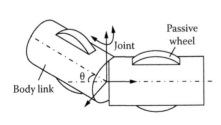
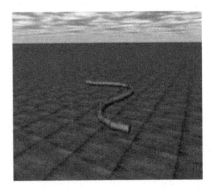

FIGURE 2.6
Simulation platform of the snake-like robot.

TABLE 2.3

Physical Parameters of the Simulated Robot

Numbers of joints	$Num = 10$
Length of link	$L_{link} = 0.13$ m
Radius of link	$R_{link} = 0.02$ m
Weight of link	$M_{link} = 0.2$ kg
Width of wheel	$L_{wheel} = 0.01$ m
Radius of wheel	$R_{wheel} = 0.03$ m
Weight of wheel	$M_{wheel} = 0.08$ kg
Friction coefficients	$\mu_N = 0.5, \mu_T = 0.02$

on the ith joint as the angle input signal. Each angle of the robot joint θ_i can be calculated by

$$\theta_i = \alpha_i y_{out,i} \tag{2.8}$$

where α_i is a gain from the control signal to the joint angle. Here, each α_i takes the same value due to the uniform CPG output (the value of α_i was considered as 1.0 with respect to the set of parameters in Table 2.1).

2.4.1 Control of the Locomotion Curvature

A snake often changes the curvature of its body to adapt to different terrain during locomotion. For instance, a large locomotion curvature is adapted for slippery ground. In the simulation, we found that if the amplitude of CPG output increased, the curvature of the snake-like robot increased correspondingly. Thus, due to the linear relation between the CPG output amplitude and the parameter driving input u_0, a different locomotion curvature can be obtained by adjusting u_0. Figure 2.7a shows the average curvature, which is

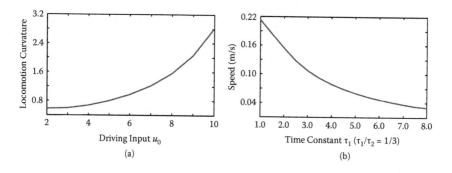

FIGURE 2.7
(a) Locomotion curvature with respect to CPG driving input and (b) motion speed with respect to CPG time constant.

derived from the reciprocal value of the snake-like robot axial distance $1/l_{axis}$ (l_{axis} is the distance of the snake-like robot along its axial axis), changed with respect to increased driving input. Here we take one *S*-shape for locomotion and the other parameters are fixed at the values given in Table 2.1.

2.4.2 Control of the Locomotion Speed

Robot speed is mainly affected by locomotion frequency. As stated in Section 2.3.2, the period of CPG output maintains a linear relationship with the time constant. Thus, the speed of the robot can be controlled by proportionally adjusting the time constant. Herein, time constant τ_1 and τ_2 are adjusted with the value of τ_1/τ_2 kept at a constant. From the result of the simulation shown in Figure 2.7b, we find that the motion speed decreases with an increasing in the time constant, because this increase makes the period of the CPG output become longer.

2.4.3 Control of the Number of S-Shapes

The number of *S*-shapes is an important motion parameter in snake-like locomotion and describes the number of periods of the sinusoidal wave existing in a snake-like locomotion shape. Based on the above analysis, we changed the CPG network by different feedback connections to obtain the desired number of locomotive *S*-shapes. For a snake-like robot with thirteen joints in the simulation, when connecting the twelfth CPG module with the first one, the robot can generate only one *S*-shape, shown in Figure 2.8a; when connecting the sixth CPG module with the first one, it can generate

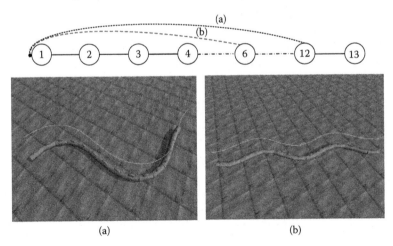

FIGURE 2.8
Number of *S*-shapes changed through feeding different CPG modules: (a) one *S*-shape and (b) two *S*-shapes.

two *S*-shapes, shown in Figure 2.8b. The same results can also be obtained from Equation (2.7) where $n = 13$ and $r = 12$ and 6, respectively.

2.4.4 Control of the Turning Motion

A common behavior of most robots when they meet an obstacle in the forward direction is to turn left or right to avoid the barrier. The snake-like robot can also perform a turn motion to avoid the obstacles. However, due to the characteristics of the creep motion of the snake-like robot generated by swinging the joints from side to side, the mechanism for performing a turn motion is totally different from that in wheeled drive robots (Wu and Ma 2009).

When the rhythmic excitations exerted on each joint of the snake-like robot are sinusoidal waves, a symmetrical undulatory locomotion will be obtained. Because the winding angles to the left and right balance out, the robot proceeds in a straight line of travel on balance. However, as shown in Figure 2.9, if the amplitude of a wave in the half period is altered from A to B, this change will be transmitted to the next joint successively after a constant interval Δt and thus the balance state will be shifted accordingly. Subsequently, the overall direction of the snake-like robot will be changed. Here, interval Δt should be the same value as the phase difference between the CPGs so that the change of the parameters can be continuous. This can be calculated from Equation (2.5). Due to the linear relation between the output amplitude and the driving input u_0 of the CPG, the value of the bias ΔA can be adjusted by driving input u_0 directly. Thus, a right or left turning motion can be executed by exerting a positive or negative bias Δu_0 on the amplitude of the joint angles from the head to the tail.

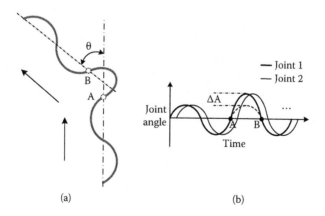

(a)   (b)

FIGURE 2.9
(a) Trajectory of a turn motion for the snake-like robot and (b) change of the angle signals of the joints during the turn motion.

TABLE 2.4

Relation between the Direction of the Robot and the
Controlled Bias Input

Orientation of the Head	$\Delta u_0 > 0$	$\Delta u_0 < 0$
Right	Turn left	Turn right
Left	Turn right	Turn left

It is difficult to apply a uniform rule such as a left or right turn for wheeled drive robots to the snake-like robot. The turn direction of the creeping motion is mainly determined by two factors: the sign of bias Δu_0 and the direction of the head module at the time when the signal begins shifting. If the orientation of the head is toward the right, a positive value of bias Δu_0 will carry out a left turn, whereas a negative value of bias Δu_0 will cause a right turn. A reverse situation occurs when the orientation of the head is toward the left. The principle for controlling the direction of a snake-like robot is shown in Table 2.4.

2.4.5 Control of the Round Motion

With an elongated and limbless body, a snake can perform not only turn motions to avoid an obstacle but also round motions to escape from irregular terrain. This is one of the most important characteristics of the snakes that is different from other animals. Utilizing this advantage of the snake, the snake-like robot can also creep through barriers conveniently.

In order to achieve this kind of motion, the frequency of the excitation signal for the first joint angle is altered from A to B in the half period, as shown in Figure 2.10. This change is transmitted to the next joint consecutively in the same way as that in turning motion. From Figure 2.10b, we can see that the increment of the signal period has resulted in a smaller phase difference between two adjacent joint angles. Thus, the locomotion curve of the snake-like robot will have larger motion amplitude. Consequently, an asymmetric forward locomotion to pass around the obstacle is achieved. From the above discussion of the linear relation between the output period and the time constant (τ_1 and τ_2) of the CPG, the desired output can be generated by changing the time constant. This means that the round motion can be performed while the time constant is changed from the head joint to the tail joint one joint at a time with a constant interval.

2.5 Experiments

To verify the validity of the CPG-based control system, some experiments were carried out on our snake-like robot (Figure 2.11). The robot model is composed

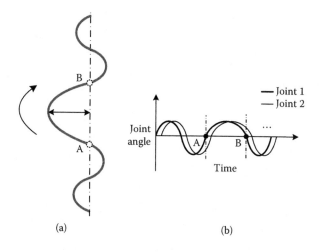

(a) (b)

FIGURE 2.10
(a) Trajectory of a round motion for the snake-like robot and (b) change of the angle signals of the joints during the round motion.

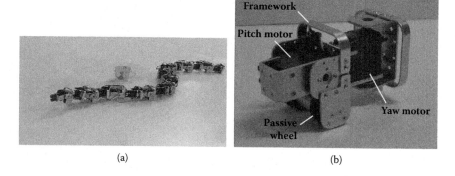

(a) (b)

FIGURE 2.11
(a) Overview of our snake-like robot and (b) mechanical structure of one module.

of ten segments that are connected serially. A two-degrees-of-freedom joint that can rotate on a vertical axis (yaw) and a horizontal axis (pitch) is located between each link. Herein, we will only consider the snake-like robot moving on a two-dimensional horizontal plane. The mechanical structure of the joint unit is shown in Figure 2.11b. At the bottom of the robot, two passive wheels are mounted to realize asymmetric friction in normal and tangential directions.

The control system design of the snake-like robot is shown as Figure 2.12. One module corresponds to one driving motor at each joint. Herein, inter-intergrated circuit (I2C) communication has been adopted to realize the closed-loop CPG network connection. All of the control modules are connected together by an I2C communication bus. The direction of information

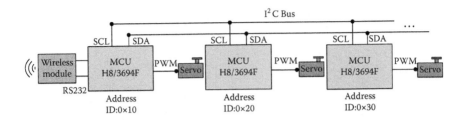

FIGURE 2.12
Design of the control system.

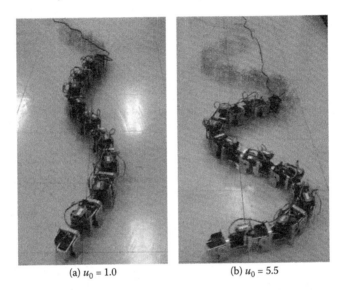

(a) $u_0 = 1.0$ (b) $u_0 = 5.5$

FIGURE 2.13
Movement with different locomotion curvatures: (a) motion trajectory with $u_0 = 1.0$ and (b) motion trajectory with $u_0 = 5.5$.

transmission is based on the ID address of each microprogrammed control unit (MCU). A wireless module using a 2.4-GHz band is installed on the head module to receive the signal for online control. By using outputs derived from the CPG-based control system, the snake-like robot successfully exhibits meandering locomotion.

According to the above discussion of CPG-based control of the snake-like robot, we evaluated the simulation result. As shown in Figure 2.13, the locomotion curvature of the snake-like robot changed with respect to the driving input u_0. With the same setting of the CPG network as that in Figure 2.13, the robot performs meandering locomotion with different S-shapes, as shown in Figure 2.14. It must be pointed out that, due to the limited the number of links in the snake-like robot, the robot mechanism restricts the increment of the number of locomotive S-shapes. Herein, the largest number of S-shapes

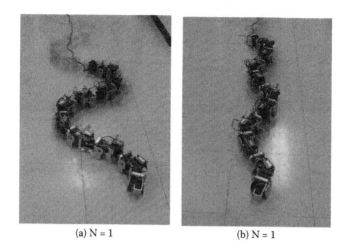

(a) N = 1   (b) N = 1

FIGURE 2.14
Movement with different numbers of S-shapes: (a) motion trajectory with one S-shape and (b) motion trajectory with two S-shapes.

of our ten-link snake-like robot is limited to two. Moreover, the method for changing motion speed by adjusting locomotion frequency was verified by experiment. Though the snake-like robot keeps the same curvature and S-shape as shown in Figure 2.13b, the motion velocity of the robot becomes 0.0839 and 0.1694 m/s with respect to the different time constant of the CPG (τ_1, τ_2) of (4.0, 12.0) and (2.0, 6.0). Because the robot will slip more frequently with the increase of speed of motion, the frequency of locomotion cannot be set too high.

By implementing the proposed control method in Sections 2.4.4 and 2.4.5, the snake-like robot can exhibit a changed locomotion for obstacle avoidance. As shown in Figure 2.15, when the robot encounters an obstacle, a command of turn motion can be sent to the CPG controller by the wireless module, and then an asymmetric locomotion is perform to avoid the obstacle. A round motion of the snake-like robot is also conducted experimentally as shown in Figure 2.16. In the experiments, a continuous locomotion curve of the snake-like robot was performed during the transmission of angle signals from the head joint to the tail joint.

2.6 Summary

In this chapter, a bio-inspired system imitating the CPG neural network has been proposed as the control method for a snake-like robot. The CPG network with a feedback connection does not necessitate additional adjustments

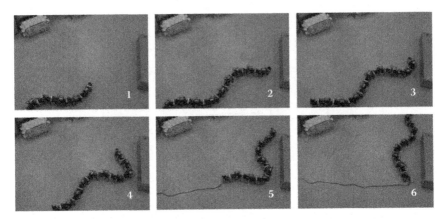

FIGURE 2.15
Experimental view of the snake-like robot avoiding an obstacle with a turning motion.

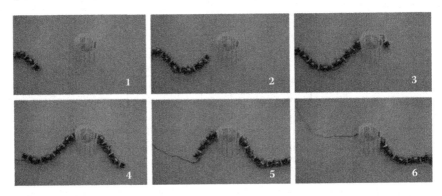

FIGURE 2.16
Experimental view of the snake-like robot avoiding an obstacle with a round motion.

of the CPG output due to its uniform outputs with the same amplitude and specific phase difference. The influence of CPG parameters on the rhythmic output was investigated and the relation curves were also obtained. By implementing CPG neural oscillators into the simulation platform, the CPG-based locomotion control of a snake-like robot has been analyzed. It was shown that the locomotion curvature of the robot and the motion velocity can be changed by adjusting the CPG parameters driving input and time constant. If these two parameters are changed from the head to tail joint with a constant interval as the phase difference, a turn motion or round motion can be performed. Furthermore, a desired number of locomotive S-shapes can be achieved by using a different feedback connection in the CPG network. Experiments have been conducted to verify the proposed CPG-based control method.

One of the important features of the CPG-based neural system is that it can not only receive inputs from a higher level of the central nervous system but also from peripheral receptors (Mattia, Paolo, and Luigi 2004). Thus, its functioning results from an interaction between central commands and local reflexes (Heliot and Espiau 2008). This concept allows us to achieve coordination between the snake's joints and environmental information by using a neural oscillator network-based controller. How to utilize this feature to achieve adaptive locomotion control of the snake-like robot will be an interesting research topic.

References

Conradt, J. and Varshavskaya, P. 2003. Distributed central pattern generator control for a serpentine robot. *Proceedings of Artificial Neural Networks and Neural Information Processing*, pp. 338–341.

Crespi, A. and Ijspeert, A.J. 2008. Online optimization of swimming and crawling in an amphibious snake robot. *IEEE Transactions on Robotics*, 24(1): 75–87.

Ekeberg, O. 1993. A combined neuronal and mechanical model of fish swimming. *Biological Cybernetics*, 69(5–6): 363–374.

Fukuoka, Y., Kimura, H., and Cohen, A.H. 2003. Adaptive dynamic walking of a quadruped robot on irregular terrain based on biological concepts. *International Journal of Robotics Research*, 22(3–4): 187–202.

Heliot, R. and Espiau, B. 2008. Multisensor input for CPG-based sensory-motor coordination. *IEEE Transactions on Robotics*, 24(1): 191–195.

Hirose, S. 1993. *Biologically Inspired Robots: Snake-Like Locomotors and Manipulators*. New York: Oxford University Press.

Inoue, K., Ma, S., and Jin, C. 2004. Neural oscillator network-based controller for meandering locomotion of snake-like robot. *Proceedings of the International Conference on Robotics and Automation*, pp. 5064–5069.

Kimura, H., Akiyama, S., and Sakurama, K. 1999. Realization of dynamic walking and running of the quadruped using neural oscillator. *Autonomous Robots*, 7(3): 247–258.

Lu, Z., Ma, S., Li, B., and Wang, Y. 2005. Serpentine locomotion of a snake-like robot controlled by cyclic inhibitory CPG model. *Proceedings of the International Conference on Intelligent Robots and Systems*, pp. 3019–3024.

Lu, Z., Ma, S., Li, B., and Wang, Y. 2006. 3D Locomotion of a snake-like robot controlled by cyclic inhibitory CPG model. *Proceedings of the International Conference on Intelligent Robots and Systems*, pp. 3897–3902.

Ma, S. 2001. Analysis of creeping locomotion of a snake-like robot. *Advanced Robotics*, 15(2): 205–224.

Matsuo, T., Yokoyama, T., and Ishii, K. 2007. Development of neural oscillator based motion control system and applied to snake-like robot. *Proceedings of the International Conference on Intelligent Robots and Systems*, pp. 3697–3702.

Matsuoka, K. 1985. Sustained oscillations generated by mutually inhibiting neurons with adaptation. *Biological Cybernetics*, 52(6): 367–376.

Matsuoka, K. 1987. Mechanisms of frequency and pattern control in the neural rhythm generators. *Biological Cybernetics*, 56(5–6): 345–353.

Mattia, F., Paolo, A., and Luigi, F. 2004. *Bio-Inspired Emergent Control of Locomotion Systems*. World Scientific Publishing.

McIsaac, K. and Ostrowski, J. 2000. Motion planning for dynamic eel-like robots. *Proceedings of the IEEE International Conference on Robotics and Automation*, pp. 1695–1700.

Mori, M. and Hirose, S. 2002. Three-dimensional serpentine motion and lateral rolling by active cord mechanism ACMR3. *Proceedings of the International Conference on Intelligent Robots and Systems*, pp. 829–834.

Sfakiotakis, M. and Tsakiris, D. 2008. Neuromuscular control of reactive behaviors for undulatory robots. *Neurocomputing*, 70(10–12): 1907–1913.

Williamson, M.M. 1998. Rhythmic robot arm control using oscillators. *Proceedings of the International Conference on Intelligent Robots and Systems*, pp. 77–83.

Wu, X. and Ma, S. 2009. CPG-controlled asymmetric locomotion of a snake-like robot for obstacle avoidance. *Proceedings of the International Conference on Robotics and Biomimetics*, pp. 69–74.

Wu, X. and Ma, S. 2010. CPG-based control of serpentine locomotion of a snake-like robot. *Mechatronics*, 20(2): 326–334.

Xu, W.L., Clara Fang, F., Bronlund, J., and Potgieter, J. 2009. Generation of rhythmic and voluntary patterns of mastication using Matsuoka oscillator for a humanoid chewing robot. *Mechatronics*, 19(2): 205–217.

3

Analysis and Design of a Bionic Fitness Cycle

Jun Zhang, Ying Hu, Haiyang Jin, and Zhijian Long
Shenzhen Institutes of Advanced Technology
Chinese Academy of Sciences
Shenzhen, China
and
The Chinese University of Hong Kong
Hong Kong, China

Jianwei Zhang
University of Hamburg
Hamburg, Germany

CONTENTS

3.1   Introduction..34
3.2   Bionic Analysis and Scheme 36
  3.2.1   Bionic Analysis of the System 36
  3.2.2   Mechanism Scheme-Based Multidrive Modes...........38
3.3   Ergonomic Analysis and Mechanism Design 39
  3.3.1   Design of the Pedal Crank and Hand Crank..............40
  3.3.2   Design of the Saddle Pole 41
  3.3.3   Handle Design...43
3.4   Design of the Compound Resistance System 44
  3.4.1   Analysis of Driving Characteristics.............................44
  3.4.2   Principle of the Compound Resistance System...........46
  3.4.3   Detection of Exercise Motions 47
3.5   Development and Test...51
3.6   Conclusions..51
References...53

Abstract

As the quality of life is rising constantly, the fitness industry has developed quickly, and the innovation and development of fitness equipment has been in high demand. In this chapter, a new type of fitness cycle is introduced, the so-called Bionic Fitness Cycle (Bio-Cycle), which can be driven using either hands or legs or any combination of any hand and leg. By changing the riding mode, the user can do many different exercises such as stair-climbing, cheetah-like running, horse-like walking, and so on, as well as cycling. The new motion modes and unique transmission mechanism are analyzed, followed by the design of a four-drive transmission system. After the ergonomical design of the structure, a compound resistance system based on electromagnetic principles is analyzed and its principle for control and exercise motion determination is introduced. Finally, a Bio-Cycle prototype is developed and tested.

3.1 Introduction

Due to the high amount of stress that people are under in their daily lives and work, more attention is given to physical exercise and relaxation. In this trend, there is a high demand for innovation in the fitness industry; many institutes and companies have been involved in the research and development of fitness equipment. By increasing the exercise mode of the fitness apparatus and improving their interaction, the new generations of fitness apparatus are more intersting and effective (Wang 2008).

The fitness cycle is a popular kind of fitness equipment both at home and in the gym. It derives from a road bike and follows the bike's exercise form. At present, by the style of its structure, the fitness cycle can be classified into three types: upright cycle, recumbent cycle, and hand cycle, as shown in Figure 3.1. The upright cycle and recumbent cycle use two different riding postures of the normal fitness cycle. In contrast to the former two, the hand cycle is driven by hand and is only for hand exercise; however, its transmission mechanism is the same as that of the traditional bike. Many different fitness cycles have been developed in the past years; however, most improvements have focused on comfort and safety rather than on their drive mechanism and riding form.

The Bio-Cycle introduced in this study provides a brand new sports concept. With a four-drive transmission system, it can be driven by either hands or legs or any combination of any hand and leg. When riding the Bio-Cycle, the user can change the riding mode easily. Its most prominent feature is that users can ride it using the bionic mode of cheetah-like riding. Different from traditional fitness cycles, it can be driven by hands and legs to imitate a cheetah or a horse's run. Its novelty is not only that it can

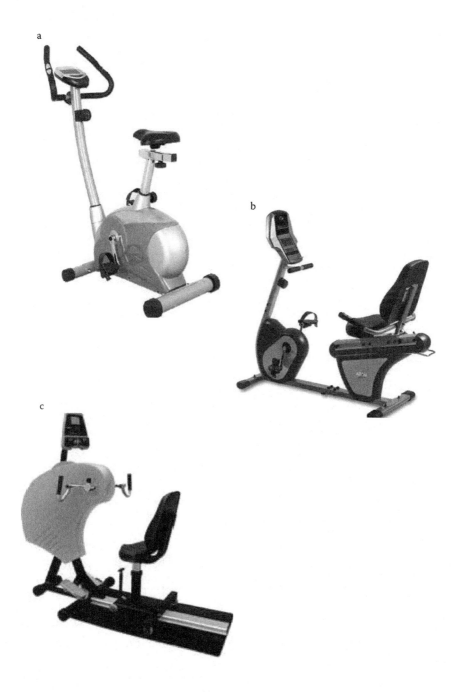

FIGURE 3.1
The types of fitness cycle: (a) upright cycle, (b) recumbent cycle, and (c) hand cycle.

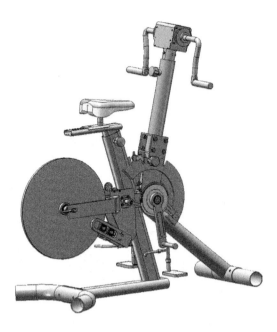

FIGURE 3.2
Three-dimensional design of the Bio-Cycle.

enhance the muscle strength of the upper limbs, lower limbs, chest, back, and abdomen but that the multiriding modes add a lot of fun to exercise. A three-dimensional design of the Bio-Cycle is shown in Figure 3.2.

3.2 Bionic Analysis and Scheme

3.2.1 Bionic Analysis of the System

The Bio-Cycle was inspired by the cheetah as well as other four-legged animals. As a member of the big cat family, the cheetah is the best runner in the animal world. When running at a high speed, the cheetah jumps forward by treading the ground with both of its forelegs at the same time and alternately pushing with both of its hind legs. Figure 3.3 shows the two states in a cycle of the cheetah's run. In this mode, the cheetah's powerful legs provide it with great strength and enable it to run at a speed of more than 100 km per hour. Different from running, when walking at a normal speed, the cheetah alternately uses one side of its foreleg and hind leg together to walk first, and then the other side, as shown in Figure 3.4.

To imitate this running motion, we designed the Bio-Cycle with a four-drive structure. In the bionic riding mode of cheetah-like running, the user's legs are treading and two hands are pushing forward at the same time. This

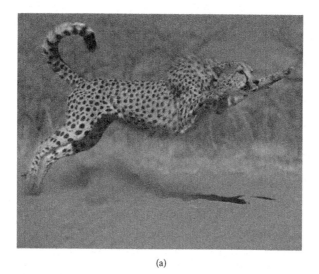

(a)

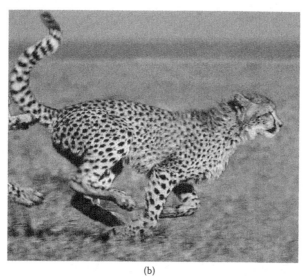

(b)

FIGURE 3.3
Two states in a cheetah's running cycle: (a) and (b).

makes the user's body stretch adequately. Almost all muscle groups of the upper limbs, lower limbs, and abdomen are balanced and exercised all over. Combined with a virtual reality scene and sound system, it can make the user feel as if he were running freely in the wild.

Furthermore, because the Bio-Cycle can be driven by either hands or legs or any combination of any hand and leg, users will be able to carry out a variety of exercise motions that cannot be achieved by a traditional fitness cycle. Theoretically, there are fourteen running modes for the Bio-Cycle

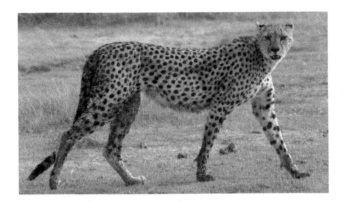

FIGURE 3.4
Walking motion of the cheetah.

TABLE 3.1

Main Exercise Modes of the Bio-Cycle

Exercise Mode	Ride Mode	Trained Muscles
One drive	The user can exercise only with a hand or leg	
Two drive	Alternate riding: Just like a traditional bike, the user exercises with the feet at a 180-degree angle	Gastrocnemius, gluteus, rectus femoris, and biceps femoris muscles
	Stair-climbing: The user does a treading exercise with one leg, and the other leg can relax	Gluteus and rectus femoris muscles
	Cheetah-like walking: The user exercises by using either hand and foot alternately	
Four drive (bionic riding)	The user exercises with both hands and legs at the same time	Gastrocnemius, gluteus, rectus femoris, biceps femoris, abdomen, and upper limb muscles

and the main exercise modes include alternate riding, stair-climbing, and bionic riding, as shown in Table 3.1. Also, the exercise motions can be freely changed any time so that the user can realize aerobic and anaerobic training.

3.2.2 Mechanism Scheme-Based Multidrive Modes

The mechanism scheme of a multidrive system is mainly applied with a set of overrunning clutches, which is a special kind of mechanically controlled clutch. In the mechanical transmission, when the relative rotation speed or direction changes, the clutch will transfer to the other mode; for example, from engage to disengage. Taking a two-drive unit as an example, when drive A is

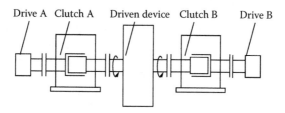

FIGURE 3.5
Mechanism scheme of a double-drive unit.

rotating in the direction as shown in Figure 3.5, overrunning clutch A engages to make the driven device rotate in the same direction. At the same time, overrunning clutch B automatically disengages (overrun) to put drive B out of action. Conversely, when drive B is rotating in the direction shown, clutch B engages to make the driven device rotate, and clutch A disengages (overrun).

Because the handles of the Bio-Cycle can carry out a 360-degree rotation motion, which differentiates them from the fixed handles designed for the common fitness cycle, a transmission system to transfer the power created by the hands to the spindle and to combine four independent transmission units to drive the fitness cycle is designed.

The common transmission mode for fitness cycles is belt driven or chain driven, but it is usually applied when the transmission distance is fixed. As to the supporting bar of the handles, the function of distance adjustment between the upper limbs and lower limbs should be considered to adapt to different users. Problems of the transmission process such as torque, stability, and noise should also be considered. Therefore, the torque transmission system uses a spur bevel gear with a spline shaft. Considering the volume of the gear and its impact on the whole design, the ratio of this gear transmission is selected to be 1:1.

As shown in Figure 3.6, the power offered by hands is transmitted to bevel gear 1 by the respective overrunning clutch. Bevel gear 2 is fixed on the external spline shaft and bevel gear 3 is fixed on the internal spline. To adapt to different users, the spline shaft is used to change the transmission distance between the hands and feet without affecting the transfer efficiency. By the transmission of bevel gear and spline shafts, output power is transmitted to the spindle efficiently. The power of the users' feet can also be transmitted to the spindle through overrunning clutches. Thus, the purpose of simultaneously driving with both hands and feet can be achieved.

3.3 Ergonomic Analysis and Mechanism Design

The size and the relative position of the Bio-Cycle should be designed to guarantee comfort and safety, and a convenient dimension adjusting function must be considered to adapt to different users. Ergonomics provides human scale

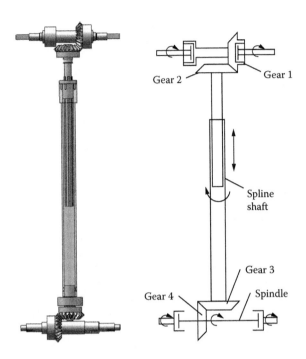

FIGURE 3.6
Design of the transmission unit.

parameters, the range and angle of physical activity, and so on (Z. Q. Zhang 2008), which is very helpful in our design. *Ergonomics* is concerned with letting people get closest to their natural state when effecting an operation.

3.3.1 Design of the Pedal Crank and Hand Crank

As shown in Figure 3.7, the structure of the pedal crank corresponds to a crank-rocker mechanism. The pedal crank l_1 is the crank that can do a cycle rotation, the shank of user l_2 is the connecting rod, leg l_3 is the rocker, and the body of Bio-Cycle l_4 is a pedestal that is fixed and unmovable. Therefore, leg l_3 is the active part for this crank-rocker mechanism. As is well known, when people exercise on a bike, the distance that the pedal crank covers in one round is equivalent to the walking step of an average person (Xu 2004). Thus, the most optimal diameter for a crank is equal to the walking step length of people in a natural state. If we do a trigonometrical analysis, we obtain an inequality of $l_2 \geq l_1$, $l_3 \geq l_1$, $l_4 \geq l_1$. Generally, the walking step length of adults is about 300–400 mm in a natural state. Therefore, the crank length of l_1 ranges from 150 to 200 mm. To satisfy most users, the median value of 170 mm is applied as the optimum.

This new fitness cycle's hand crank can also carry out a 360-degree rotation motion. The length of the pedal crank is designed to be equivalent to

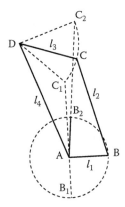

FIGURE 3.7
Crank-rocker mechanisms formed by pedal movement.

the step of people in their natural state, and the bionic riding motion, which is driven by both hands and legs, imitates the running methods of animals; thus the hand crank's length should be kept the same as the pedal crank length; that is, 170 mm.

3.3.2 Design of the Saddle Pole

There are two main parameters for the saddle pole: the tilt angle and the length adjustment range.

1. Analysis of the tilt angle

   When the user rides a fitness cycle, the relationship of the plane location of the user's thigh, shank, pedal crank, and saddle pole is shown in Figure 3.8a (N. Y. Zhang 2001). The limit location as shown in Figure 3.8b is taken to determine the tilt angle of the saddle pole; that is, the location where the user's legs are straight and the pedal crank is horizontal. The first human template provided by the GB/T 15759-95 standard form is adopted (General Administration of Quality Supervision, Inspection and Quarantine of China, 1995). That is, the female minimum perineum height $h = 673$ mm is selected as the design standard; therefore, most users will not need to unbend their legs and almost all will be able to tread the pedal crank to the bottom of its motion. According to physiological characteristics, angle α should not be greater than 90 degrees (Das and Behara 1998); $\alpha = 90$ degrees was chosen.

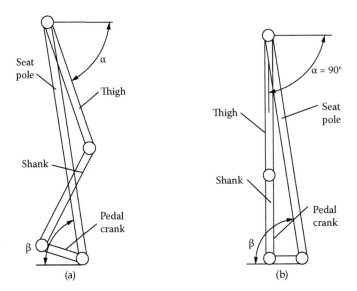

FIGURE 3.8
Relationship of the plane location of the lower limb: (a) normal location and (b) limit location.

Then, the tilt angle of the saddle pole β is

$$\beta = \arctan\left(h/l\right) = \arctan\left(673/170\right) = 75.8° \tag{3.1}$$

According to the working condition of the saddle, the ideal angle of β is 90 degrees. The smaller β is, the higher the requirement of material strength is on the pole. The seat is designed to move horizontally, and the effect of the seat moving backwards horizontally is similar to increasing the tilt angle of the saddle pole. Therefore, β = 75 degrees is used.

2. Analysis of the length adjustment range

The lower limb movement is equivalent to a crank-rocker mechanism. As shown in Figure 3.9, part of the bike $O_1 O_2$ stands for the frame, pedal crank L_0 stands for the crank for the mechanism, shank L_2 stands for the connecting rod, and thigh L_1 stands for the rocker. The rocker constitutes the active part of the crank-rocker mechanism. The comfort angles of human joints correspond to a shoulder joint of 35–90 degrees, an elbow joint of 95–180 degrees, and a knee joint of 60–130 degrees (Hu, Jiang, and Wu 1997).

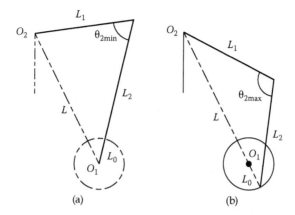

FIGURE 3.9
Diagram of the lower limb movement: (a) the location of θ_{2min} and (b) the location of θ_{2max}.

When the feet are at the top dead center, that is, when the crank and shank are in line, as shown in Figure 3.9a, the knee joint has the minimum value; that is, θ_{2min} = 60 degrees. According to the cosine theorem, the minimum value L_{min} of the saddle pole can be obtained.

$$L_{min}^2 = L_1^2 + (L_0 + L_2)^2 - 2L_1(L_0 + L_2)\cos\theta_{2min} \tag{3.2}$$

When the crank and $O_1 O_2$ are in line, as shown in Figure 3.9b, the knee joint has the maximum value, that is, θ_{2max} = 130 degrees, and the maximum value L_{max} of the saddle pole can be obtained.

$$(L_{min} + L_0)^2 = L_1^2 + L_2^2 - 2L_1 L_2 \cos\theta_{2max} \tag{3.3}$$

3.3.3 Handle Design

The handles of the Bio-Cycle are designed to adjust the height to the saddle. The adjusting method of rotating the support bar around the shaft is also part of this fitness cycle. This enables most users to exercise in comfort.

The greater the height difference between the handles and seat, the worse the manipulation, and the greater the pressure on the arms. In order to make the fitness cycle more comfortable, the handle should not be too low—it should be designed to be higher than the seat.

In the horizontal direction, the space of the handle must be in the size range of the user's upper limbs. It should not be too far from the saddle; otherwise, it will exceed the maximum forward angle of 45 degrees at which the

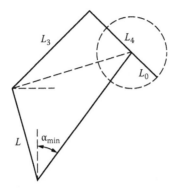

FIGURE 3.10
Solution of the maximum elevation angle for the tap.

human body maintains a comfortable sitting posture. The distance should not be more than that of the largest upper limbs of the first human example. The forward angle of almost all the users is less than 45 degrees and they can exercise in a comfortable range. Thus, the first human example with the forward angle of 45 degrees is used as a design standard to determine the maximum tilt angle of the support bar.

According to the first human example, thigh length L_1 is 402 mm and shank length L_2 is 313 mm. Then the length of the saddle pole can be retrieved from the above analysis: 448 mm < L < 479 mm. In order to obtain the maximum tilt angle, L_{min} = 450 mm is used as the length of the saddle pole. The other data can be retrieved from the first human example: shoulder height L_3 is 518 mm and upper limb length L_4 is 455 mm. The hand crank L_0 is 170 mm. Under the cosine theorem, as shown in Figure 3.10, the maximum tilt angle α_{min} is about 37 degrees.

3.4 Design of the Compound Resistance System

As one of the most important parts of a fitness cycle, the resistance system provides the resistance necessary to build a condition that makes the user feel like he is riding a bike on a real road. Furthermore, it should be able to adjust to meet the user's requirement automatically or manually. Considering the characteristics of the Bio-Cycle, we designed a resistance system called a *compound resistance system*, which is based on the electromagnetic principles of the eddy current (Huang 1999).

3.4.1 Analysis of Driving Characteristics

The motion of the pedal crank can be divided into four areas in one cycle (Figure 3.11; He et al. 2005; Li and Liu 2005; Wu, Yuan, and Wu 2007). For

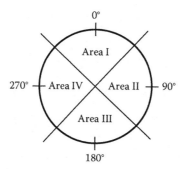

FIGURE 3.11
Distribution area of the crank position.

traditional fitness cycles, the pedal can only fit the treading motion, and the feet do not produce a driving effect while lifting because the two pedals are fixed at a 180-degree angle. Thus, when the foot on one side is treading, the pedal will drive the foot on the other side to lift at the same time. Finally, a circular motion is completed.

For the Bio-Cycle, the driving force in a cycle of motion has its own characteristics. Because they are driving separately, the two feet need to produce a driving force in both treading and lifting motions. The driving force in the whole circular motion is always positive and has two peak values as shown in Figure 3.12. One peak value is in area II for treading motion, and another peak value is in area IV for lifting motion. The lifting motion is rarely used in normal human sport, so the lifting peak value is much smaller than the treading peak value and will cause discomfort while riding. Therefore, the range of such cyclical fluctuation must be reduced.

In addition, the Bio-Cycle can achieve many motion modes, and different motions have different driving characteristics. So when the user changes

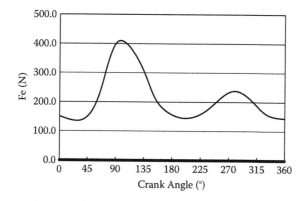

FIGURE 3.12
Driving force in one cycle.

from one riding mode to another, the balance between resistance and former driving force will be broken. This will cause the user an uncomfortable feeling and the phenomenon of no-load running.

3.4.2 Principle of the Compound Resistance System

In order to adapt the driving characteristics, three kinds of resistance methods are considered in the system. The compound resistance system includes the following:

- *Basic resistance* refers to the exercise intensity, the level of which can be selected by the user.
- *Position resistance* R_p is normally used when using the bionic riding mode to counteract the cyclical fluctuation, and a designed cam mechanism is used to adjust the position resistance automatically.
- *Speed resistance* R_s is an adjustment parameter to avoid driving fluctuation, which always occurs when speeding up.

$$R_c = f_{i1}R_b + f_{i2}R_p + f_{i3}R_s \tag{3.4}$$

where f_{ij} (j = 1,2,3) stands for the weighing factor based on different motion modes, j represents different resistances, and i refers to different exercise modes; f_{ij} can be acquired through experiments.

For the driving fluctuation caused by the change of the riding mode, a method to avoid the phenomenon of no-load running must be considered.

The speed of the inertia wheel goes through two stages. In the first stage, the driving force is constant and the output power of the user increases from 0 to P_{max}. The speed of the inertia wheel can be brought up to ω_p. In the second stage, the output power will keep the maximum value P_{max}. According to formulas (3.5) and (3.6), when the speed increases from ω_p to ω_{max}, the driving momentum M will decrease because of the reduction of the inertia force $J\Delta\dot{\omega}$.

$$\omega = \frac{P_{max}}{M} \tag{3.5}$$

$$M = J(\dot{\omega} - \Delta\dot{\omega}) + M_r \tag{3.6}$$

When the speed reaches ω_{max}, the inertia wheel rotates in a constant speed, the inertia force decrease to 0, and the driving momentum $M = M_r$. The phenomenon of no-load running will occur when $M < M_{min}$, where M_{min} is

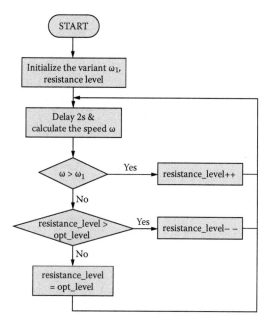

FIGURE 3.13
Flowchart of the automatic control of the resistance system.

the limit value of the occurrence of no-load running. Therefore, the limit speed ω_l can be obtained.

$$\omega_l = \frac{P_{max}}{M_{min}} \tag{3.7}$$

In order to avoid the phenomenon of no-load running, when $\omega < \omega_l$, the speed resistance can be increased by controlling the angle of the steering engine.

A flowchart of the automatic resistance control system is shown in Figure 3.13.

3.4.3 Detection of Exercise Motions

The system of exercise motions can be determined by the relative position of arms and legs. The typical exercise motion of the Bio-Cycle is alternate riding and bionic riding. These two motions can be classified by the system of exercise motions. An infrared photoelectric switch has been used as a sensor and a code wheel has been designed.

For the upper limbs, one sensor has been used and an interstice of the code wheel has been designed as a circular arc of about 45 degrees, as

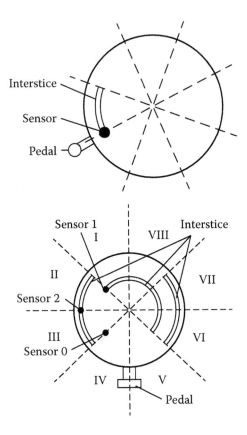

FIGURE 3.14
Arrangement of the sensors and design of the code wheel: for (a) upper limbs and (b) lower limbs.

shown in Figure 3.14a. The signal is 11 when two hands are pushing or pulling simultaneously.

For the lower limbs, motions such as alternate riding or bionic riding must be determined, so the position of the pedal crank should be determined accurately. Three sensors for one side have been used and the code wheel has been designed as shown in Figure 3.14b. Two legs are considered to be synchronous when the phase difference of the legs is less than 45 degrees. Two legs are considered to be alternately riding when the phase difference of the legs is between 135 and 180 degrees. The corresponding signal for the different places of the pedal crank is shown in Table 3.2.

According to the arrangement of the sensors and the design of the code wheel, an algorithm for the determination of exercise motions has been achieved, and a flowchart on the determination of exercise motions is shown in Figure 3.15.

TABLE 3.2

Corresponding Signals for the Place
of the Pedal Crank

Place of Pedal Crank	Corresponding Signal
Area I	101
Area II	001
Area III	000
Area IV	100
Area V	110
Area VI	010
Area VII	011
Area VIII	111

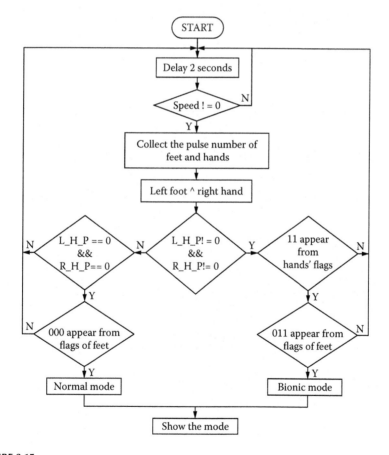

FIGURE 3.15
Flowchart on the determination of exercise motions.

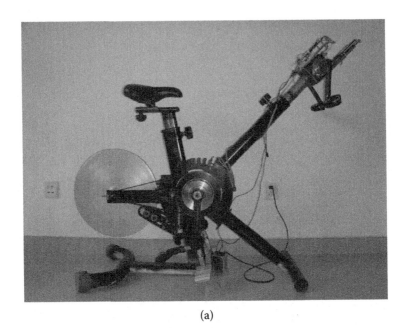

(a)

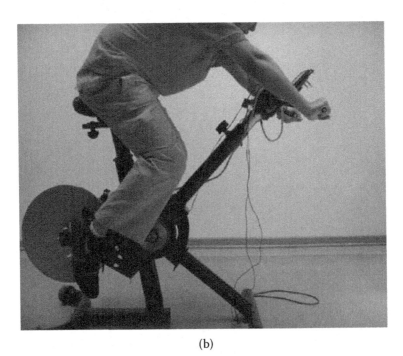

(b)

FIGURE 3.16
Prototype of the Bio-Cycle: (a) picture of the prototype, and (b) a typical posture for riding the Bio-Cycle.

3.5 Development and Test

At present, the first prototype (Figure 3.16) has been developed and has been used to determine the scheme and to design the mechanical structure. Through several debugs and the corresponding experiments on the prototype, the feasibility of the Bio-Cycle has been proven. Each adjustment range according to the ergonomic design was in line with the requirements of comfort. As for the resistance system, the adjustment range can be set by programming and initializing the steering engine, and the test has shown that its resistance torque ranges from about 10 to 25 Nm, which is sufficient for different people's needs. We also invited a couple of people to test the resistance control in different exercise motions, as shown in Figure 3.17.

Most test persons felt the training of the lumbar muscles to be relatively strong at a larger tilt angle of the supporting bar, which was set while testing the mode of bionic riding. In comparison, the training of the limb muscles was felt to be stronger at a smaller tilt angle of the supporting bar. This shows that that the changes in the depression angle have a great influence on the effect of the exercises.

3.6 Conclusions

In this study, we analyzed the principle of a bionic fitness cycle and its new characteristics. A four-drive transmission system and a compound resistance system have been developed. We planned the overall size and designed the structure to meet the requirement of ergonomics in order to render the riding more comfortable for different groups of people. We also developed an interactive interface so that the user could obtain the exercise information in real-time and control it accurately. As a new riding motion was created, we analyzed the characteristics of its resistance system and designed a compound resistance system to adequately fulfill the requirements of comfort and safety. This new fitness cycle puts forward a completely new exercise concept and brings the users a more enjoyable riding experience. We hope it will provide new impulses to the fitness industry and to bicycle sports.

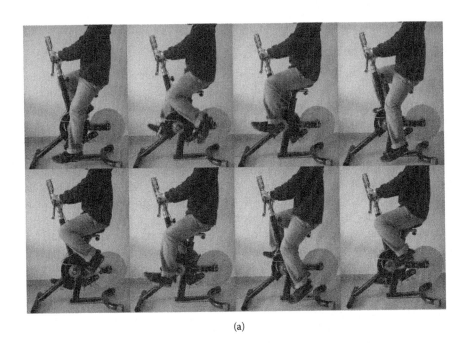

(a)

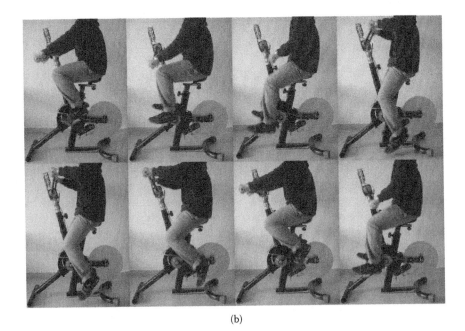

(b)

FIGURE 3.17
Demonstration of all riding modes: (a) alternate riding, (b) bionic riding.

(continued)

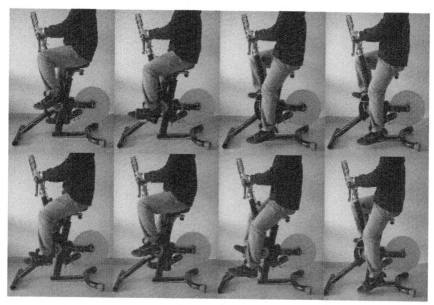

(c)

FIGURE 3.17 (Continued)
Demonstration of all riding modes: (c) stair-climbing.

References

Das, B. and Behara, D.N. 1998. Three-dimensional workspace for industrial workstations. *Human Factors*, 40(4): 633–646.

General Administration of Quality Supervision, Inspection and Quarantine of China. 1995. The size template for the body shape of human, GB/T 15759-95, Beijing.

He, Q.C., Fan, X.M., Ma, D.Z., et al. 2005. An investigation of force feedback in interactive bicycle simulator. *Journal of System Simulation*, 17(4): 795–797.

Hu, Z.W., Jiang, Y.S., and Wu, Z.M. 1997. A study on the riding model of bicycle with computer simulation. *Journal of Da-Yeh University*, 6(1): 119–125.

Huang, K.M. 1999. Magnetic damping system of magnetically controlled bicycle. *Journal of Magnetic Materials and Devices*, 30(4): 15–17.

Li, Q. and Liu, W.G. 2005. Biomechanical research on domestic and foreign present condition of cycle event. *Journal of Anhui Sports Science*, 26(3): 54–56.

Wang, Z.H. 2008. The current situation and development countermeasure of sports goods industry in China. *Journal of Beijing Sport University*, 31(3): 300–302.

Wu, C.E., Yuan, P., and Wu, G.X. 2007. Investigation of pedaling force at different cadence in cycle-ergometer. *Journal of Sports and Science*, 28(1): 72–75.

Xu, H.W. 2004. Research on the product design and simulation based on human engineering. M.S. thesis, Wuhan University.

Zhang, N.Y. 2001. Application of ergonomics in the design of bicycle products. *China Bicycle*, 1: 25–29.

Zhang, Z.Q. 2008. Ergonomics analysis and study about the home fitness equipment. M.S. thesis, Shandong University.

4

Human-Inspired Hyper Dynamic Manipulation

Aiguo Ming and Chunquan Xu

The University of Electro-Communications
Tokyo, Japan

CONTENTS

4.1 Introduction 56
4.2 Basic Concept 57
    4.2.1 Utilization of Dynamically Coupled Driving 57
    4.2.2 Utilization of Structural Joint Stop 63
    4.2.3 Case Study: Mechanism Design of a Golf Swing Robot 65
4.3 Method to Utilize Dynamically Coupled Driving and Joint Stops 67
    4.3.1 Motion Generation and Control Method 68
        4.3.1.1 Motion Generation 68
        4.3.1.2 Control Method 70
    4.3.2 Case Study: Motion Generation and Control of a Golf
        Swing Robot 70
4.4 Simulation and Experimental Results for the Golf Swing Robot 74
    4.4.1 Simulation 74
    4.4.2 Experiments 77
4.5 Conclusion 82
References 83

Abstract

Hyper dynamic manipulation is defined as highly skilled manipulation with hyper motion specifications, as performed by some athletes. Though hyper dynamic manipulation has been realized in some conventional robots, how to realize hyper dynamic manipulation by a smart structure still remains an interesting and challenging topic to be studied in the robotics field. The purpose of this work is to realize human-inspired hyper dynamic manipulations by a smart manipulator. Based on the analysis results from human hyper dynamic motion, we propose a solution to the realization of hyper dynamic manipulation by robots through utilizing dynamically coupled driving and structural joint stops. This chapter gives the basic idea for utilizing dynamically coupled driving and structural joint stops in a hyper dynamic manipulator. The implementation method shows how to realize the manipulation, and the simulations and experimental results provide verification of the overall effectiveness of this proposal.

4.1 Introduction

Hyper dynamic manipulation is defined here as highly skilled manipulation with hyper motion specifications, as performed by some athletes. Realization of such hyper dynamic manipulation by a robot is an interesting and challenging topic in robotics, because the need for the capability of dynamic manipulation is increasing.

Although some robots have been developed to perform hyper dynamic manipulation, these robots conform to the conventional robot design method, that of designing the robot by satisfying the specifications of velocity and acceleration of individual joints (Shimon 1999).

The revolute joint of a manipulator usually cannot rotate 360 degrees due to the structural limitation. The rotation range of the joint is limited by a mechanical structure, namely, the joint stop. Conventional manipulators provide protection against collision or contact between an arm and the joint stop by employing a software barrier based on the rotation range of each joint and an electronic hardware barrier using a proximity sensor and a control circuit. That is, the passive torque between the joint stop and the arm is not utilized by conventional manipulators.

Recent advances in the mechanical design of manipulators have produced a new generation of lightweight manipulators (Hirzinger et al. 2001). Such work focused on how to design compact mechanisms for a manipulator. The research and development on manipulators has provided the foundation for work on humanoids (Kagami et al. 2001). Though humanoids can do some dynamic manipulations, such as some kinds of slow dancing and running (Nagasaka et al. 2004), they are still limited in their dynamic manipulation capability due to conventional robot design methods.

Compared to conventional manipulators, human beings can perform hyper dynamic manipulations while in a smart structure. The motion control skill, namely, efficiently utilizing dynamically coupled driving in hyper dynamic manipulation, has been presented in previous work (Ming et al. 2001). That successful motion is due to the smart structure of humans, in which the joints near the body are more powerful than those near the end of the arm. To produce a hyper dynamic action, the power of the joint near the body must be transferred to the parts near the palm by multistep acceleration due to dynamically coupled driving. In addition, a human's arthrosis cannot rotate all around like conventional manipulators due to limitations of the body's structure (joint stop).

Such limitations are often utilized by humans to improve their capability of dynamic manipulation. For example, in the downswing phase of a high-speed golf swing motion, the joint stop in the wrist joint is utilized by professional golfers to accelerate the golf club (Ming, Kajitani, and Shimojo 2002; Ming et al. 2001; Ming et al. 2003).

As a human-inspired approach to improve the capability of a manipulator for hyper dynamic manipulations by a smart structure, we propose to utilize dynamically coupled driving and the joint stop in the manipulator. That is, to make the joint stop in the manipulator available and utilize the structural joint stops effectively by a unique control method based on dynamically coupled driving. This will lead to a large improvement on the dynamic capability.

This chapter gives the basic idea and expected effects of utilizing dynamically coupled driving and structural joint stops in a manipulator in Section 4.2. The control method to utilize dynamically coupled driving and joint stops is described in Section 4.3. Simulation and experimental results and discussion are given in Section 4.4. Section 4.5 concludes.

4.2 Basic Concept

4.2.1 Utilization of Dynamically Coupled Driving

As mentioned before, humans can utilize dynamically coupled driving while performing hyper dynamic manipulation, which provides a useful suggestion of realizing hyper dynamic manipulation by a manipulator with a smart structure. There have been some works about the positioning control of manipulators with passive joints using dynamically coupled driving (Arai and Tachi 1991; DeLuca and Oriolo 2002; Nakamura, Koinuma, and Suzuki 1996). Here, we consider how to utilize dynamically coupled driving to design a hyper dynamic manipulator with a smart structure.

For a planar *n*-degrees-of-freedom (DOF) open-chained multijoint manipulator, the dynamics equation is (Murry, Li, and Sastry 1994):

$$\tau = \mathbf{M}(\theta)\ddot{\theta} + \mathbf{C}(\theta, \dot{\theta})\dot{\theta} + \mathbf{N}(\theta, \dot{\theta}) \tag{4.1}$$

where

$\quad\quad\theta$ = generalized driving torque
$\quad\quad\theta$ = generalized coordinate
$\quad\mathbf{M}(\theta)$ = inertia matrix

$\mathbf{C}\left(\theta,\dot{\theta}\right)$ = Coriolis matrix determining the Coriolis force and the centrifugal force

$\mathbf{N}\left(\theta,\dot{\theta}\right)$ = gravity force and frictional/damping force

The scalar form of the equation is as follows:

$$\begin{cases} \tau_1 = \displaystyle\sum_{j=1}^{n} M_{1j}\left(\theta\right)\ddot{\theta}_j + \sum_{j,k=1}^{n}\Gamma_{1jk}\dot{\theta}_j\dot{\theta}_k + N_1\left(\theta,\dot{\theta}\right) \\[4pt] \hspace{1cm}\cdots\cdots\cdots\cdots\cdots\cdots\cdots\cdots\cdots\cdots\cdots\cdots \\[4pt] \tau_i = \displaystyle\sum_{j=1}^{n} M_{ij}\left(\theta\theta\right)\ddot{\theta}_j + \sum_{j,k=1}^{n}\Gamma_{ijk}\dot{\theta}_j\dot{\theta}_k + N_i\left(\theta,\dot{\theta}\right) \\[4pt] \hspace{1cm}\cdots\cdots\cdots\cdots\cdots\cdots\cdots\cdots\cdots\cdots\cdots\cdots \\[4pt] \tau_n = \displaystyle\sum_{j=1}^{n} M_{nj}\left(\theta\theta\right)\ddot{\theta}_j + \sum_{j,k=1}^{n}\Gamma_{njk}\dot{\theta}_j\dot{\theta}_k + N_n\left(\theta,\dot{\theta}\right) \end{cases} \tag{4.2}$$

where

$$\Gamma_{ijk} = \frac{1}{2}\left\{\frac{\partial M_{ij}\left(\theta\right)}{\partial\theta_k} + \frac{\partial M_{ik}\left(\theta\right)}{\partial\theta_j} - \frac{\partial M_{kj}\left(\theta\right)}{\partial\theta_i}\right\}$$

$$C_{ij}\left(\theta,\dot{\theta}\right) = \sum_{k=1}^{n}\Gamma_{ijk}\dot{\theta}_k$$

$\displaystyle\sum_{j=1}^{n} M_{ij}\left(\theta\right)\ddot{\theta}_j$ is inertia force.

$\displaystyle\sum_{j,k=1}^{n}\Gamma_{ijk}\dot{\theta}_j\dot{\theta}_k$ is Coriolis force and centrifugal force.

Obviously, there are dynamic coupling relations among the different equations of the set in Equation (4.2). To analyze these relations more clearly, we subtract τ_{i+1} from τ_i ($i = 1,\cdots, n - 1$) and write it in the world coordinate frame, resulting in the following equation:

$$\tau_i - \tau_{i+1} + \tau_{id} = \left(J_i + m_i l_{gi}^2 + l_i^2 \sum_{j=i+1}^{n} m_j \right) \ddot{\varphi}_i + \left(m_i l_{gi} + l_i \sum_{j=i+1}^{n} m_j \right) g \cos \varphi_i \tag{4.3}$$

$$(i = 1, 2, \cdots, n-1)$$

where

$$\tau_{id} = -\sum_{j=1, j\neq i}^{n-1} P_j \left(\mathbf{M}, \mathbf{L}, \mathbf{L_g} \right) \left[\ddot{\varphi}_j \cos\left(\varphi_i - \varphi_j \right) + \dot{\varphi}_j^2 \sin\left(\varphi_i - \varphi_j \right) \right]$$

J_i is the moment of inertia of link i about the center of mass, m_i is the mass of link i, l_i is the length of link i, l_{gi} is the length from the centroid to joint of link i, φ_i is the angular position of link i referring to the world coordinate, $P_j \left(\mathbf{M}, \mathbf{L}, \mathbf{L_g} \right)$ is the coefficient function, and g is acceleration due to gravity. In particular, for the end-effector the following equation holds:

$$\tau_n + \tau_{nd} = \left(J_n + m_n l_{gn}^2 \right) \ddot{\varphi}_n + m_n g l_{gn} \cos \varphi_n \tag{4.4}$$

where

$$\tau_{nd} = -m_n l_{gn} \sum_{j=1}^{n-1} \ddot{\varphi}_j l_j \cos\left(\varphi_n - \varphi_j \right) + \dot{\varphi}_j^2 l_j \sin\left(\varphi_n - \varphi_j \right)$$

It is very clear that both terms on the right-hand side of Equations (4.3) and (4.4) represent the motion equation of a single pendulum. According to this characteristic, the multi-joint manipulator can be regarded as a dynamic system consisting of single pendulums connected serially. The whole motion of the manipulator is the compound motion of the single pendulums. On the other hand, according to the terms on the left-hand side of Equations (4.3) and (4.4), all of the links are driven by not only the active torque from the actuators but also the torque τ_{id} due to coupling. We call this *dynamically coupled driving torque*.

Therefore, due to the existence of dynamically coupled driving in a planar open-chained manipulator, we hope to utilize it to improve the capability of hyper dynamic manipulation of a manipulator. Further, if there are nonperpendicular joints in a spatial manipulator, there is still dynamically coupled driving torque among these joints. Thus, it can be utilized as such in a planar manipulator.

As an example, we discuss a simplified two-joint manipulator shown in Figure 4.1 in detail. According to Equations (4.3) and (4.4), its dynamics can be written as:

$$\tau_1 - \tau_2 + \tau_{1d} = \left(m_1 l_{g1}^2 + m_2 l_1^2 + J_1 \right) \ddot{\varphi}_1 + \left(m_1 g_y l_{g1} + m_2 g_y l_1 \right) \cos \varphi_1 \tag{4.5}$$

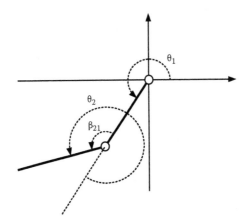

FIGURE 4.1
Model of a two-joint manipulator.

$$\tau_2 - 0 + \tau_{2d} = \left(m_2 l_{g2}^2 + J_2 \right) \ddot{\varphi}_2 + m_2 g_y l_{g2} \cos \varphi_2 \tag{4.6}$$

where

$$\tau_{1d} = m_2 l_1 l_{g2} (\ddot{\varphi}_2 \cos \beta_{21} - \dot{\varphi}_2^2 \sin \beta_{21})$$

$$\tau_{2d} = m_2 l_1 l_{g2} (\ddot{\varphi}_1 \cos \beta_{21} + \dot{\varphi}_1^2 \sin \beta_{21})$$

$\varphi_1 = \theta_1$ and $\varphi_2 = \theta_1 + \theta_2$, which represent the angular positions of joints 1 and 2 in their world coordinates, and $\beta_{21} = \theta_2 - \pi$ represents the angular position of link 2 relative to link 1. τ_{1d}, τ_{2d} are dynamically coupled driving torques. τ_{2d} consists of two parts:

$$\tau_{2d} = \tau_{2dv} + \tau_{2da} \tag{4.7}$$

where:

$$\tau_{2dv} = m_2 l_1 l_{g2} \dot{\varphi}_1^2 \sin \beta_{21}$$

$$\tau_{2da} = m_2 l_1 l_{g2} \ddot{\varphi}_1 \cos \beta_{21}$$

We define τ_{2dv} as velocity coupling torque and τ_{2da} as acceleration coupling torque. The velocity coupling torque is always positive and helps the active torque to accelerate joint 2 should the relative angular position $\beta_{21} \in [0, \pi]$. The acceleration coupling torque is rather complex and is determined by both acceleration of joint 1 $\ddot{\varphi}_1$ and relative angular position β_{21}. Only if both $\ddot{\varphi}_1$ and $\cos \beta_{21}$ are positive or negative does τ_{2da} contribute to the acceleration of joint 2. Figure 4.2 shows the effect of dynamically coupled driving

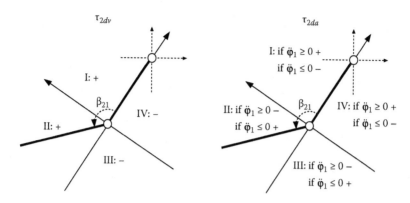

FIGURE 4.2
Effect of dynamically coupled driving torque in joint 2.

torque in joint 2. The "+" represents an acceleration effect and "−" represents a deceleration effect.

In accordance with Equation (4.7) and Figure 4.2, we can utilize the dynamically coupled driving torque to accelerate joint 2. However, to accelerate joint 2, joint 1 must accelerate first to a very high angular velocity; that is, it must obtain a large velocity coupling torque and acceleration coupling torque when link 2 is in quadrant I ($\beta_{21} \in [0, \pi/2]$). But, when link 2 is in quadrant II ($\beta_{21} \in [\pi/2, \pi]$), joint 1 must decelerate in order to maintain the acceleration effect of the acceleration coupling torque in joint 2.

Utilizing the same analysis method, we can define:

$$\tau_{1d} = \tau_{1dv} + \tau_{1da} \tag{4.8}$$

where

$$\tau_{1dv} = -m_2 l_1 l_{g2} \dot{\phi}_2^2 \sin \beta_{21}$$

$$\tau_{1da} = m_2 l_1 l_{g2} \ddot{\phi}_2 \cos \beta_{21}$$

The effect of dynamically coupled driving torque in joint 1 is shown in Figure 4.3.

By comparing Figures 4.2 and 4.3, we conclude that (1) the effects of velocity coupling torque on joint 1 and joint 2 are opposite at any position; and (2) the acceleration of joint 2 results in the same acceleration effect on joint 1 in quadrants I and IV but results in the opposite deceleration effect on joint 1 in quadrants II and III. Therefore, to utilize the dynamically coupled driving to accelerate joint 2, the deceleration effect on joint 1 is inevitable in quadrant II.

Actually, the effect of dynamically coupled driving is due to the power transfer from joint 1 to joint 2 by multistep acceleration. Because it is possible to use the dynamically coupled driving torque instead of the active torque

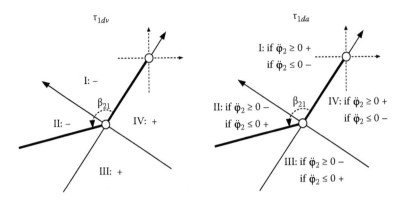

FIGURE 4.3
Effect of dynamically coupled driving torque in joint 1.

as the main driving torque, a light, low-power actuator can be used near the end-effector (joint 2) to lighten the structural weight of a manipulator. This benefits the dynamic manipulation. On the other hand, a more powerful actuator can be used on the base (joint 1) to overcome the deceleration effect of the dynamically coupled driving torque resulting from joint 2; that is, to supply more power to joint 1 so that more power will be transferred to joint 2. In so doing, the capability of dynamic manipulation is improved.

Similarly, due to the existence of dynamically coupled driving in an n-DOF open-chained manipulator, it is possible to utilize it to improve the capability of dynamic manipulation of the whole manipulator. According to the analysis of the two-link model, dynamically coupled driving torque, rather than active torque, can be utilized to drive joints of an n-DOF manipulator. Hence, all of the joints except the one on the base are driven by lighter, low-power actuators compared to those of conventional manipulators. Further, the actuator in joint i can be selected so that its load capability is only a little greater than the static torque due to the weight of the mechanism from link i to the end-effector. To supply power to be transferred to the end-effector, a more powerful actuator is selected and mounted on the base to drive the first link. By selecting lighter, low-power actuators, the links can also become lighter. Then the weight of such a structure is significantly lighter than that of conventional manipulators, and it is beneficial to the improvement of the capability of dynamic manipulation. Only one high-power actuator is required to realize hyper dynamic manipulation.

Because of the utilization of low-power actuators, the active torque is strictly limited. It is necessary to develop a method to utilize dynamically coupled driving to improve the capability of hyper dynamic manipulation of a manipulator subject to such active torque limitation. According to Equations (4.3) and (4.4) and the discussion above, the dynamically coupled driving torque is determined by the motion states of manipulators. One rational way to utilize dynamically coupled driving is planning a special motion trajectory that can utilize it effectively during the whole motion phase. However, the complicated relation between the effect of dynamically coupled driving and the motion states and the strict active torque limitation make it difficult to find such a motion trajectory directly. We deal with this problem by adopting an optimization method. The trajectory of hyper dynamic manipulation is generated subject to the active torque limitation and motion equation. If the motion can be generated under this condition, then dynamically coupled driving is to be utilized to drive the manipulator in the motion rather than the active torque.

4.2.2 Utilization of Structural Joint Stop

The other key point for human hyper dynamic manipulation is the structural joint stop utilized by humans. Much work has already been done investigating the elastic and damping characteristics of the joint stop. Some work (Hogan 1985) has focused on realizing the desired compliance by controlling the joint actuators, whereas others (Hayakawa et al. 1996; Katsurashima et al. 1998; Laurin-Kovitz, Colgate, and Carnes 1991; Mizuuchi et al. 1998; Morita et al. 1998; Okada, Nakamura, and Ban 2001) tried to utilize special mechanisms in order to meet the compliance requirements. All of the work previously mentioned is based on an assumption that the load is within the load capability of all actuators in the joints.

Our proposal is different. We propose the passive elastic and damping characteristics of the structural joint stop within the stop positions of the joint to be utilized to improve the capability of dynamic manipulation of manipulators, in addition to the elastic and damping characteristics realized by controlling the actuators or supplied by some mechanisms within the rotation range of a joint.

The reasons for using the structural joint stop in a manipulator are as follows:

- *Large load capability*: The load capability of a mechanical joint stop depends on its structural strength, instead of the load capability of an actuator. This will be useful to transfer high power from the joints near the base to the joints near the end of the manipulator.
- *Easy realization by simple and compact mechanism*: The structure of the joint stop can be built into the joint as a simple module, instead of a conventional stiff joint stop.
- *Power savings*: The configuration of a manipulator, in which some or all joints are in joint stop positions, can be used as a rest configuration. By switching off the servo loops of the joints in joint stop positions, power savings is possible.

Therefore, it is possible to realize efficient dynamic manipulations by utilizing the joint stop, compared to conventional manipulators limited by the load capability of actuators.

Considering the utilization of joint stops, the dynamics of an open-chained multijoint manipulator (Equation (4.2)) is modified to be

$$
\left\{
\begin{aligned}
\tau_1 + \tau_{1p} &= \sum_{j=1}^{n} M_{1j}(\theta\theta)\ddot{\theta}_j + \sum_{j,k=1}^{n} \Gamma_{1jk}\dot{\theta}_j\dot{\theta}_k + N_1(\theta,\dot{\theta}) \\
&\cdots\cdots\cdots\cdots\cdots\cdots\cdots\cdots\cdots \\
\tau_i + \tau_{ip} &= \sum_{j=1}^{n} M_{ij}(\theta\theta)\ddot{\theta}_j + \sum_{j,k=1}^{n} \Gamma_{ijk}\dot{\theta}_j\dot{\theta}_k + N_i(\theta,\dot{\theta}) \\
&\cdots\cdots\cdots\cdots\cdots\cdots\cdots\cdots\cdots \\
\tau_n + \tau_{np} &= \sum_{j=1}^{n} M_{nj}(\theta\theta)\ddot{\theta}_j + \sum_{j,k=1}^{n} \Gamma_{njk}\dot{\theta}_j\dot{\theta}_k + N_n(\theta,\dot{\theta})
\end{aligned}
\right.
\tag{4.9}
$$

Equations (4.3) and (4.4) are then modified to be Equations (4.10) and (4.11), respectively.

$$
\tau_i + \tau_{ip} - \tau_{i+1} - \tau_{(i+1)p} + \tau_{id} = \left(J_i + m_i l_{gi}^2 + l_i^2 \sum_{j=i+1}^{n} m_j \right)\ddot{\varphi}_i + \left(m_i l_{gi} + l_i \sum_{j=i+1}^{n} m_j \right) g \cos\varphi_i
$$

$$(i = 1, 2, \cdots, n-1)$$

$$\tag{4.10}$$

$$
\tau_n + \tau_{np} + \tau_{nd} = \left(J_n + m_n l_{gn}^2 \right)\ddot{\varphi}_n + m_n g l_{gn} \cos\varphi_n
\tag{4.11}
$$

where,

$$
\tau_{ip} =
\begin{cases}
\tau_{iminp}(\theta_i), & \theta_{ilb} \le \theta_i \le \theta_{imin} \\
0, & \theta_{imin} < \theta_i < \theta_{imax} \\
\tau_{imaxp}(\theta_i), & \theta_{imax} \le \theta_i \le \theta_{iub}
\end{cases}
$$

is the passive torque generated by the joint stop mounted on joint *i*. $(\theta_{imin}, \theta_{imax})$ is the free rotation range of joint *i*. $[\theta_{ilb}, \theta_{imin}]$ and $[\theta_{imax}, \theta_{iub}]$

are the action ranges of joint stops in clockwise and counterclockwise directions, respectively.

According to Equations (4.10) and (4.11), it is possible to utilize the passive torque resulting from the joint stop as part of the driving torque in the joint, similar to the utilization of dynamically coupled driving to improve the capability of hyper dynamic manipulation for the whole manipulator. Actually, this is also due to the transference of power from the base to the end-effector through the contact of joint stops. Additionally, the load capability of the end-effector can be improved to exceed the limitation of the active torque of actuators when the link is in contact with the joint stop.

Another useful method is forming the joint stop by the mechanism configuration of a manipulator itself. That is, by contacting one arm with another arm, this contact can be regarded as an available joint stop. In this case, some flexible skin on the arm is necessary to supply elastic and damping characteristics. This is especially useful for the redundant manipulator. Because the utilization of this kind of joint stop is similar to the aforementioned joint stop, the following discussions are limited to the case of the structural joint stop.

4.2.3 Case Study: Mechanism Design of a Golf Swing Robot

As a case study to utilize dynamically coupled driving and joint stops in a manipulator, a golf swing robot with a smart structure is considered that can imitate the golf swing motion by a human.

Figure 4.4 shows an overview of the developed prototype of the golf swing robot and its configuration. The robot consists of a base frame, the first joint (shoulder joint), an arm, the second joint (wrist joint), and a club. The first joint is to realize the equivalent function of shoulder in human and is driven by a direct drive (DD) motor, which is suitable for dynamically coupled driving. In the second joint a small DD motor with two joint stops to realize the function of wrist in human is used. The small DD motor in the wrist joint is selected so that its load capability is only a little greater than the static torque due to the weight of the club. Because a small DD motor is used in the wrist joint, the structure of the wrist joint, as well as that of the whole manipulator, becomes very compact and light; that is, smart. Distribution of the actuators is an important point to realize hyper dynamic manipulations in a smart structure. On the other hand, the small DD motor in the wrist joint does not directly contribute to the acceleration of the wrist joint in a high-speed swing motion. Therefore, in this mechanism, the dynamic manipulation is mainly realized by the power of the DD motor in the shoulder joint; that is, dynamically coupled driving is to be utilized for hyper dynamic manipulations.

The detailed structure of the joint stops is shown in Figure 4.5. Each joint stop consists of a pair of magnets and a shock absorber. The elastic force is derived from the repelling force between two magnets, and the viscous force

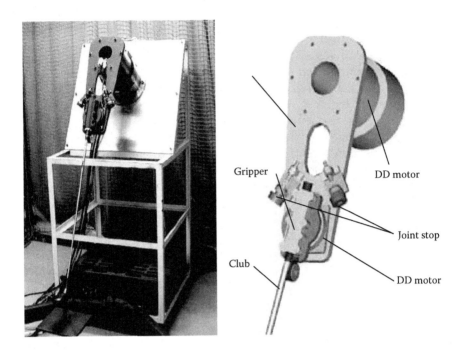

FIGURE 4.4
Prototype of golf swing robot.

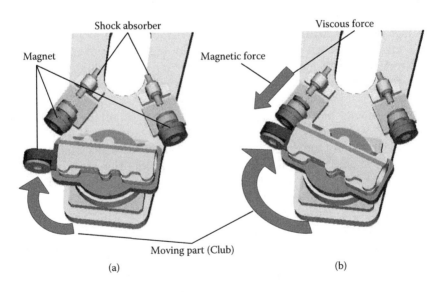

FIGURE 4.5
Detailed structure of the joint stop.

is generated by the absorber. The approximate equation of the elastic characteristic of the joint stops is shown in Equation (4.12).

$$\tau_{2stop\_char}\left(\theta_{2s}\right) = a_0 + a_1\theta_{2s} + a_2\theta_{2s}^2 + a_3\theta_{2s}^2 + a_4\theta_{2s}^4 + a_5\theta_{2s}^5 + a_6\theta_{2s}^6 \qquad (4.12)$$

$a_0 = 1.164 \times 10$, $a_1 = -2.915 \times 10$, $a_2 = 3.724 \times 10^{-1}$, $a_3 = -2.675 \times 10^{-2}$

$a_4 = 1.060 \times 10^{-3}$, $a_5 = -2.141 \times 10^{-5}$, $a_6 = 1.715 \times 10^{-7}$

The action range of the joint stops is from $\theta_{2s} = 0\left[\text{deg}\right]$ to $\theta_{2s} = 20\left[\text{deg}\right]$. The
role of the shock absorber is to absorb the collision between the arm and the
club, and the shock absorber used here can absorb a velocity difference up
to 9.3 rad/s.

Therefore, the passive torque in the wrist joint generated by the joint stops
can be represented by the following equation:

$$\tau_{2p} = \begin{cases} \tau_{2minp}, & \theta_{2lb} \leq \theta_2 \leq \theta_{2min} \\ 0, & \theta_{2min} < \theta_2 < \theta_{2max} \\ \tau_{2maxp}, & \theta_{2max} \leq \theta_2 \leq \theta_{2ub} \end{cases} \qquad (4.13)$$

where

$$\tau_{2minp} = \tau_{2stop\_char}\left(20° - \left|\theta_{2min} - \theta_2\right|\right)$$

$$\tau_{2maxp} = -\tau_{2stop\_char}\left(20° - \left|\theta_2 - \theta_{2max}\right|\right)$$

When the club rotates in the clockwise direction, the passive torque will be
generated after the club enters the action range of the joint stop from θ_{2min} to
θ_{2lb}. Likewise, when the club rotates in the counterclockwise direction, the
passive torque will be generated after the club enters the action range of the
joint stop from θ_{2max} to θ_{2ub}.

4.3 Method to Utilize Dynamically Coupled Driving and Joint Stops

Some methods for controlling a manipulator with a passive joint using
dynamically coupled driving have been proposed (Arai and Tachi 1991; De
Luca and Oriolo 2002; Nakamura, Koinuma, and Suzuki 1996). The proposed
methods are interesting and effective for the manipulator with a complete

passive joint. For the hyper dynamic manipulator proposed in this chapter, these methods cannot be applied directly. Herein, we use a control method based on motion generation.

According to the foregoing statements, to improve the capability of dynamic manipulation, dynamically coupled driving must be made use of efficiently by adopting light and low-power actuators in a manipulator and one special motion trajectory, and the joint stop must be made available in the manipulator and utilized correctly in the motion. Obviously, the utilization of both dynamically coupled driving and the joint stop depends on the motion planning. Unfortunately, to the best of our knowledge, there is no mature analytical method to generate such motion for a nonlinear system. We solve this problem by adopting a constrained optimization method.

4.3.1 Motion Generation and Control Method

4.3.1.1 Motion Generation

Many related works have been reported regarding the motion generation of a manipulator (Wang, Timoszyk, and Bobrow 2001). Most of these optimal motion generation methods were based on joint trajectory approximation with a performance index and some constraints. In addition, general motion generation methods mainly generate the joint trajectory according to the specifications for velocity, acceleration, etc., of different joints in their joint space separately (Shimon 1999).

However, as mentioned previously, the features of this proposal are utilizing dynamically coupled driving and joint stops in a hyper dynamic manipulator to realize a smart structure like a human. Therefore, it is necessary to generate hyper dynamic manipulation of a manipulator while considering the constraints on maximum active torque and the power of the actuators, the characteristics of joint stops, etc., in addition to the boundary conditions such as motion specifications. If a motion trajectory satisfies both constraints and boundary conditions, dynamically coupled driving and joint stops will be utilized automatically. However, because the nonlinearity and coupling are strengthened by those constraints, the problem of motion planning becomes more difficult. Among the constraints, the hard constraint on active torque is the most pivotal factor for motion generation. It was found that joint trajectory-based methods are difficult to use to solve such kinds of motion generation problems.

To deal with such motion generation problems, time-dependent active torque functions of joint $i(i = 1, \cdots, n)$ during the whole period from initial position to finish position are used as inputs. If the active torque functions of joint $i(i = 1, \cdots, n)$ are known, the motions of these joints can be derived by solving direct dynamics by satisfying the hard constraints on active torque and actuator power and the characteristics of joint stops. We assign active torque functions of joint $i(i = 1, \cdots, n)$ as the sum of a series of basis functions multiplied by coefficients and transform the optimal motion planning problem into a problem of obtaining coefficients of the basis functions, the time (t_m) when the manipulator has the specified motion specifications and finish time (t_f). Therefore, the hyper dynamic manipulation that utilizes dynamically coupled driving and joint stops efficiently becomes the solution of such a constrained optimization problem.

$$\tau_i(t) = \sum_{j=1}^{p} c_{ij}B_j(t), \ (i = 1, \cdots, n) \tag{4.14}$$

where $0 \leq t \leq t_f$, $B_j(t)$ is the basis function, and c_{ij} is the coefficient of basis function.

The coefficients of the basis function and the time durations to satisfy the boundary conditions

$$(\theta(0), \dot{\theta}(0), \ddot{\theta}(0), \theta(t_m), \dot{\theta}(t_m), \ddot{\theta}(t_m), \theta(t_f), \dot{\theta}(t_f), \ddot{\theta}(t_f)$$

with different cost functions (J) can be derived by numerical iterative calculation shown in Equation (4.15) ($\mathbf{w}_1$, $\mathbf{w}_2$, and $\mathbf{w}_3$ are weighting factors). Then the solution of torque inputs for optimal motion and optimal motion itself can be generated simultaneously by calculation. Motion generation is performed by considering the hard constraints on the load capability of actuators and the constraints of two-direction joint stops.

$$\min \ C\left(\boldsymbol{\tau}, t_m, t_f\right) \tag{4.15}$$

subject to dynamics Equation (4.9), the initial conditions

$$\boldsymbol{\theta}(0) = \boldsymbol{\theta}_0, \dot{\boldsymbol{\theta}}(0) = 0, \ddot{\boldsymbol{\theta}}(0) = 0$$

and the hard constraints on the active torque $|\tau_i| \leq \tau_{imax}$, $(i = 1, \cdots, n)$, where

$$C\left(\boldsymbol{\tau}, t_m, t_f\right) = \mathbf{e}\left(\boldsymbol{\tau}, t_m\right)^{\mathrm{T}} \mathbf{w}_1 \mathbf{e}\left(\boldsymbol{\tau}, t_m\right) + \mathbf{e}\left(\boldsymbol{\tau}, t_f\right)^{\mathrm{T}} \mathbf{w}_2 \mathbf{e}\left(\boldsymbol{\tau}, t_f\right) + \mathbf{w}_3 J\left(\boldsymbol{\tau}\right)$$

$$\mathbf{e}\left(\boldsymbol{\tau}, t_m\right) = \mathbf{e}\left(\boldsymbol{\theta}\left(t_m\right), \dot{\boldsymbol{\theta}}\left(t_m\right), \ddot{\boldsymbol{\theta}}\left(t_m\right), \boldsymbol{\theta}_m, \dot{\boldsymbol{\theta}}_m, \ddot{\boldsymbol{\theta}}_m\right)$$

is the error function of the motion specifications at time t_m.

$$\mathbf{e}\left(\boldsymbol{\tau}, t_f\right) = \mathbf{e}\left(\boldsymbol{\theta}\left(t_f\right), \dot{\boldsymbol{\theta}}\left(t_f\right), \ddot{\boldsymbol{\theta}}\left(t_f\right), \boldsymbol{\theta}_f, \dot{\boldsymbol{\theta}}_f, \ddot{\boldsymbol{\theta}}_f\right)$$

is the finish conditions of the motion.

$$\theta = \left[\theta_1, \cdots, \theta_n\right]^T$$

4.3.1.2 Control Method

Generally, a computed torque method with linear feedback compensation can be adopted to realize trajectory tracking, based on the linearization and decoupling of a nonlinear and coupled system. However, for a hyper dynamic manipulator, because of the assumption of utilizing dynamically coupled driving and the ultra-high-motion speed, the real-time problem of control becomes more difficult compared to that of conventional manipulators even when adopting a computed torque method with linear feedback compensation. Therefore, a simplified feedforward system with a proportional-derivative (PD) controller is adopted instead of computed torque method.

4.3.2 Case Study: Motion Generation and Control of a Golf Swing Robot

As a study case, herein we discuss the motion generation and control of the real golf swing robot shown in Figure 4.4. For simplicity, we assume that the motion of the golf swing robot is on a plane, called a *swing plane*, and consider the motion of the arm and the club only. According to the above assumption, a simple model of the golf swing robot is used as shown in Figure 4.6.

The motion equation of the model can be represented by Equation (4.16), where the driving torque of the wrist joint is the sum of the active torque by the actuator and the passive torque by the joint stops shown in Equation (4.17). As the characteristics of the joint stop, a mathematical model of the passive torque shown by Equation (4.18) is considered. The hard constraints on the active torque are represented in Equation (4.19).

$$\tau_1 = M_{11}\ddot{\theta}_1 + M_{12}\ddot{\theta}_2 + h_{122}\dot{\theta}_2^{\,2} + 2h_{112}\dot{\theta}_1\dot{\theta}_2 + g_1$$

$$\tau_2 + \tau_{2p} = M_{21}\ddot{\theta}_1 + M_{22}\ddot{\theta}_2 + h_{211}\dot{\theta}_1^{\,2} + g_2$$

(4.16)

where

$$\tau_{2p} = \begin{cases} \tau_{2minp}, & 240° = \theta_{2lb} \le \theta_2 \le \theta_{2min} = 260° \\ 0, & 260° = \theta_{2min} < \theta_2 < \theta_{2max} = 460° \\ \tau_{2maxp}, & 460° = \theta_{2max} \le \theta_2 \le \theta_{2ub} = 480° \end{cases}$$

(4.17)

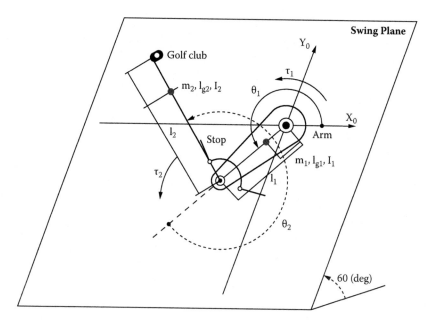

FIGURE 4.6
Model of a two-joint golf swing robot.

$$\tau_{2minp} = \tau_{2stop\_char}\left(20° - \left|\theta_{2min} - \theta_2\right|\right)$$

$$\tau_{2maxp} = -\tau_{2stop\_char}\left(20° - \left|\theta_{2max} - \theta_2\right|\right)$$

(4.18)

$$\left|\tau_1\right| \le \tau_{1max}$$

$$\left|\tau_2\right| \le \tau_{2max}$$

(4.19)

$\left(\theta_{2min}, \theta_{2max}\right)$ is the free rotation range of joint 2.

The main specifications of the DD motor (DR1130E00(H), Yokogawa Precision Co., Japan) used in the shoulder joint and the DD motor (D100-30, Nikki Denso Co., Japan) used in the wrist joint are shown in Table 4.1. The boundary conditions for motion specifications are shown in Table 4.2.

Here, we assign the active torque functions of joint 1 and joint 2 as a Fourier time series.

TABLE 4.1

Main Specifications of DD Motors

	Shoulder Joint	Wrist Joint
Max. torque (Nm)	110	9.8
Max. speed (rps)	4.3	5
Max. power (W)	3,000	70
Resolution of resolver (PPR)	31,9488	338,840
Weight (kg)	32	1.6

TABLE 4.2

Boundary Conditions

	$t = t_0 = 0$ (Address Time)	$t = t_m$ (Impact Time)	$t = t_f$ (Finish Time)
θ (deg)	$\theta_{10} = 270$	$\theta_{1m} = 270$	N/A
	$\theta_{20} = 0$	$\theta_{2m} = 0$	
$\dot{\theta}$ (rad/s)	$\dot{\theta}_{10} = 0$	$v_{ym} = 0\,(\text{m/s})$	$\dot{\theta}_{1f} = 0$
	$\dot{\theta}_{20} = 0$		$\dot{\theta}_{2f} = 0$
$\ddot{\theta}$ (rad/s^2)	$\ddot{\theta}_{10} = 0$	N/A	$\ddot{\theta}_{1f} = 0$
	$\ddot{\theta}_{20} = 0$		$\ddot{\theta}_{2f} = 0$

$$\begin{cases} \tau_1(t) = a_0 + \displaystyle\sum_{n=1}^{p} a_{2n\text{-}1} \cos\left(nt/kt_f + a_{2n}\right) \\[2mm] \tau_2(t) = b_0 + \displaystyle\sum_{n=1}^{q} b_{2n\text{-}1} \cos\left(nt/kt_f + b_{2n}\right) \end{cases} \tag{4.20}$$

where $0 \le t \le t_f$, $k > 0$.

Considering the motion specifications shown in Table 4.2, the detailed motion generation model is expressed by Equation (4.21). Herein, t_m is the time to realize the desired motion specifications, t_f is the finish time, v_x is the translational speed of the club head in the X_0 direction, v_y is the translational speed in the Y_0 direction, v_{xm} and v_{ym} are the desired impact speeds in the X_0 and Y_0 directions, and θ_m is the desired impact position. $\dot{\boldsymbol{\theta}}_f = \mathbf{0}$ and $\ddot{\boldsymbol{\theta}}_f = \mathbf{0}$ are the stop conditions of the manipulator without considering the stop position.

$$\min \; C\left(\boldsymbol{\tau}, t_m, t_f\right) \tag{4.21}$$

subject to Equations (4.16), (4.17), (4.18), (4.19) and the initial conditions $\boldsymbol{\theta}(0) = \boldsymbol{\theta}_0, \dot{\boldsymbol{\theta}}(0) = 0, \ddot{\boldsymbol{\theta}}(0) = 0$,

where

$$C\left(\boldsymbol{\tau}, t_m, t_f\right) = \mathbf{e}\left(\boldsymbol{\tau}, t_m\right)^{\mathrm{T}} \mathbf{w}_1 \mathbf{e}\left(\boldsymbol{\tau}, t_m\right) + \mathbf{e}\left(\boldsymbol{\tau}, t_f\right)^{\mathrm{T}} \mathbf{w}_2 \mathbf{e}\left(\boldsymbol{\tau}, t_f\right) + \mathbf{w}_3 J\left(\boldsymbol{\tau}\right)$$

$$\mathbf{e}\left(\boldsymbol{\tau}, t_m\right) = \left[\boldsymbol{\theta}\left(t_m\right) - \boldsymbol{\theta}_m; v_x\left(t_m\right) - v_{xm}; v_y\left(t_m\right) - v_{ym}\right]$$

$$\mathbf{e}\left(\boldsymbol{\tau}, t_f\right) = \left[\dot{\boldsymbol{\theta}}\left(t_f\right) - \dot{\boldsymbol{\theta}}_f; \ddot{\boldsymbol{\theta}}\left(t_f\right) - \ddot{\boldsymbol{\theta}}_f\right]$$

$$\boldsymbol{\theta} = \left[\theta_1, \theta_2\right]^{\mathrm{T}}$$

The other parameters for simulation are determined according to the average values of human beings and are omitted here.

The following cost function toward minimizing the total work consumed by the actuators of joint 1 and joint 2 is used.

$$J = \int_0^{t_f} \left|\tau_1(t) \cdot \dot{\theta}_1(t)\right| dt + \int_0^{t_f} \left|\tau_2(t) \cdot \dot{\theta}_2(t)\right| dt \tag{4.22}$$

DD motors are set to torque mode and are controlled by torque (voltage) reference from the computer. Angular positions of joints are measured through resolvers and counters by a board computer.

As characteristics of DD motors, coulomb friction torque and viscous friction torque must be compensated for because they cannot be neglected in the case of DD motors. Coulomb friction torque is calculated according to the relation between the reference voltage input to the motor driver and the output torque produced by the motor and is calibrated by experiments. Viscous friction coefficients are also calculated according to the experimental results of the relation between the voltage reference and the angular velocity.

As an implementation of the control system to the real manipulator, we constructed a controller shown in Figure 4.7. Considering the features of the robot, such as high speed, strong nonlinearity, and dynamic coupling, a feed-forward compensation is introduced with a PD controller. That is, the torque feed-forward compensations of joints combined with PD controllers for the angular positions of joints are used. The torques of joints for feed-forward compensation and the reference motions of joints for PD controller are generated by offline calculation according to the method described previously, before the swing starts. Sampling time for a feed-forward and feedback loop is 1 ms.

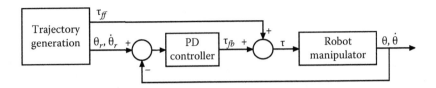

FIGURE 4.7
Control system.

4.4 Simulation and Experimental Results for the Golf Swing Robot

4.4.1 Simulation

Using the above-discussed motion generation method, simulations of the golf swing motion with joint stops for an impact speed of 25 m/s are implemented and the results are shown in Figure 4.8.

From Figure 4.8, the following features can be concluded.

1. In the backswing phase from the address position to the top position, the arm and the club are taken back by their motors just like in conventional motion control, because the angular velocity in this period is not so high.

2. During the downswing phase, the shoulder joint is accelerated first, and the wrist joint is accelerated later. At the beginning of the downswing, the wrist joint is kept in contact with the joint stop and a large constraint (passive) torque by the joint stop is generated (Figures 4.8b and 4.8d). This passive torque plays an important role in the initial acceleration of the wrist joint, because the active torque by the wrist joint is too small to accelerate the wrist joint itself at the beginning of the downswing. Just before the impact time, the shoulder joint is decelerated first, but the wrist joint is still accelerated rapidly to realize a very high head speed at the impact time (Figure 4.8b). This multistep acceleration is due to the utilization of dynamically coupled driving in joint 2, as discussed in Section 4.2. From Figure 4.8e, it can be observed that the dynamically coupled driving torque of joint 2 is mainly utilized to accelerate the golf club (Figure 4.6) in the downswing phase.

3. In the follow-through phase from impact position to finish position, an inverse behavior to that in the downswing period can be observed. That is, the wrist joint is decelerated and stopped mainly by dynamically coupled driving torque and passive torque

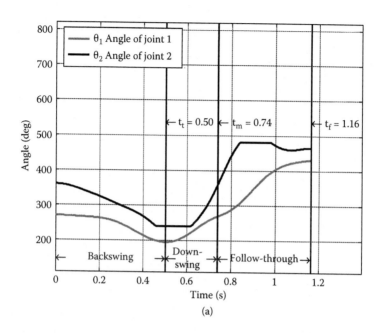

(a)

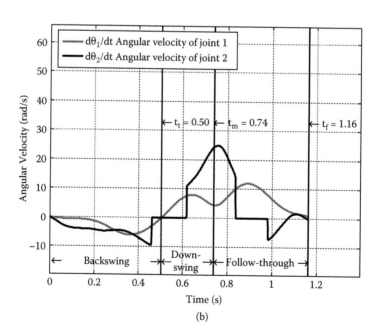

(b)

FIGURE 4.8
Simulation results with joint stops for V_{xm} = 25 m/s: (a) angle, (b) angular velocity. (*continued*)

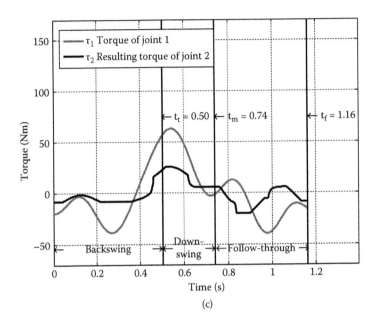

(c)

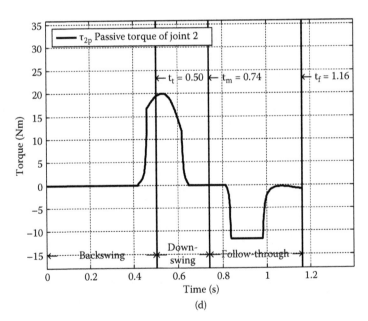

(d)

FIGURE 4.8 (Continued)
Simulation results with joint stops for $V_{xm} = 25$ m/s: (c) torque; (d) passive torque of joint 2.
(continued)

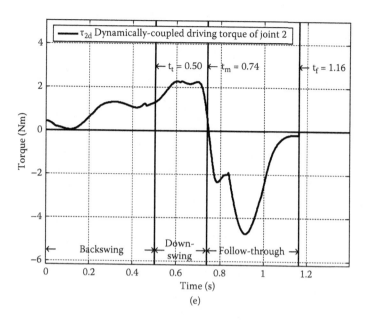

FIGURE 4.8 (Continued)
Simulation results with joint stops for V_{xm} = 25 m/s: (e) dynamically coupled driving torque of joint 2.

(Figures 4.8d and 4.8e). Then the shoulder joint is decelerated and stopped by its motor.

4.4.2 Experiments

By using the developed prototype shown in Figure 4.4 and the control system shown in Figure 4.7, experiments in various conditions have been done to validate the simulation results. As an example, a comparison between the swing without the joint stops (the joint stops are removed from the robot) and the swing with the joint stops is shown.

The experimental results of angle, angular velocity, and torques of each joint during the swing are shown in Figures 4.9 and 4.10. The case of not using the joint stops is presented in Figure 4.9, and Figure 4.10 presents the results obtained when using the joint stops. It is important to note that these experimental results are consistent with those obtained through the simulation (Figure 4.8).

By comparing Figures 4.9 and 4.10 the following can be concluded:

1. A compact swing can be realized by using joint stops (Figure 4.10a). That is, the angular displacement from the address position to the top position of the shoulder joint becomes smaller.

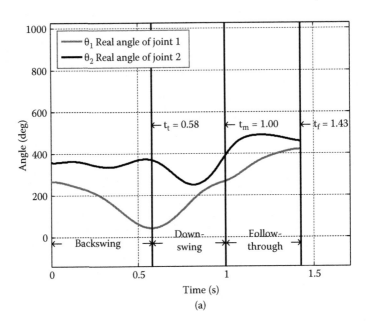

(a)

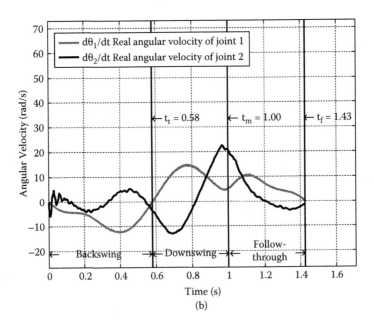

(b)

FIGURE 4.9
Experimental result without joint stop for $V_{xm} = 25$ m/s: (a) angle, (b) angular velocity.

(*continued*)

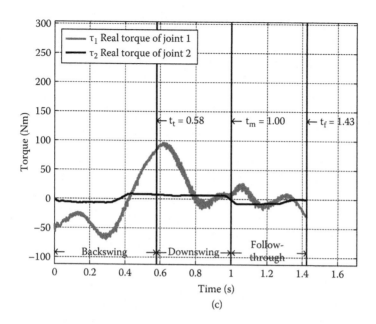

(c)

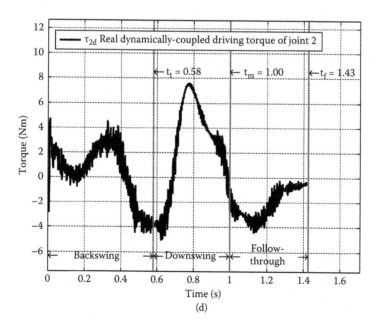

(d)

FIGURE 4.9 (Continued)
Experimental result without joint stop for V_{xm} = 25 m/s: (c) torque, (d) dynamically coupled driving torque of joint 2.

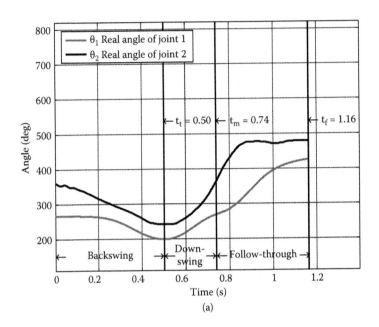

(a)

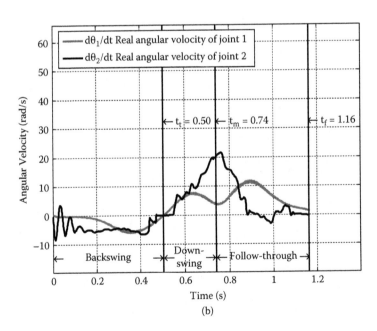

(b)

FIGURE 4.10
Experimental result with joint stop for $V_{xm} = 25$ m/s: (a) angle, (b) angular velocity.

(continued)

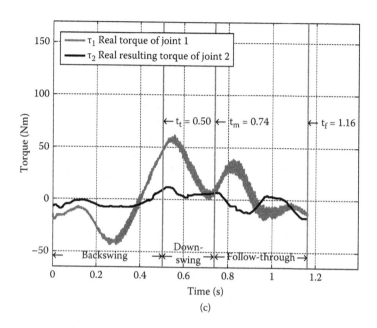

(c)

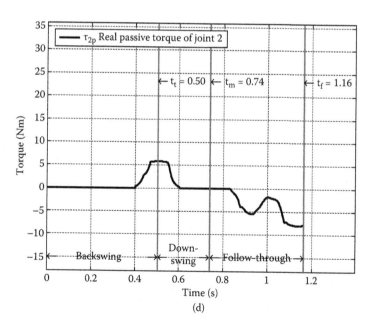

(d)

FIGURE 4.10 (Continued)
Experimental result with joint stop for $V_{xm} = 25$ m/s: (c) torque, (d) passive torque. (*continued*)

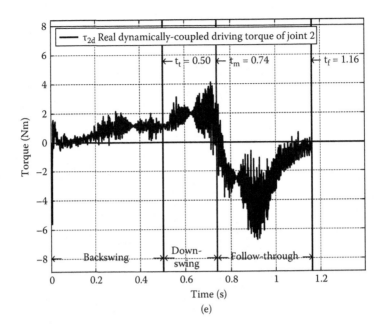

FIGURE 4.10 (Continued)
Experimental result with joint stop for $V_{xm} = 25$ m/s: (e) dynamically coupled driving torque of joint 2.

2. The maximum torque of the shoulder joint becomes much smaller due to the joint stop (Figure 4.10c).

Therefore, it is concluded that an efficient hyper dynamic manipulation is achieved by way of using dynamically coupled driving and joint stops in the smart structure manipulator.

4.5 Conclusion

To improve the capability of a manipulator, especially the capability for hyper dynamic manipulation, a basic concept of utilizing dynamically coupled driving and structural joint stops in a manipulator inspired by humans has been proposed. To show the feasibility of this proposal, a prototype of a hyper dynamic manipulator, namely, a golf swing robot, has been developed.

Experimental results show that hyper dynamic manipulation can be realized efficiently by the smart structure manipulator, through using such disposition of actuators and joint stops in the manipulator. It can be expected that this approach will serve as a general way toward realizing hyper dynamic manipulations for robots; for example, humanoid robots.

References

Arai, H. and Tachi, S. 1991. Position control system of a two degree of freedom manipulator with a passive joint. *IEEE Transactions on Industrial Electronics*, 38(1): 15–20.

De Luca, A. and Oriolo, G. 2002. Trajectory planning and control for planar robots with passive last joint. *The International Journal of Robotics Research*, 21(5–6): 575–590.

Hayakawa, Y., Kawamura, S., Goto, T., and Nagai, K. 1996. Development of a revolving drive mechanism for a robot manipulator by using pneumatic bellows actuators with force sensing ability. *Journal of the Robotics Society of Japan*, 14(2): 271–278. (in Japanese)

Hirzinger, G., Albu-Schaffer, A., Hahnle, M., Schaefer, I., and Spofer, N.. 2001. On a new generation of torque controlled light-weight robots. Paper read at the IEEE International Conference on Robotics and Automation, Seoul, Korea, May 21–26.

Hogan, N. 1985. An approach to manipulation. *ASME Journal of Dynamics, Systems, Measurement and Control*, 107: 1–24.

Kagami, S., Nishiwaki, K., Sugihara, T., Kuffner, J. J., Jr., Inaba, M., and Inoue, H. 2001. Design and implementation of software research platform for humanoid Robotics: H6. Paper read at the IEEE International Conference on Robotics and Automation, Seoul, Korea, May 21–26..

Katsurashima, W., Kikuchi, H., Abe, K., and Uchiyama, M. 1998. Design and development of a robot arm with flexible joints. Paper read at the RSJ Annual Conference, Hakkaido, Japan, September 18–20. (in Japanese)

Laurin-Kovitz, K. F., Colgate, J. E., and Carnes, S. D. R. 1991. Design of components for programmable passive impedance. Paper read at the IEEE International Conference on Robotics and Automation, Sacremento, CA, April 9–11.

Ming, A., Harada, N., Shimojo, M., and Kajitani, M. 2003. Development of a hyper dynamic manipulator utilizing joint stops. Paper read at the International Conference on Intelligent Robots and Systems, Las Vegas, NV, October 27–31.

Ming, A., Kajitani, M., and Shimojo, M. 2002. A proposal for utilizing structural joint stop in a manipulator. Paper read at the International Conference on Robotics and Automation.

Ming, A., Mita, T., Dhlamini S., and Kajitani, M. 2001. Motion control skill in human hyper dynamic manipulations—An investigation on the golf swing by simulation. Paper read at the IEEE International Symposium on Computational Intelligence in Robotics and Automation, Alberta, Canada, July 29–August 1.

Mizuuchi, I., Matsuki, T., Kagami, S., Inaba, M., and Inoue, H. 1998. An approach to a humanoid that has a variable flexible torso. Paper read at the RSJ Annual Conference, Hakkaido, Japan, September 18–20.. (in Japanese)

Morita, T., Tomita, N., Ueda, T., and Sugano, S. 1998. Development of force-controlled robot arm using mechanical impedance adjuster. *Journal of the Robotics Society of Japan*, 16(7): 1001–1006. (in Japanese)

Murray, R.M., Li, Z., and Sastry, S.S. 1994. *A Mathematical Introduction to Robotic Manipulation*. Boca Raton, FL: CRC Press.

Nagasaka, K., Kuroki, Y., Suzuki, S., Itoh, Y., and Yamaguchi, J. 2004. Integrated motion control for walking, jumping and running on a small bipedal entertrainment robot. Paper read at the IEEE International Conference on Robotics and Automation, New Orleans, LA, April 26–May 1.

Nakamura, Y., Koinuma, M., and Suzuki, T. 1996. Chotic behavior and nonlinear control of a two-joint planar arm with a free joint-control of noholonomic mechanisms with drift. *Journal of the Robotics Society of Japan*, 14(4): 602–611.

Okada, M., Nakamura, Y., and Ban, S. 2001. Design of programmable compliance for humanoid shoulder. *Experimental Robotics VII*, 31–40.

Shimon, N.Y. 1999. *Handbook of Industrial Robotics*, 2nd ed. New York: John Wiley & Sons.

Wang, C.-Y.E., Timoszyk, W.K., and Bobrow, J.E. 2001. Payload maximization for open chained manipulators: Finding weightlifting motions for a Puma 762 robot. *IEEE Transaction on Robotics and Automation*, 17(2): 218–224.

5

A School of Robotic Fish for Pollution Detection in Port

Huosheng Hu, John Oyekan, and Dongbing Gu
University of Essex
Colchester, UK

CONTENTS

5.1 Introduction 86
5.2 Inspired from Nature 87
5.3 Biologically Inspired Design 89
5.4 Layered Control Architecture 90
    5.4.1 Cognitive Layer 92
    5.4.2 Behavior Layer 92
    5.4.3 Swim Pattern Layer 93
5.5 Robotic Fish for Pollution Detection at Port 95
    5.5.1 System Configuration 95
    5.5.2 Bio-Inspired Coverage of Pollutants 97
5.6 Summary 101
Acknowledgments 102
References 103

Abstract

Natural selection has made fish beautiful swimmers with high efficiency and perfect maneuvering abilities. No man-made aquatic systems are currently able to match such performance. To build a robot to realize fish-like propulsion and maneuvering abilities requires a full understanding of fish muscle structure, hydrodynamics, and how to mimic. This chapter overviews the robotic fish research at Essex, which is focused on the biologically inspired design of autonomous robotic fish as well as their applications to pollution detection in port. Our efforts and experience in building a number of generations of robotic fishes to navigate in a three-dimensional unstructured environment are described, including the successful launch of an EU FP7 project SHOAL since March 2009. Finally, a brief summary and future research directions are outlined.

5.1 Introduction

In nature, fish propel themselves by bending their bodies and/or using their fins and have gained astonishing swim and maneuvering abilities after thousands years of evolution. For instance, the tuna swims with high speed and high efficiency, the pike accelerates in a flash, and the eel can swim skillfully into narrow holes. This has inspired many robotics researchers to build new types of aquatic man-made systems, namely, robotic fish. Instead of the conventional rotary propeller used in ships or underwater vehicles, a robotic fish relies on undulation or oscillatory movements to generate the main propulsion energy. It is clear that this kind of propulsion is less noisy and more maneuverable than man-made underwater vehicles.

RoboTuna was the first robotic fish developed at the Massachusetts Institute of Technology in 1994 (Streitlien, Triantafyllou, and Triantafyllou 1996) to explore and understand the biology of aquatic creatures. Since then, many kinds of robotic fishes have been developed worldwide. A robotic lamprey using shape memory alloy (SMA; Jalbert, Kashin, and Ayers 1995) was built at Northwestern University, with the aim to realize mine countermeasures. In Japan, a micro-robotic fish was developed at Nagoya University using an ionic conducting polymer film (ICPF) actuator (Guo et al. 1998) and Tokai University constructed a robotic Blackbass (Kato 2000) to research the propulsion of pectoral fins. The National Maritime Research Institute (NMRI) has developed many kinds of robotic fish prototypes, from PF300 to PPF-09, to exploit the effective swimming mode. Mitsubishi Heavy Industries built a robotic fish to mimic an extinct fish, namely, coelacanth (Yamamoto and Terada 2003). Most of the current robotic fish can only operate in the laboratory, swimming on the water surface, and are not robust enough for daily operation in the real world.

The Essex Robotics Research Group has worked on robotic fish research since 2003, aiming to design and build autonomous robotic fish that would have three major features: to (1) swim like a real fish; (2) realize autonomous navigation; and (3) be deployed in real-world applications (Liu and Hu 2010). Most important, the robotic fish we built should be able to swim in three dimensions within an unknown and dynamically changing environment and should be fully autonomous in daily operations. Also, it will be able to be deployed for real-world applications such as water pollution monitoring and security surveillance. This chapter is focused on the biologically inspired design of our autonomous robotic fish; that is, how the basic fish swimming behaviors have been realized in our robotic fish, as well as its application to pollution detection in a seaport.

The rest of this chapter is organized as follows. Inspired from nature, Section 5.2 describes fish swimming behaviors and their division in terms of propulsion mechanism and temporal features. Section 5.3 presents the biologically inspired design of Essex robotic fish and Section 5.4 describes novel layered control architecture for the realization of fish swim behaviors in our robotic fish. Section 5.5 presents a brief introduction of our robotic fish used in pollution detection. Finally, a brief summary is presented in Section 5.6.

5.2 Inspired from Nature

Today, biological fish exhibit a large variety of swimming behaviors that are generated by undulatory or oscillatory movements of their body or fins, as shown in Figure 5.1. In general, fish swimming motion can be viewed from two different angles. One is propulsion mechanisms and another is temporal features. This has inspired robotics researchers to build robotic fish that can mimic the swimming behaviors of real fish.

In terms of propulsion mechanisms, some fish bend their bodies and/or caudal fins (BCF) and other fish use their median and/or paired fins (MPF). Both BCF and MPF propulsion can be further divided into undulatory and oscillatory propulsion. Four types of undulatory BCF propulsion (anguilliform, subcarangiform, carangiform, thunniform) and one type of oscillatory BCF propulsion (ostraciiform) are shown in Figure 5.2 (Sfakiotakis, Lane, and Davies 1999). In undulatory BCF propulsion, the propulsive wave traverses the fish body in a direction opposite to the overall movement and at a speed greater than the overall swimming speed. Apart from caudal fins, some fish use more bodies to generate the propulsive wave and others use less bodies.

Anguilliform in Figure 5.2a is highly undulatory, and thunniform in Figure 5.2d is toward oscillatory. Subcarangiform in Figure 5.2b and carangiform in Figure 5.2c are in between. Their wavelength, wave amplitude, and the way in which thrust is generated are all different. For instance, the fish body shows large-amplitude undulation in anguilliform, but undulation decreased gradually from subcarangiform to carangiform to thunniform.

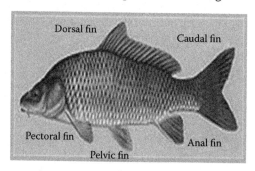

FIGURE 5.1
Typical fin configuration of fish.

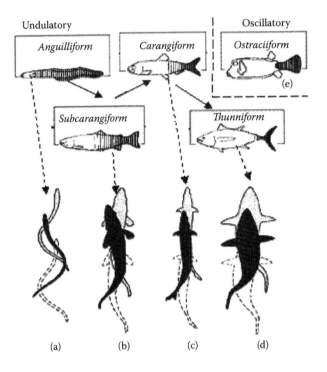

FIGURE 5.2
Fish with BCF propulsion.

The oscillatory BCF propulsion, which ostraciiform, is characterized by the pendulum oscillation of its stiff caudal fin. The fish body is essentially rigid, as shown in Figure 5.2e. On the other hand, both undulatory and oscillatory MPF propulsion are routinely adopted by many fish as auxiliary propulsors for stabilization and maneuvering, although some fish may use them as main locomotion means at low speeds. The temporal features of fish swimming behaviors can be classified as:

- Steady/sustained swimming, which is characterized by a cyclic repetition of the propulsive movements for a long distance at a roughly constant speed.
- Unsteady/transient swimming, which is typically for catching prey or avoiding predators, including fast starts, sharp turns, bursts, and escape maneuvers (Sfakiotakis, Lane, and Davies 1999).

Steady swimming behaviors of fish have been widely investigated by biologists, mathematicians, and robotics researchers. In fact, unsteady swimming behaviors of fish also play an important role in fish life, in which body movements are very significant and characterized by high accelerations. Some biologists have recently studied unsteady swimming motion of fish;

for example, the kinematics of fish. It should be noticed that both steady and unsteady swimming behaviors of fish can be realized by BCF and MPF propulsions or their combination. This reflects the complexity of fish swimming movements (Drucker and Lauder 2002).

To mimic fish swimming abilities, current robotic fish projects have been focused on three aspects: (1) fish locomotion and hydrodynamics, (2) artificial muscle technologies, and (3) sensor-based control mechanisms. Most researchers have worked on one of these aspects. Man-made ships and underwater vehicles are based on steady-state hydrodynamics for the high stability and high loading capability and are unable to match the turning and maneuvering capability of real fish. Therefore, the construction of the robotic fish relies on a full understanding of undulatory or oscillatory movements of real fish, corresponding hydrodynamics, new materials, and advanced control mechanisms.

Different from most previous research, we focus on two levels of complexity of fish locomotion systems; that is, swimming patterns for propulsion and multiple behaviors for temperate features. Layered control architecture has been developed at Essex by Liu, Hu, and Gu (2006) to realize fish-like swimming behaviors, especially unsteady behaviors such as sharp turning and fast starts. Our research has focused on undulatory BCF propulsion, that is, carangiform, in order to realize it in our robotic fish and study its advantages in the engineering field. Other types of BCF and MPF will be investigated gradually in our future research.

5.3 Biologically Inspired Design

We have built a number of generations of robotic fishes at Essex. Figure 5.3 shows six generations. In general, these robotic fish are about 50 cm long and have three or four powerful R/C servo motors and 2 DC motors. Servo motors are concatenated together in the tail to act as joints, as shown in Figure 5.4. Additionally, one DC motor is fixed in the head to change center of gravity of the fish for diving and another DC motor controls the micropump. On the back of the fish body, a dorsal fin is fixed vertically to keep the fish from swaying. The high quality of the servo motors and the very soft structure of the tail make it possible for the robotic fish to bend its body at a large angle in a short time, which is novel, and nobody, as far as we know, has done this before us.

Each robotic fish has over ten embedded sensors: one gyroscope, one pressure sensor, two position sensors, two current sensors, one voltmeter, four infrared sensors, and one inclinometer. These embedded sensors enable the fish to detect its depth, the yaw/roll/pitch angle of its body, and the distance to the obstacle in front of it. Additionally, the servo position and current consumption information can be obtained. Bluetooth and RS232 serial ports

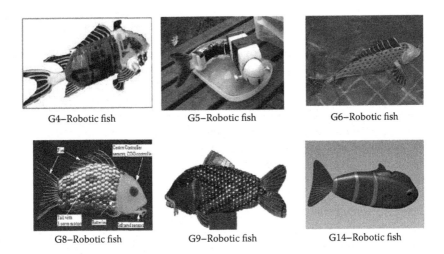

G4–Robotic fish   G5–Robotic fish   G6–Robotic fish

G8–Robotic fish   G9–Robotic fish   G14–Robotic fish

FIGURE 5.3
Robotic fish built at Essex (*G* means generation).

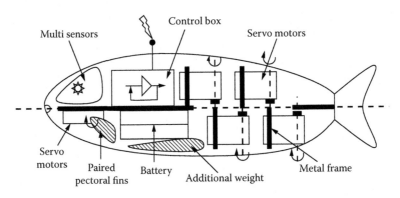

FIGURE 5.4
Configuration of Essex robotic fish.

are used to communicate with an external PC, which is used to program Gumstix and peripheral interface controller (PIC) and collect the sensor log. Figure 5.5 shows one of the Essex robotic fish that operated in the London Aquarium in 2005. The fish demonstrated an extremely fish-like motion and attracted much attention worldwide.

5.4 Layered Control Architecture

Figure 5.6 presents the layered control architecture for our robotic fish, which consists of three layers: the cognitive layer, behavior layer, and swim

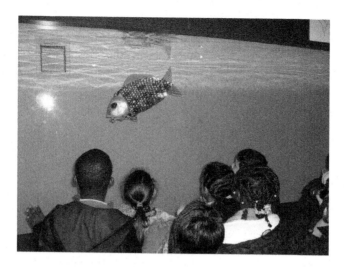

FIGURE 5.5
Essex robotic fish operated in the London Aquarium.

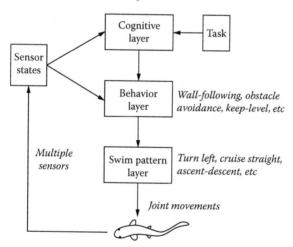

FIGURE 5.6
Layered control architecture.

pattern layer (Liu, Hu, and Gu 2006). Compared with traditional plan-based approaches, it has the advantages of easy design, fast response, and robustness. The swim pattern layer is particularly designed for the special propulsion feature of the robotic fish. In the behavior layer, states and actions are directly related to the robot physical sensors and swim patterns. In the cognitive layer, states related to high-level activities are abstracted and used to direct the behavior coordination in the behavior layer.

Within this layered architecture, parameter optimization can be conducted separately at each layer. For instance, in the swim pattern layer, each swim pattern is optimized to achieve the best performance. In the behavior layer, behaviors are optimized according to the encoding method of behaviors. If behaviors are encoded by fuzzy logic controllers, fuzzy rulers and fuzzy function parameters will be optimized. In the cognitive layer, optimization also could be designed for the parameters of reasoning and planning tasks (Liu, Hu, and Gu 2006).

5.4.1 Cognitive Layer

The cognitive layer extracts the robotic fish status from the sensor states and then performs task-oriented reasoning and planning. It makes decisions on how to coordinate fish behaviors to achieve a given task. Rather than providing a detailed objective for the behavior layer, for example, a particular trajectory for the robotic fish to follow, the cognitive layer adjusts the contribution weights of individual behaviors for the emergent behavior. In addition, the cognitive layer will adjust the parameters for some individual behaviors, such as the depth level for keep-level behaviors.

In a known environment with available models, planning can be done offline, and solutions can be found and evaluated prior to execution. However, in dynamically changing environments, models and policies need to be adaptively revised online at this layer. Trial-and-error processes are normally carried out. As can be seen from Figure 5.6, the raw sensor data are converted into sensor states so that individual behaviors take sensor states as stimulus and calculate responses concurrently. The cognitive layer extracts the abstracted states from the sensor states. The parameters for behavior coordination are transferred into the behavior layer after reasoning and planning.

5.4.2 Behavior Layer

The behavior layer is located in the middle of the proposed layered control architecture for the reactive control of our robotic fish. It firstly converts the sensor raw data into sensory states by fuzzy membership functions and then inputs these states into individual behaviors. Fuzzy logic controllers are designed for individual behaviors to process these states. The responses of all behaviors are coordinated together by the behavior coordination function, which is defined by the parameters from the output of the cognitive layer. The subsumption architecture is adopted for this layer because of its simplicity. Here the stimulus is the sensor states and the response is the action. Stimulus–response (SR) diagrams (Arkin 1998) are used for the design of specific behavioral configurations. Eight behaviors are designed for the generic purpose in this layer, namely:

1. Avoid obstacles behavior to avoid both stationary and moving objects based on infrared (IR) sensors. The possible action is selected from all swim patterns.

2. Follow-wall behavior to keep the robotic fish at a certain distance from the wall based on the information gathered by IR sensors. The possible actions are cruise straight, cruise in left/right turn.

3. Wander behavior to explore the tank randomly. No sensor states are necessary. Possible actions include cruise straight, cruise in left/right turn, and ascend/descend.

4. Keep-level behavior to keep the robotic fish swimming at a desired depth level specified by the cognitive layer. It monitors the pressure sensor data and controls whether the fish ascend or descend.

5. Seek-goal behavior to direct the robotic fish to swim toward the goal; the possible actions are cruise straight and cruise in right turn.

6. Noise behavior using a random swim pattern to avoid the local minima and go out from a trap situation by trying all kinds of swim patterns.

7. Feed behavior for a robotic fish to return to a charging station when its battery is low.

8. Rescue behavior for emergency and self-protection action when robotic fish face unexpected situations such as motors malfunction, extreme high internal temperature, etc.

The behavior layer not only decides which swim pattern will be selected next but adjusts some key parameters for the selected swim pattern. Each swim pattern has tens of parameters in its function to specify its performance. However, to simplify the control loop, the behavior layer only adjusts two parameters. More details can be found in Liu and Hu (2010).

5.4.3 Swim Pattern Layer

Our project aims to design and build an autonomous navigation robotic fish that would swim like a real fish and realize autonomous navigation. To realize the fish-like motion, we have designed three or four tail joints for our robotic fish. The added-mass hydrodynamic theory is adopted here to achieve seven fish-like swim patterns as follows.

1. *Cruise straight*: The fish swims along a straight line at a constant speed, possibly with small acceleration/deceleration.

2. *Cruise in turning*: Fish is turning in a small angle and at a constant speed.

3. *Burst*: The fish shows sudden straight acceleration; that is, cyclic fast undulation. The burst-and-coast swim pattern is commonly used in fish life for energy savings expected up to 50%.

4. *Sharp turn*: Generates a sudden angular acceleration for avoiding predators or obstacles, including two types: C-shaped and S-shaped.

5. *Brake*: The fish generates a sudden straight deceleration by its special tail motion, usually in combination with pectoral and pelvic fins.

6. *Coast*: A kind of motion in which the fish body is kept motionless and straight.

7. *Ascend–descend*: A kind of motion in which a robotic fish can change its depth in water.

A detailed description of these swimming patterns can be found in Hu et al. (2006). Here we only explain two swimming patterns for simplicity.

The motion of the fish tail in cruise straight could be described by a traveling wave shown in Equation (5.1), which was originally suggested by Lighthill (1960). Its original point is set at the conjunction point between the fish head and its tail. The parameter vector $E = \{c_1, c_2, k, \omega\}$ is the key element to determine the kinematics of the fish tail.

$$y_{body}(x, t) = (c_1 x + c_2 x^2)\sin(kx + \omega t)w \tag{5.1}$$

where y_{body} is transverse displacement of a tail unit; X is displacement along the main axis; $k = 2\pi/\lambda$ is the wave number; λ is the wavelength; c_1 is the linear wave amplitude envelope; c_2 is the quadratic wave amplitude envelope; $\omega = 2\pi f$ is wave frequency; f is the oscillating frequency of the tail; and t is time.

The sharp turn sequence includes the *shrink stage*, in which the tail bends to one side very quickly, and the *release stage*, in which the tail unbends in a relatively slow speed from the middle section of the body to the tail tip (Liu and Hu 2004). A circle function shown in Equation (5.2) is deployed to describe the joint-end trajectory, which is tangential to the *x*-axis. The center of the circle changes with respect to time.

$$[x - Cx(t)]^2 + [y - Cy(t)]^2 = Cy^2(t) \tag{5.2}$$

where

$$Cx(t) = \begin{cases} (cx_1 - cx_0)(t - t_0)/(t_1 - t_0) + cx_0 & t \in [t_0, t_1) \\ cx_2(t - t_1/t_2 - t_1)^2 & t \in [t_1, t_2] \end{cases}$$

$$Cy(t) = \begin{cases} \min(cy_0, cy_1 \cdot e^{-k(t-t_1)}) & t \in [t_0, t_1) \\ (cy_1 - cy_2)(t - t_2)/(t_1 - t_2) + cy_2 & t \in [t_1, t_2] \end{cases}$$

where $cx_i, cy_i, t_i, (i = 1, 2, 3), k$ are parameters to decide the feature of the sharp turn swim pattern such as shape, bending speed, maximum bending angle, etc.

5.5 Robotic Fish for Pollution Detection at Port

5.5.1 System Configuration

Funded by the European Union FP7 grant, the SHOAL project (Search and monitoring of Harmful contaminants Other pollutants And Leaks in vessels in part using a swarm of robotic fish) aims to design and create advanced robotic fish that are able to navigate the port environment autonomously. These robotic fish will be fitted with underwater communications in order to communicate with each other and broadcast their information to the shoreline. They will be fitted with chemical sensors in order to detect different pollutants in the water, and they will have embedded intelligence allowing them to search and monitor pollution as a swarm.

To develop a technique to control the robotic fish swarm for their sensors to monitor a port environment, we face some technical challenges. The first challenge is how to quickly find the source of pollutant, and the second challenge is how to effectively control the agents so that collision between them is avoided. Researchers have been investigating various approaches to provide coverage to the environment. This includes the use of deterministic approaches such as multispanning trees for multiple robots and cellular decomposition (Gabriely and Rimon 2001; Zheng et al. 2005). However, it has been proven that the performance of deterministic approaches approaches that of stochastic approaches in the presence of noise from the environment (Balch 2000; Nikolaus and Alcherio 2007).

Figure 5.7 shows the general architecture of the SHOAL system being developed by the SHOAL consortium. A swarm of robotic fish will be built at Essex and communicated through an underwater sonar system developed by the project partner, Thales Safare in France. Robotic fish receive the signals from a network of four pingers in order to calculate their position. When a robotic fish is surfacing, it is able to receive a Global Positioning System (GPS) signal from satellites to update its position and its clock.

Figure 5.8 presents the control software architecture for SHOAL robotic fish. As can be seen, it has three layers and is based on the layered control architecture shown in Figure 5.6. The addition of three modules, such as

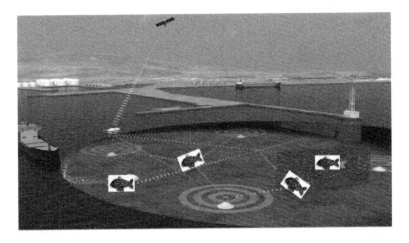

FIGURE 5.7
Description of EU SHOAL project.

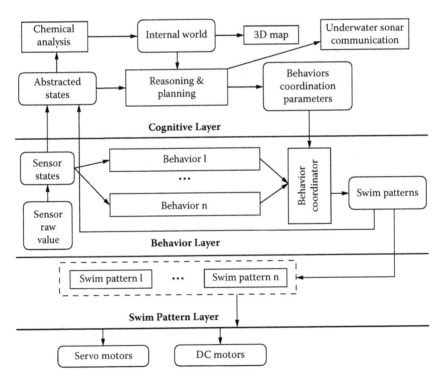

FIGURE 5.8
Control software architecture for SHOAL robotic fish.

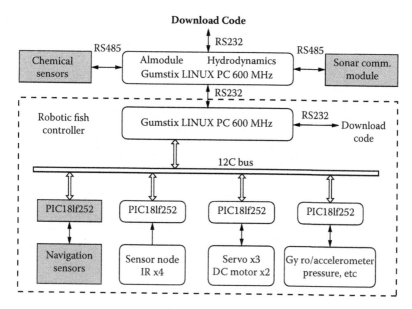

FIGURE 5.9
Hardware configuration of SHOAL robotic fish.

chemical analysis, underwater sonar communication, and a three-dimensional map, is to implement the pollution monitoring tasks as well as pollution mapping. The hardware configuration of the control system for SHOAL robotic fish is shown in Figure 5.9, in which two small Gumstix PCs with a Linux operating system are deployed. The design of a SHOAL-1 robotic fish, which is about 80 cm long and 30 cm high, is presented in Figure 5.10. It was displayed at the Science Museum in London between June 2010 and February 2011.

5.5.2 Bio-Inspired Coverage of Pollutants

We have developed a novel bacterial chemotaxis algorithm to find the source of the pollution in a port. A flocking algorithm is deployed to position the robotic fish optimally, avoid collisions, and ensure group foraging. The key idea is to place our robotic fish in a port environment based upon the density profile of the pollutant to be monitored so that areas of high environmental pollutant concentration receive more attention than areas of low pollutant concentration. In this way, densely polluted areas are monitored more close than the sparsely polluted areas, which is computationally efficient and cost-effective.

A bacterium chemotaxis motion is composed of a combination of tumble and run phases. The frequency of these phases depends on the measured concentration gradient in the surrounding environment. The run phase is

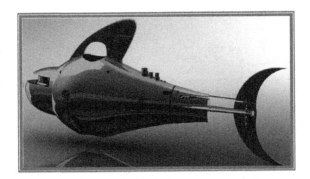

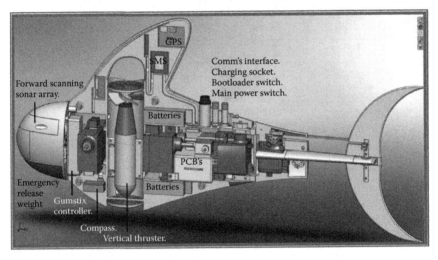

FIGURE 5.10
SHOAL fish for pollution detection: (a) run length = 2 and (b) run length = 30.

generally a straight line, whereas the tumble phase is a random change in direction with a mean of about 68 degrees in the *Escherichia coli* bacterium. If the bacterium is moving up a favorable gradient, it tumbles less, thereby increasing the length of the run phase and vice versa if going down an unfavorable gradient. This behavior was modeled by Berg and Brown by fitting the results of their experimental observations in Brown and Berg (1974) with a best fit equation in Berg and Brown (1972). This model is shown below:

$$\tau = \tau_0 \exp(\alpha \, dP_b/dt) \tag{5.3}$$

$$\frac{dP_b}{dt} = \frac{k_d}{(k_d + C)^2} \frac{dC}{dt} \tag{5.4}$$

$x_i P_b$ where τ is the mean run length and τ_0 is the mean run length in the absence of concentration gradients, α is a constant of the system based on the chemotaxis sensitivity factor of the bacteria, and P_b is the fraction of the receptor bound at concentration C. In this work, C is taken as the present reading taken by the robotic agent. k_d is the dissociation constant of the bacterial chemoreceptor, and dP_b/dt is the rate of change of P_b.

The following modified flocking controller is used to realize the flocking control for agent x_i.

$$x_i^f(t) = -K(dist(t) - d)(x_i(t) - x_j(t)) + B \qquad (5.5)$$

where $D(t) = |x_i(t) - x_j(t)|$; $B = H(x_i(t) - x_h(t))$; $x_h(t)$ is the position of the agent with the highest measurement in the neighborhood of x_i. The neighborhood is determined by the communication radius of each robot agent. $K > 0$ is the magnitude of the repulsion force between agent x_i and agent x_j. Constant H is the attractant gain for the force between agent x_i and the agent x_h with the highest environmental quantity measurement in the neighborhood.

The two behaviors are then combined and the new position of the agent x_i calculated using x_i:

$$x_i(t+1) = \beta(t) + (Fx_i^f(t) + Bx_i^b(t)) \qquad (5.6)$$

where both constants $F = 0.01$ and $B = 0.94$ are gains for the flocking and the bacteria behavior, respectively.

Before combining the two behaviors together, the bacterial chemotaxis controller was subjected to tests using two metrics of environmental exploration and source convergence. Fifty robots were used in our simulations for each change in parameter value to gain an accurate view of the effects of the parameter value change. Each parameter was increased from 2 to 30 in increments of two and results were recorded from each investigation. Each robot moved independently without knowing about other robots in the environment.

In addition, each simulation ran for a short time of 2.5 minutes because given a long enough time, all robots would eventually find the source and would not give an opportunity to investigate the effect of parameter changes. The source was placed at coordinates of $(x, y) = (400, 400)$ and the agents were randomly placed at $(x, y) = (250, 150)$ with a standard deviation of 5. In the bacteria chemotaxis experiments, the velocity was kept constant.

As shown in Figure 5.11, the larger the standard run length is, the larger the area covered by the robots is and the longer it takes to converge at the source. The reason for this is that greater run length values tend to reduce

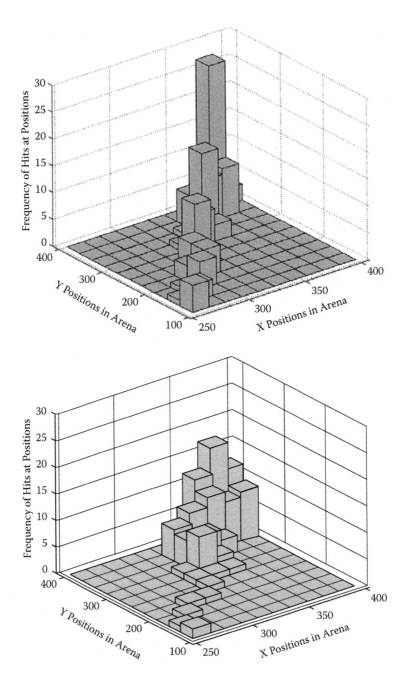

FIGURE 5.11
Pollutant coverage at different run length values.

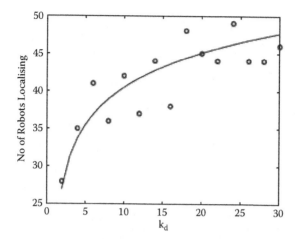

FIGURE 5.12
Relation between k_d and the number of robots at $\alpha = 30$.

the rate of tumble taking place in the environment according to Equation (5.1). The k_d value is responsible for the chemosensory sensitivity of the receptors on the bacteria as mentioned above. As shown in Figure 5.12, a higher k_d results in more robots localizing at the source. As a result, the areas with higher k_d are covered more often by the robots that seek rich pollutant concentrations.

By combining the bacteria behavior with the flocking behavior, a swarm of robots is able to cover the environmental pollution. As can be seen in Figure 5.13, the mean of the distribution of the flock of robots is close to the mean of the distribution of the pollutants. By changing the control parameters, it is possible to change the spread of the robots in the pollutants. This feature is very useful in real-world applications.

5.6 Summary

This chapter overviews our research work on the design and construction of autonomous robotic fish at Essex. Our research has been focused on two levels of complexity of fish locomotion by building a layered control architecture. A number of robot behaviors have been developed to realize autonomous navigation and a number of fish swimming patterns were designed to realize the fish-like swimming motion as a carangiform fish does, including cruise straight, cruise in turning, sharp turn, and ascend–descend. Our robotic fish has a number of computers embedded in it (one Gumstix and three PIC microcontrollers) and over ten sensors. It can cope

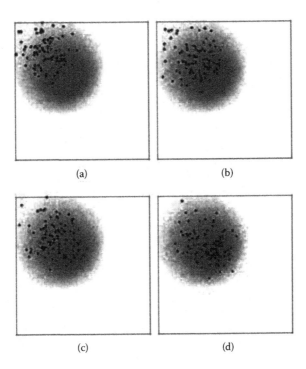

FIGURE 5.13
Sequence of the flock distribution in pollutants.

with unexpected obstacles and can swim in a three-dimensional unstructured environment as a real fish does.

Currently we are working on the construction of SHOAL robotic fish for pollution monitoring at port. The field testing will be carried out at Gijón in Spain in 2012, as shown in Figure 5.14. These robotic fish could be potentially useful in many other marine and military applications such as investigating deep-sea fish behaviors, demining, seabed exploration, oil pipe leakage detection, military reconnaissance, etc. To reach this goal, we will develop an efficient strategy for a school of robotic fish to cooperate on a common mission task. Our future research will be focused on how to make our robotic fish more robust and adaptive like a real fish. Different types of fish swimming behaviors will be added gradually. Also, our robotic fish should be able to find the charging station similar to the way in which real fish look for food.

Acknowledgments

This project was financially sponsored by the European Union FP7 program, ICT-231646, SHOAL. Thanks to the other members of the EU SHOAL

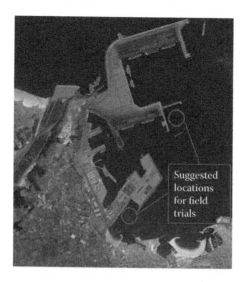

FIGURE 5.14
Test site at the Port of Gijón, Spain.

consortium, namely, BMT (Coordinator), Tyndall, THALÈS-SAFARE, The University of Strathclyde, and The Port Authority of Gijón. Our thanks also go to the current team members at Essex, Ian Dukes, George Francis, and Bowen Lv, as well as previous team members Jindong Liu and Robert Knight, for their excellent contributions to the project.

References

Arkin, R. 1998. *Behaviour Based Robotics*. Cambridge, MA: MIT Press.

Balch, T. 2000. The case for randomized search. Paper read at the Workshop on Sensors and Motion, IEEE International Conference on Robotics and Automation, San Francisco, CA, April 24–28, 2000..

Berg, H.C. and Brown, D.A. 1972. Chemotaxis in *Escherichia coli* analysed by 3D tracking. *Nature*, 239.

Brown, D.A. and Berg, H.C. 1974. Temporal stimulation of chemotaxis in *Escherichia coli*. *Proceedings of the National Academy of Sciences, USA*, 71(4): 1388–1392.

Drucker, E.G. and Lauder, G.V. 2002. Experimental hydrodynamics of fish locomotion: Functional insights from wake visualization. *Journal of Integrative and Comparative Biology*, 42: 243–257.

Gabriely, Y. and Rimon, E. 2001. Spanning-tree based coverage of continuous areas by a mobile robot. *Annals of Mathematics and Artificial Intelligence*, 31: 77–98.

Guo, S., Fukuda, T., Kato, N., and Oguro, K. 1998. Development of underwater micro-robot using ICPF actuator. Paper read at the IEEE Conference on Robotics and Automation, Leuven, Belgium, May 16–20, 1998.

Hu, H., Liu, J., Dukes, I., and Francis, G. 2006. Design of 3D swim patterns for autonomous robotic fish. Paper read at the IEEE/RSJ International Conference on Intelligent Robots & Systems, Beijing, China, October 9–15, 2006.

Jalbert, J., Kashin, S., and Ayers, J. 1995. A biologically-based undulatory lamprey-like AUV. Paper read at the Autonomous Vehicles in Mine Countermeasures Symposium. Naval Postgraduate School, Monterey, CA.

Kato, N. 2000. Control performance in the horizontal plane of a fish robot with mechanical pectoral fins. *IEEE Journal of Oceanic Engineering*, 25(1): 121–129.

Lighthill, M.J. 1960. Note on the swimming of slender fish. *Journal of Fluid Mechanics*, 9: 305–317.

Liu, J. and Hu, H. 2004. A 3D simulator for autonomous robotic fishes. *International Journal of Automation and Computing*, 1(1): 42–50.

Liu, J. and Hu, H. 2010. Biological inspiration: From carangiform fish to multi-joint robotic fish. *Journal of Bionic Engineering*, 7(2): 35–48.

Liu, J., Hu, H., and Gu, D. 2006. A layered control architecture for robotic fish. Paper read at the IEEE/RSJ International Conference on Intelligent Robots and Systems, 9–15 October, Beijing, China.

Nikolaus, C. and Alcherio, M. 2007. Robust distributed coverage using a swarm of miniature robots. Paper read at the IEEE/RSJ International Conference on Robotics and Automation, San Diego, CA, October 29–November 2, 2007.

Sfakiotakis, M., Lane, D.M., and Davies, J.B.C. 1999. Review of fish swimming modes for aquatic locomotion. *IEEE Journal of Ocean Engineering*, 24(2): 237–252.

Streitlien, K., Triantafyllou, G.S., and Triantafyllou, M.S. 1996. Efficient foil propulsion through vortex control. *AIAA Journal*, 34(11): 2315–2319.

Yamamoto, I. and Terada, Y. 2003. Robotic fish and its technology. Paper read at the SICE Annual Conference in Fukui, Fukui University, Japan.

Zheng, X., Jain, X., Koenig, S., and Kempe, D. 2005. Multi-robot forest coverage. Paper read at the IEEE International Conference on Robotics and Automation, Barcelona, Spain, April 18–22, 2005.

6

Development of a Low-Noise Bio-Inspired Humanoid Robot Neck

Bingtuan Gao
Southeast University
Nanjing, China
and
Michigan State University
East Lansing, Michigan

Ning Xi, Jianguo Zhao, and Jing Xu
Michigan State University
East Lansing, Michigan

CONTENTS

6.1 Introduction 106
6.2 Low-Motion–Noise Robotic Head/Neck System 107
    6.2.1 System Overview 107
    6.2.2 Hardware Development 108
    6.2.3 Programming Head Movements 111
6.3 Inverse Kinematics and Statics Analysis 111
    6.3.1 Neck Mechanism 111
    6.3.2 Cable and Housing 114
6.4 Control Strategy 116
    6.4.1 Rigidity Maintenance 116
    6.4.2 Motion Control 117
6.5 Implementation 118
    6.5.1 Experimental Setup and Motion Control of the Robotic Neck. 118
    6.5.2 Motion Noise Test 118
6.6 Summary 120
Acknowledgment 120
References 123

Abstract

105

A humanoid neck system that can effectively mimic the motion of a human neck with very low motion noises is presented in this chapter. The low-motion–noise humanoid neck system is based on the spring structure and is cable driven, which can generate 3 degrees of freedom of neck movement. To guarantee the low-noise feature, no noisemakers like motors, gearboxes, and electrodriven parts are embedded in the head–neck structure. Instead, the motions are driven by six polyester cables, and the actuators winching the cables are sealed in a sound insulation box. Statics analysis and control strategy of the system is discussed. Experimental results clearly show that the head–neck system can greatly mimic the motions of human head with an A-weighted noise level of 30 dB or below.

6.1 Introduction

The use of donning respirators or chemical-resistant jackets for some emergent conditions or during performing some special tasks is required. Most current donning respirators or chemical-resistant jackets unavoidably generate acoustic noises when the user moves his head/neck. These noises strongly interfere with the user's hearing even when using head-worn wireless communication equipment. Thus, it is necessary to develop a testing wearable audio system. Many companies have created systems for testing headphones and cell phones such as KEMAR manikins (G.R.A.S. Sound & Vibration, www.gras.dk). But the movements of the manikins are very limited and cannot be used to test the interaction of the audio system with other systems such as overcoats. This chapter will focus on the design and control of a low-noise biomimetic humanoid neck system, which can be used to investigate the level of acoustic noises produced by the interactive motion between wearable equipment and the human head/neck to facilitate the use of head-worn communication devices.

Although many humanoid neck mechanisms have been developed by different institutions, they can be divided into two categories; that is, the serial neck and parallel neck. Serial necks are the more common mechanisms due to their simple structure and the ease of DC motor control. The HRP-2 (Hirukawa et al. 2004) has a two-degrees-of-freedom (DOF) serial neck including pitch and yaw. The Albert HUBO (Park et al. 2008), the Dav (Han et al. 2002), and the iCub (Beira et al. 2006) have 3-DOF serial necks. The WE-4 (Miwa et al. 2002), the ARMAR-III (Albers et al. 2006), the WABIAN-RIV (Carbone et al. 2006), and the ROMAN (Hirth, Schmitz, and Berns 2007) have 4-DOF serial necks. The parallel neck can be divided into three subcategories; that is, Stewart-like necks, spring-based necks, and spherical necks. The main structure of Stewart-like necks is a Stewart platform (Beira et al. 2006), which needs a passive spine and is controlled by several legs with a combination of universal, prismatic, and spherical joints. The actuators for the parallel necks can be DC motors or pneumatic cylinders. Parallel mechanisms have the characteristics of rigidity, high load capacity, and high precision; however, it is hard to achieve a large range of motion and they are not suitable for use in limited neck space. The motion of a spherical neck is based on a spherical joint. Using screw theory, Sabater et al. (2006) designed and analyzed a spherical humanoid neck. A spring neck uses a spring as the spine to support the head and facilitate its motion. A spring neck is usually driven by motors (Beira et al. 2006; Nori et al. 2007) and artificial muscles (Hashimoto et al. 2006). According to previous investigations, a spring neck is similar to a real human neck and it is economical to build; however, it is hard to achieve high precision positioning control because of the complicated dynamics of the springs.

Most of the research on humanoid robotic necks provides insight into how to make the neck move similar to a real human neck. However, little research has adequately addressed how to design a robotic neck that can move quietly. Inspired by the human neck structure (White and Panjabi 1990), the main part of the developed head/neck is a compressed column spring that has a similar function to that of the spine. It supports the artificial/robotic head and can bend around the neutral axis to generate 2-DOF rotation including pitch and roll motions (bending of the head forward and backward and left and right, respectively). A cable–pulley structure mounted above the spring is used to realize the yaw motion (rotating the head to the left and right). The 3-DOF motion of the neck is realized through six cables that have similar functions of human neck muscles. These cables are pulled by the actuators sealed in a sound insulation box. Because no sound generation parts are embedded into the robotic neck, only very low motion noises are generated.

6.2 Low-Motion–Noise Robotic Head/Neck System

6.2.1 System Overview

The structure of the developed robotic system is shown in Figure 6.1. The system consists of three main parts: a humanoid robotic unit, a sound insulation box, and a personal computer. The robotic unit has a movable robotic head, a torso, and a height-adjustable support frame used to match humans of different heights either sitting or standing. The size of the head and torso is designed based on the head size of a human adult so that a full-size personal protective uniform fits the robotic system well. The movable robotic head has a 3-DOF neck framework to mimic human neck movements. These movements are driven by the remote motor-based actuators installed in the sound insulation box through the compound cable-and-housing group. The

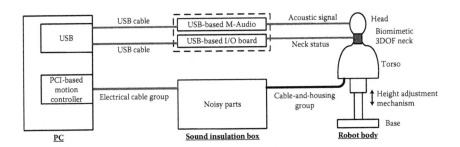

FIGURE 6.1
Overview of the robot system.

motor-based actuators are controlled by a PC via a peripheral component interconnect (PCI)-based motion controller board, and the control/driven strategy of the motor system is developed and conducted using the PC. Two Omni microphones are installed in the robot head to mimic human ears that can collect the sound information around the robot head effectively. Sensors embedded in the robot neck are capable of measuring its absolute rotation along three orthogonal axes. Signals from the microphones and sensors are collected by the PC through two USB-based data acquisition boards. The main task is to design and develop a humanoid head, sound insulation box, and PC-controller system.

In the system, cable housings are used to guide the drive cables or to transmit the outputs of actuators from the sound insulation box to the robot head. We found at least three advantages for utilizing a cable-and-housing group in this system: (1) it simplified the mechanical transmission design significantly, (2) few noises were generated by the cable-and-housing group, and (3) it facilitated the sealing issue for the sound insulation box. The materials of the drive cables are braided polyester. The housings are typical bicycle brake cable housings. Because the innermost layer is lubricated in the cable housing, the friction coefficient is relatively low between the cable and its housing. It should be noted that the steel drive cables can transmit noise outside of the sound insulation box, in which motors, gearboxes, and corresponding electrical parts are installed, to the robotic head/neck.

6.2.2 Hardware Development

The computer assisted design (CAD) assembly model of the 3-DOF robotic neck is shown in Figure 6.2. A compressive spring connecting two plates serves as the main mechanical structure of the robotic neck. The fixed plate is mounted onto the torso and the movable plate together with all parts mounted on it can be bent by the four symmetrically distributed drive cables. Thus, the movable plate can realize 2-DOF rotation including pitch and roll (the single-axis motions corresponding to the head motions flexion, extension, bending left, and bending right). As shown in Figure 6.2, four small pulleys mounted on the bottom surface of the movable plate are used to enhance the bending force exerted by the four cables. Note that one end of the four cables is fastened to the fixed plate. These four cables are guided to the robotic neck by their cable housings, and one end of the cable housing is also fastened to the fixed plate.

The yaw motion of the robotic head mimicking a human head's yaw motion can be achieved by using a cable-and-pulley structure, which is connected to the movable plate via a shaft and ball bearing group. As a result, the yaw motion of the robotic head is designed to be realized by the structure located on the top of the robotic neck. This design is in accordance with the fact that most of the yaw motion of a human head is generated between the C1 and C2 cervical vertebrae (White and Panjabi 1990). The shaft and ball bearing group in the structure can effectively reduce the friction and motion noises of the rolling shaft during the yaw motion. Because the cable housings used to guide the yaw drive cables cannot be mounted with a small curvature radius within the small space between the movable slate and the pulley, they are fixed into the movable plate. Instead, two small pulleys are used to guide the two cables to realize yaw motion.

In addition, two sensors for monitoring the motion of the 3-DOF neck are used, as shown in Figure 6.2. One is a two-axis inclinometer that measures the pitch and roll angles and is mounted on the top surface of the movable plate. The other is a potentiometer for measuring the yaw motion angle. The shaft of the potentiometer is fixed with the yaw pulley through the

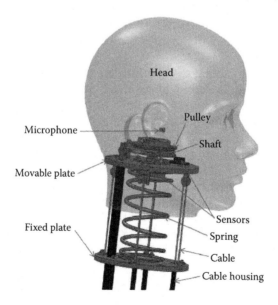

FIGURE 6.2
CAD assembly model of 3-DOF robotic neck.

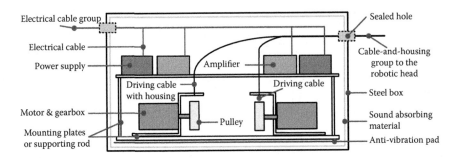

FIGURE 6.3
Overview of the sound insulation box.

shaft and bearing group. Two Omni microphones for collecting the acoustic information around the robot head are embedded into the two ears of the robotic head.

The sound insulation drive box is an important part of the whole system. The noisy parts such as motors and their gearboxes are installed in the sealed space within the box. An overview of the sound insulation box can be seen in Figure 6.3. There is a mounting frame with two layers; that is, two mounting plates connected by rods. On the top plate, power supplies, motor drivers, a power switch, fuses, and other electrical parts are mounted and the motor-based drive mechanisms are mounted on the bottom plate. The drive cables are wound and unwound by pulleys connected to the output shafts of the gearboxes. The other ends of the cable housings are fixed to the mounting frame. The drive cables within the housings and electrical cables are guided out of the box in bunches through two well-sealed holes in the side walls of the box.

There are two ways to passively eliminate the noise. One is sound insulation and the other is sound absorption. Sound insulation eliminates the sound path from a source. Usually high-density materials are the best choice for sound insulation. Sound absorption works when some or all of the incident sound energy is either converted into heat or passes through an absorber such as porous foams. To prevent sound transmission from the box, sound insulation and sound absorption techniques are both adopted. As shown in Figure 6.3, the box itself is made of a heavy, 12-gauge cold-rolled steel with a sound insulation technique. The six inner walls of the box are covered by 10-mm-thick butyl rubber, which has good acoustic absorption effects. The rubber helps to absorb the noises with frequencies between 30 and 4,000 Hz. The mounting frame is actually floated in the box, and between the butyl rubber on the bottom wall of the box and the mounting frame, an anti-vibration pad is employed to isolate the sound propagation paths.

In summary, because (1) no noisy gears and electrodriven parts are embedded in the biomimetic head/neck structure, (2) sound generation parts are sealed in the sound insulation box, and (3) the drive system is dominated by the low-friction and highly efficient cable-and-housing group, the humanoid head/neck system can mimic well the motion of a human head without generating unacceptable motion noises.

6.2.3 Programming Head Movements

The 3-DOF neck motion can fulfill six single movements including head flexion, head extension, bending head left, bending head right, rotating head left, and rotating head right. The instructions for each movement have two programmable parameters: movement range and movement time. In other words, the position and velocity of each movement can be defined. All nonconflicting multi-axis combined movements and sequences of movements are able to be performed by the robotic system. This means that all complex movements associated with a human neck can be conducted by the robotic head/neck.

6.3 Inverse Kinematics and Statics Analysis

6.3.1 Neck Mechanism

A general configuration of the spring-based, cable-driven mechanism corresponding to Figure 6.2 is shown in Figure 6.4, in which Figures 6.4a–c show the parallel mechanism of pitch and roll motions, general lateral bending of the compressive spring, and yaw motion by the rotating pulley, respectively. The yaw motion driven by two cables as shown in Figure 6.4c is straightforward; thus, we are mainly interested in analysis of the parallel mechanism and compressive spring.

As shown in Figure 6.4a, a fixed coordinate frame $OXYZ$ is attached to the fixed plate, with the origin at the bottom center of the spring, and a body frame $oxyz$ is attached to the moving plate, with the origin at the top center of the spring. Four flexible cables with negligible mass and diameter are connected to the moving platform at points B_i ($i = 1, 2, 3, 4$) and pulled from the base plate at point A_i. Denote the force value along the cable as T_i and the cable length between two plates as l_i. $\mathbf{u}_i$ is the unit vector for the force direction pointing to the base plate, thus $T_i \mathbf{u}_i = T_i$. The compressive spring produces a force/torque between the fixed base and the moving platform to support the robot head and facilitate the head motion. If the cables are actuated, the spring will bend in a plane formed by O, o, and o', where o' is the vertical projection of o onto the fixed base. In this plane, a planar body frame Oph is attached to this spring.

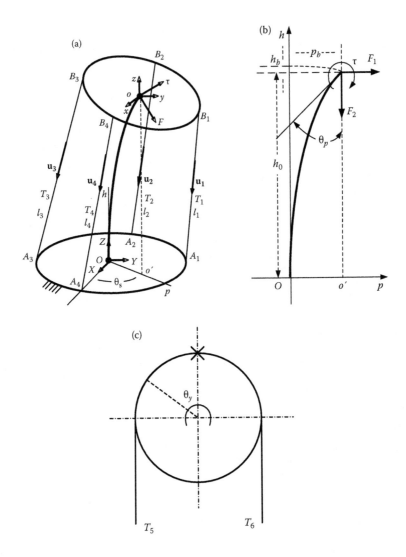

FIGURE 6.4
General configuration of the neck mechanisms: (a) configuration of the parallel mechanism for pitch and roll motions, (b) configuration of lateral bending of the compressive spring, and (c) configuration of the yaw motion by the rotating pulley.

This parallel mechanism has 3 DOF: the vertical translation DOF and two rotational DOFs. For the rotational DOFs, we use θ_s and θ_p to parameterize them where θ_s is the rotation direction and θ_p is the rotation amplitude. For the vertical DOF, we use h_0 to denote the coordinate in frame Oph. For the inverse kinematics, we want to obtain the driven cable length given the desired DOF value. Thus, the inverse kinematics is to find the mapping $f : (\theta_s, \theta_p, h_0) \rightarrow (l_1, l_2, l_3, l_4)$. However, unlike traditional parallel mechanism, this is not trivial because of the dependent motion characteristic of the spring bending, which in turn is related to the static force along the cables. Therefore, we should combine the inverse kinematics and statics in order to obtain a solution.

By the equivalence of force systems, all of the forces along the four cables can be transformed into the bending plane Oph; otherwise, the spring will not bend in that plane. Therefore, we convert all of the forces to two perpendicular forces F_1 and F_2, and a momentum τ at the top center of the spring in the plane as shown in Figure 6.4b. For the force and momentum balance, we have:

$$\sum_{i=1}^{4} \mathbf{T}_i = \sum_{i=1}^{4} (T_i \mathbf{u}_i) = \left[F_1 \cos\theta_s, F_1 \sin\theta_s, -F_2 \right]^{\mathrm{T}} \tag{6.1}$$

$$\sum_{i=1}^{4} (\mathbf{r}_i \times \mathbf{T}_i) = \left[-\tau \sin\theta_s, \tau \cos\theta_s, 0 \right]^{\mathrm{T}} \tag{6.2}$$

where $\mathbf{r}_i$ corresponds to the vector $\overline{OB_i}$ expressed in the fixed frame $OXYZ$ and the unit vector $\mathbf{u}_i$ can be expressed as

$$\mathbf{u}_i = \frac{\mathbf{l}_i}{l_i} = \frac{\overline{OA_i} - \mathbf{r}_i}{\left\| \overline{OA_i} - \mathbf{r}_i \right\|} \tag{6.3}$$

We take the compressive helical spring as a flexible bar to investigate lateral bending characteristics of the spring, but it is necessary to consider the change in length of the spring due to compression, because the change is not negligible in the case of compressed bars (Timoshenko 1936). Consider the practical lateral bending of the neck as in Figure 6.4b. The spring-based mechanism will be bent by forces F_1 and F_2 plus τ. Because the motion of the head is usually no more than 15 degrees buckled in all roll, pitch, and yaw axes (Sterling et al. 2008), it is feasible to use a linear equation to calculate the statics model of lateral bending for the cable-driven robotic head/neck in this application:

$$\beta \frac{d^2 p}{dh^2} = F_1(h_0 - h) + F_2(p_b - p) + \tau \tag{6.4}$$

where β is the flexural rigidity of the spring under compression, and it is inversely proportional to the number of coils per unit length of the spring (Timoshenko 1936); hence,

$$\beta = \frac{h_0}{H_0}\beta_0$$

where H_0 is the original length of the spring, and β_0 can be calculated based on physical parameters of the compressive spring.

The initial conditions at the two ends of the spring are

$$(p)_{h=0} = 0, (p')_{h=0} = 0; (p)_{h=h_0} = p_b, (p')_{h=h_0} = \theta_p \tag{6.5}$$

By neglecting the corresponding vertical displacement h_b of the spring under small bending, as shown in Figure 6.4b, the spring length under compression is calculated as

$$F_2 = K(H_0 - h_0) \tag{6.6}$$

where K is the spring stiffness and L_0 is the initial length of the spring.

Based on Equations (6.1)–(6.6), for a configured cable-driven, spring-based parallel mechanism as shown in Figures 6.4a and 6.4b, both the inverse kinematics and statics can be solved analytically.

6.3.2 Cable and Housing

The drive cable used in this application is braided extra-strength polyester twine. Because the length of the drive cable is longer than 2 m, the extension of the cable has to be considered. While a cable is pulled in a curved housing, friction force is unavoidable. Here it is assumed that the shape of the cable and housing is unchanged for each robot motion control, and we can depict a cable and housing with n turns as shown in Figure 6.5.

The coefficient of static friction and kinetic friction between the cable and the inner wall of its hose is taken as the same μ. Each turn in the curving path can define a plane and we define the hose bends counterclockwise away from the velocity of the cable as its turn angle Λ_j. As in this application, the turn angles are defined as $\Lambda_j \in [0, 2\pi] \setminus \pi, j = 1, \cdots, n$. We use F_j and l_j to denote the cable force and hose length of each segment. Note that the j here is in $[1, n-1]$. The F_0 and F_n are the input driving force and output driving force of the cable-hose drive mechanism. The l_0 denotes the cable length measured

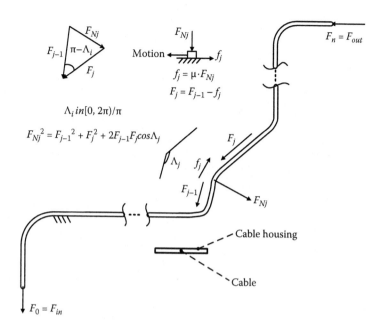

FIGURE 6.5
Sketch of the cable and housing.

from a fixed point of the output of the motor to the first turn of the hose and l_n denotes the cable length measured from the last turn of the hose to a fixed point on the robot head.

Because the diameter of the drive cable is very close to the inner diameter of the cable hose, we take the turn angles of the cable as the same as the turn angles of the cable hose. The relationship between the input force and output force in each segment can be derived as

$$F_j = \frac{1 + \mu^2 \cos \Lambda_j - \sqrt{(1 + \mu^2 \cos \Lambda_j)^2 - (1 - \mu^2)^2}}{1 - \mu^2} F_{j-1} = \lambda_j F_{j-1} \quad (0 < \lambda_j \le 1) \ (6.7)$$

Based on the developed relationship, we can obtain the relationship between the input force and output force for a given drive cable-and-housing path

$$F_{out} = \left(\prod_{j=1}^{n} \lambda_j \right) F_{in} \tag{6.8}$$

In this case, when the friction coefficient and turn angles are known, we can calculate the input force and output force when one of them is given.

The cable will be extended like a spring with stiffness constant k when a force is applied on it. Therefore, the absolute extended length of the cable will be

$$\Delta l = \sum_{j=0}^{n} \Delta l_j = \sum_{j=0}^{n} \left(\frac{F_j}{k} \right) \qquad (6.9)$$

Finally, we state the overall inverse kinematics from the head position to the cable winding/unwinding pulley. For given motion task parameters $(\theta_s, \theta_p, h_0)$, the cable length l_i and exerted cable force T_i, which is equivalent to the output force F_{out}, can be calculated based on Equations (6.1)–(6.6). The overall elongation length of each cable can be found based on the cable-and-housing model once the cable drive paths are given. Finally, the cable length needed to be wound/unwound by driving winches can be determined.

6.4 Control Strategy

6.4.1 Rigidity Maintenance

It is well known that cables can only generate pull force. This unilateral force constraint in drive cables has to be incorporated into the design and control procedure; otherwise, the cable-based manipulator may collapse. Therefore, maintaining positive tension (tensile force) in all of the cables is an essential requirement for the rigidity of a cable-based manipulator. Because the rigidity of a cable-based manipulator depends on the external load, it is complicated to analyze. To overcome this problem, Behzadipour and Khajepour (2006) employed *tensionability*, which only depends on the geometry to express the potential of the manipulator to be rigid. The *tensionability* is defined as: a cable-based mechanism is called tensionable at a given configuration of the movable platform if and only if for any arbitrary external load there exists a finite spine force/torque and a set of finite cable tensions to make the mechanism rigid. As a result, tensionability and large enough tensile force together provide a sufficient condition for the rigidity.

According to the static analysis in the last section, for an arbitrary positive spine force $\mathbf{F}$ and torque τ, the static equilibrium Equations (6.1) and (6.2) have a solution with all positive cable tensions T_i $(i = 1, 2, 3, 4)$. This implies that the robot head can be statically balanced (in pitch and roll DOF) under an arbitrary compressive spring force/torque. Consequently, it is tensionable and thus can stay rigid for any external force and torque with a large enough precompressed force/torque. To maintain the rigidity of the robotic head, different personal protective equipment (PPE) and their combinations as an external payload were studied together with the robotic head itself to derive the potential maximum spine force/torque (compressive force/torque of the spring). In other words, the length of the spring needed to be precompressed by the drive cables is enough to maintain the rigidity of the robotic head when different PPEs or their combinations are put on the head. In this way, we decide h_0 as in Figure 6.4 during the implementation. A bang-bang control algorithm is employed to achieve the precompressive process at the beginning of the robotic system's operation.

6.4.2 Motion Control

Although 3-DOF human head motions are always coupled, we divided the robotic head motions into two categories depending on the number of active axes in a motion: single axis motion and multi-axis motion, such as looking down and forward (flexion) and down and to the left (flexion and rotation left). We divided the robotic head motions into two categories based on the motion continuity: single motion and continuous motion, such as looking down and forward (flexion) and nodding (flexion back and forth). Before the motion execution, it is necessary to transform a continuous motion to a series of single motions and map a multi-axis motion into simultaneous single-axis motions.

Based on the movement characteristics of the human head, moving smoothly other than positioning accuracy is the first priority of the each movement. Because the robot will be used to collect the noises generated by the PPE during human head/neck movements, continuous motion is performed more frequently. For each single movement, two parameters are given as described in Section 6.2; that is, range of movement and movement time. By considering the initial position of the robotic head, trapezoidal velocities of the robotic head movement can be generated. According to the analysis in Section 6.3, these trapezoidal velocities are transformed into the cable length needed to be wound or unwound. Using this open-loop control, it is hard to achieve accurate positioning control due to the unmodeled parameters and disturbances. To ensure the positioning control of the robotic head, at the end of the motion, a simple bang-bang controller

$$
v_e = \begin{cases} +v_0 & \Delta\theta \geq \varepsilon \\ 0 & |\Delta\theta| < \varepsilon \\ -v_0 & \Delta\theta \leq -\varepsilon \end{cases}
$$

is employed to locate the robot head at the right destination, where v_e is the execution velocity, v_0 is a small velocity value, and ε is a prescribed position error threshold.

6.5 Implementation

6.5.1 Experimental Setup and Motion Control of the Robotic Neck

The low-motion–noise humanoid head/neck system developed as described in Section 6.2 is pictured in Figure 6.6. Figure 6.6a shows the overall system. In the system, an NI USB-6215 multifunction I/O board is used to acquire the sensor data and collect information to monitor the working status of electrical parts in the sound insulation box. An M-Audio interface, USB-based Fast Track Pro, is used to record the acoustic information obtained by two sensitive microphones in the robot ears during the motion of the robotic head/neck. For one of the applications, the robot body and the sound insulation box are located in one acoustic room, and the personal computer, the NI USB-6215, and M-Audio interface are located outside of the room to avoid inducing other acoustic noises. Real PPEs such as helmets, masks (respirators), and chemical-resistant suits were employed in our experiments. These PPEs were equipped with the robotic head/neck system for our further studies on acoustic noise induced by motion between the PPEs and the robotic system.

Single and combination head motions have been implemented successfully on the developed robot system. Typical single head movements demonstrated in Figure 6.6b are: flexion, extension, bending left, bending right, rotating left, and rotating right. And motion parameters of the developed robotic neck system are listed in Table 6.1.

6.5.2 Motion Noise Test

An anechoic chamber at Michigan State University was used as an acoustic room to test the noise level of the robotic head/neck system during its motion. The noise level of the system during its motions was monitored by a sound level alert from Extech Instruments. A picture of the noise level testing experiment is shown in Figure 6.7a. The experimental results showed that the maximum noise level of the system during different motions was no more than 30 dB A-weighted.

To compare the different noise generation between the motions of the robot head without and with PPE, another experiment was done in a common lab environment, where several computers and the air-conditioning system were running. The head executed a rotating left right (like shaking) motion for 17 seconds, and the PPE selected was a plastic jacket hood. The steps for audio calibration and recording were as follows: (1) place speaker 1 m away from the robot ears (microphones); (2) play a 1-kHz standard tone for 28 seconds; (3) adjust the tone volume so that when placed near each microphone, a sound level meter measures a sound level of 60 dB; (4) without changing the microphone gain settings, start to record the acoustic data generated by the robot's motion without PPE; (5) record the acoustic data

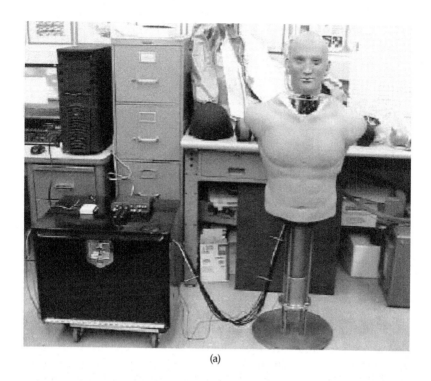

(a)

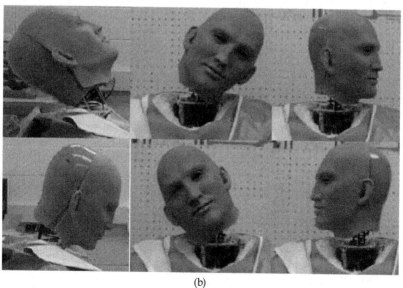

(b)

FIGURE 6.6

Pictures of the robotic system developed and its typical movements: (a) the overall system and (b) instructions for six typical movements.

TABLE 6.1

Motion Parameters of the Robotic Head Developed

Movements	Range	Maximum Velocity
Bending left/right	30°/30°	150°/s
Flexion/extension	30°/45°	150°/s
Rotating left/right	60°/60°	200°/s

generated by the same robot motion with a plastic jacket hood. A picture of the audio calibration procedure is shown in Figure 6.7b, and the recorded acoustic data were combined and are shown as Figures 6.7c and 6.7d. As we can see from the acoustic recording results, the characteristics of the noise generated by the PPE are distinct and easy to extract and analyze with the help of the low-motion bio-inspired humanoid neck.

6.6 Summary

This chapter presents our recently developed 3-DOF humanoid neck system that can effectively mimic motion of human neck with very low motion noises. Three main ideas are fulfilled to reduce noise as follows: (1) a compressive helical spring to mimic the cervical vertebrae and cables to mimic muscles, which means there are no gears and electrodriven parts that make noise, are embedded in the head/neck structure; (2) a remotely driven head/neck system using a cable-and-housing group, which guarantees low friction and low noise transmission; and (3) the noisy cable-pulling actuators are sealed in a sound insulation box. To validate the design of the system, both theoretical statics analysis and experiments were implemented. The experimental results prove the effectiveness of the head/neck system designed. The system can be effectively used to investigate the level of acoustic noises produced by the interactive motion between wearable equipment/uniforms and a human head/neck to facilitate using head-worn communication devices.

Acknowledgment

The authors thank Qi (Peter) Li, Uday Jain, and Josh Hajicek from Li Creative Technology, Inc., for helpful discussions on the robots.

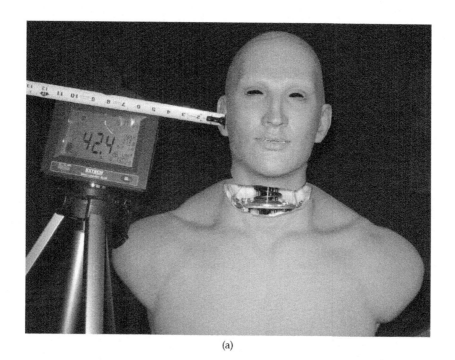

(a)

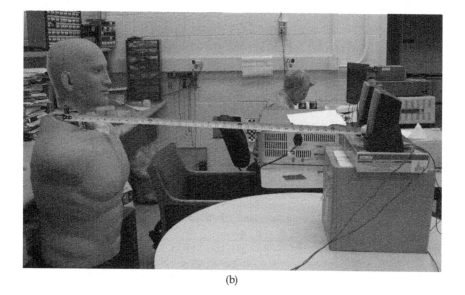

(b)

FIGURE 6.7

Typical acoustic testing of the robot system: (a) sound level experiment of the robot in an anechoic chamber, (b) audio recording experiment in a normal lab environment   (*continued*)

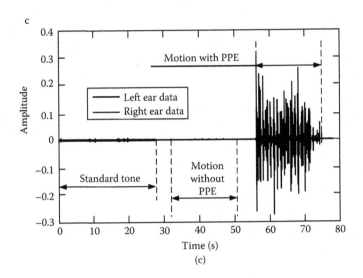

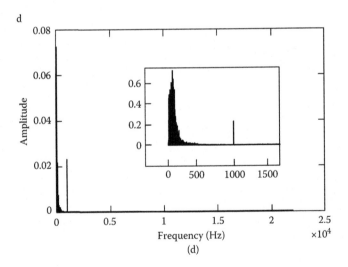

FIGURE 6.7 (Continued)
Typical acoustic testing of the robot system: (c) sound wave of the recorded audio, and (d) frequency spectrum analysis of the recorded sound data.

References

Albers, A., Brudniok, S., Ottnad, J., Sauter, C., and Sedchaicham, K. 2006. Upper body of a new humanoid robot: The design of ARMAR III. *Paper read at the IEEE/RAS International Conference on Humanoid Robots,* Genoa, Italy, December 4–6, 2006.

Behzadipour, S. and Khajepour, A. 2006. Cable-based robot manipulators with translational degrees of freedom. In *Industrial Robotics: Theory, Modeling and Control,* edited by S. Cubero. Germany: ARS/plV.

Beira, R., Lopes, M., Praca, M., Santos-Victor, J.A., Bernardino, A., Metta, G., Beechi, F., and Saltaren, R. 2006. Design of the robot-cub (iCub) head. Paper read at the IEEE International Conference on Robotics and Automation, Orlando, FL, May 15–19, 2006.

Carbone, G., Lim, H., Takanishi, A., and Ceccarelli, M. 2006. Stiffness analysis of biped humanoid robot WABIAN-RIV. *Mechanism and Machine Theory,* 41: 17–40.

Han, J.D., Zeng, S., Tham, K.Y., Badgero, M., and Weng, J. 2002. Dav: A humanoid robot platform for autonomous mental development. Paper read at the IEEE International Conference on Development and Learning.

Hashimoto, T., Hitramatsu, S., Tsuji, T., and Kobayashi, H. 2006. Development of the face robot SAYA for rich facial expressions. Paper read at the SICE-ICASE International Joint Conference. Busan, Korea, October 18–21, 2006.

Hirth, J., Schmitz, N., and Berns, K. 2007. Emotional architecture for the humanoid robot head ROMAN. Paper read at the IEEE International Conference on Robotics and Automation, Rome, Italy, April 10–14, 2007.

Hirukawa, H., Kanehiroa, F., Kanekoa, K., Kajita, S., Fujiwara, K., Kawai, Y., Tomita, F., Hirai, S., Tanie, K., Isozumi, T., Akachi, K., Kawasaki, T., Ota, S., Yokoyama, K., Handa, H., Fukase, Y., Maeda, J., Nakamua, Y., Tachi, S., and Inoue, H. 2004. Humanoid robotics platforms developed in HRP. *Robotics and Autonomous Systems,* 48: 165–175.

Miwa, H. Okuchi, T., Takanobu, H., and Takanishi, A. 2002. Development of a new human-like head robot WE-4. Paper read at the IEEE/RSJ International Conference on Intelligent Robots and Systems, Lausanne, Switzerland, September 30–October 4, 2002.

Nori, F., Janone, L., Sandini, G., and Metta, G. 2007. Accurate control of a human-like tendon-driven neck. Paper read at the IEEE/RAS International Conference on Humanoid Robots, Pittsburg, PA, November 29–December 1, 2007.

Park, I., Kim, J., Cho, B., and Oh. J. 2008. Control hardware integration of a biped humanoid robot with an android head. *Robotics and Autonomous Systems,* 56: 95–103.

Sabater, J.M., Garcia, N., Perez, C., Azorin, J.M., Saltaren, R.J., and Yime, E.. 2006. Design and analysis of a spherical humanoid neck using screw theory. Paper read at the IEEE/RAS-EMBS International Conference on Biomedical Robotics and Biomechatronics, Pisa, Italy, February 20–22, 2006.

Sterling, A.C., Cobian, D.G., Anderson, P.A., and Heiderscheit, B.C. 2008. Annual frequency and magnitude of neck motion in healthy individuals. *Spine,* 33(17): 1882–1888.

Timoshenko, S. 1936. *Theory of Elastic Stability.* New York: McGraw-Hill.

White, A.A. and Panjabi, M.M. 1990. *Clinical Biomechanics of the Spine.* Philadelphia: J.B. Lippincott.

7

Automatic Single-Cell Transfer Module

Huseyin Uvet
Yildiz Technical University
Istanbul, Turkey

Akiyuki Hasegawa
Tokyo Women's Medical University
Tokyo, Japan

Kenichi Ohara, Tomohito Takubo, Yasushi Mae, and Tatsuo Arai
Osaka University
Osaka, Japan

CONTENTS

7.1 Introduction 126
7.2 Materials and Methods 128
    7.2.1 Cell Types and Preparation 129
    7.2.2 Penicillin-Streptomycin and Bottom Surface Treatment 130
    7.2.3 Cell Suction System 130
    7.2.4 Manufacture of the Microfluidic Chip 131
    7.2.5 Valve Control Principle 132
    7.2.6 Vision Systems 133
    7.2.7 Cell Detection/Tracking and Control 134
7.3 Experimental Results 138
    7.3.1 Oocyte and Fibroblast Suction 138
    7.3.2 Direction Control 139
7.4 Discussion and Conclusion 143
References 143

Abstract

Conventional hybrid microfluidic systems have many functions such as separation, sorting, and filtering of biological particles. These hybrid systems are required for delivering particles into microfluidic chips and for their dexterous on-chip manipulation. Successful realization of these functionalities requires visual sensing of particles. However, only a limited number of studies are available on on-chip visual sensing techniques as well as on retrieval of living cells into microfluidic devices and their manipulation thereafter. Automated continuous individual cell transfer is a critical step in single-cell applications using microfluidic devices. Cells must be aspirated gently from a buffer before transferring to an operation zone to avoid artificially perturbing their biostructures. Vision-based manipulation is a key sensing technique that allows nondestructive cell detection. In this chapter, we present a design for an automated single-cell transfer module that can be integrated with complex microfluidic applications that examine or process one cell at a time such as the current nuclear transplantation method. The aim of the system is to automatically transfer mammalian fibroblasts (~15 μm) or oocytes (~100 μm) one by one from a container to a polydimethylsiloxane (PDMS) microchannel and then transport them to other modules. The system consists of two main parts: a single-cell suction module and a disposable PDMS-based microfluidic chip controlled by external pumps. The desired number of vacuumed cells can be directed into the microfluidic chip and stored in a docking area. From the batch, they can be moved to the next module by activating pneumatic pressure valves located on two sides of the chip. The entire mechanism is combined with monitoring systems that perform the detection/tracking and control program.

7.1 Introduction

Microfluidic technology and its applications are extensive and have many significant advantages, bringing the benefits of miniaturization, integration, and automation to biotechnology-related studies over the past several decades (Jager, Inganäs, and Lundström 2000; Vilkner, Janasek, and Manz 2004). Microfluidic-based technology offers a convenient platform for cellular analyses of biological systems, because the small scale of microchannels and devices allows producing scalable system architectures (Unger et al. 2000; Walker, Zeringu, and Beebe 2004). Their inexpensive composition makes them a potential candidate for large-scale production. Microfluidic technology covers not only the material phenomena but also the technology for manipulating and controlling the components as microsize particles in microsize artificial capillaries. Therefore, the integration of these technologies with microrobotic applications could be useful in the automation of cell manipulation for important areas such as single-cell analysis, manipulation, and treatment, including nuclear transplantation (Cui et al. 2001; Lee et al. 2003; Ramesham and Ghaffarian 2000; Schwarz and Hauser 2001).

Integration of cell treatment steps is crucial to developing microfluidic devices for analysis of cell constituents, cell lysis, and cell culture (Elfwing et al. 2004; Schonholzer et al. 2002). For example, experimental results show that microfluidic technology provides a significant advantage in the production of mammalian embryos. In addition to these vital concepts, cell fusion and nuclear transplantation (Skelley, Kirak, and Suh 2009; Yia et al. 2006) are important topics. Our project "Automated Nuclear Transplantation Using Micro Robotics" is a novel approach to finding a solution to overcome difficulties in the nuclear transplantation process. In this project, several cell manipulation tasks such as positioning, cutting, sorting, filtering, and fusion are performed by different interconnected modules using a so-called desktop bioplant (Arai et al. 2007). This desktop bioplant, which includes microchannels and microwells on a chip with appropriate sensors and actuators, is increasingly in demand for nuclear transplantation operations in biotechnology.

Microfluidic methodologies, however, have suffered from limited means to manipulate fluids and cells. In conventional methods, the single-cell transfer and control from a container to a polydimethylsiloxane (PDMS) microfluidic chip is carried out by the aid of a micropipette suction and manual on-chip stream manipulation by a pump. Biological cells must be picked up from the container one by one under the view of a microscope and supplied to the microfluidic chip, where single-cell operations are performed. For each single cell, an operator should repeat the same method until the desired number of cells is collected. Although this process is relatively easy for large cells (i.e., oocyte ~100 μm), it is infeasible for small cells (i.e., fibroblast ~15 μm). A skilled operator is required for such time-consuming applications. Moreover, if the pump speed does not synchronize with the manual cell supply process, bubble formation can be observed in the flow stream, which is harmful to living cells. Once the desired number of cells is delivered into the microchannel, they need to be brought into the operation area one by one. In addition, the distance between consecutive cells cannot be maintained in the microchannel by manual methods. The principle behind our proposed solution is to accomplish all of these functions (cell suction, transportation, on-chip position control, observation, and cell supply) automatically with one integrated system. For example, in the case of the cell fusion step of mammalian cloning, a microfluidic chip requires simultaneous control of the cells involved. In this process, two cells (a donor cell and an oocyte) are brought into very close contact and aligned via alternating current (AC), after which a direct current (DC) is applied for a brief period to complete the fusion (MacDonald, Spalding, and Dholakia 2003; Walker, Zeringu, and Beebe 2004). Precise cell supply and transportation are essential when performing such an operation. This has significant advantages for some microfluidic cell applications such as on-chip micro-injection (Andrea and Klavs 2008), on-chip single-cell polymerase chain reaction (PCR; Toriello et al. 2008), and cell encapsulation with microfluidic droplets (He, Edgar, and Jeffries 2005). Moreover, due to the importance of the information gathered by individual cells, several analytical techniques for chemical analysis of single cells have been proposed by different groups. These techniques include capillary electrophoresis (Huang et al. 2008; Wu, Wheeler, and Zare 2004) and fluorescent microscopy (Cookson et al. 2005), which are other popular microfluidic methods that require manipulation of living cells one at a time. To the best of our knowledge, there exists no successfully implemented nondestructive automated single-cell loading and supply system.

Our motivation in this study is to support on-chip cloning technology. Gentle cell handling and supply into a microfluidic chip one by one is the first part of a successful application, because any damage to the cells could cause experimental failure. The cells must be aspirated precisely from a container, which requires micromanipulation and accurate positioning while approaching the target cell with a glass micropipette (suction tip) attached to a micromanipulator. Secondly, the desired number of cells is stored in a dock. The snake-shaped PDMS docking zone is designed for this purpose. Once cells are sorted, they are transferred to the next module or operation zone. To do this, a "Y" character microchannel is combined with the docking side and the pneumatic pressure valves are formed at the intersection of the two. When the external pump infuses air into the valves, the membrane between the layers deflects, closing the fluidic flow. Finally, synchronization of the valves and the suction tip are handled via monitoring systems, which provide full automation and system integration. Because the intersection of PDMS chip is monitored by a compact vision system, the suction tip is monitored by a microscopic system. Instead of using two microscopic units, which requires a long tube connection between the suction tip and the microfluidic chip, we designed the compact vision system as a nondestructive sensing method in order to enable high-throughput single-cell transfer.

This chapter is divided into three main sections according to the different parts and functions of the systems: (1) materials and methods, (2) experimental results, and (3) discussion and conclusion. In the first section, the materials used to fabricate the microfluidic chip and methods for preparing cells as well as a new design of a compact vision structure are briefly described. Secondly, an automated cell detection/tracking and controlling algorithm is presented along with its applications in microfluidic chips, micromanipulators, and pumps. In the final section, experimental results indicating the efficiency and usability of the total mechanism are described.

7.2 Materials and Methods

The proposed system is able to singly pick cells from a container and transport them to a microfluidic chip. The structure allows manipulating cells in microfluidic channels and docking them in desired locations in controllable numbers. However, due to the complex physical properties of oocyte and donor cells, manipulating cells through a microfluidic chip poses certain challenges.

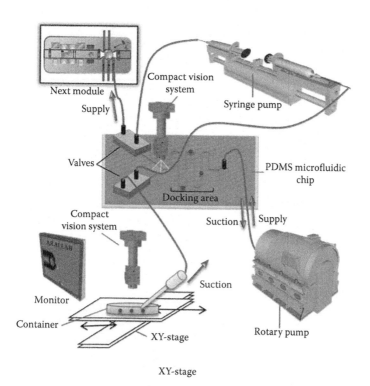

FIGURE 7.1
Schematic view of the automatic single cell transfer module. © 2009 IEEE.

This system is comprised of the parts shown in Figure 7.1. External pumps, micromanipulators, and camera systems are connected to a computer and run automatically based on a cell detection/tracking and control algorithm. All experiments were performed at room temperature and one microfluidic device was used several times, where the device was cleaned with filtered water after every experiment. A syringe filter (hydrophilic, Sartorius-Minisart, Aubagne, France) was attached to the end of a syringe to absorb impurities as the water passed through and to prevent contamination in the microchannels.

7.2.1 Cell Types and Preparation

In this chapter, we primarily focus on somatic cell cloning. Experiments were performed using fibroblasts as donor cells and oocyte cells as recipient cells. Oocytes were isolated from bovine. Ova were cultured approximately 24 hours after harvesting from the ovary. In order to detach cumulus cells from the harvested ova, cells were treated with hyaluronidase (Nacalai Tesque Inc., Kyoto, Japan). The pellucid zone of the ova was removed by pronase treatment and near-circular oocyte cells were isolated. The diameter of isolated oocytes was about 100–150 μm (Figure 7.2).

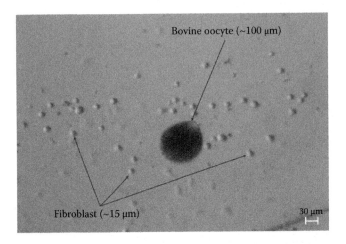

FIGURE 7.2
Bovine oocyte and fibroblasts. The fibroblasts are transparent, whereas the oocytes are easily viewable under the visible light condition.

Fibroblasts 10–30 μm in diameter were isolated from female bovine ears (Figure 7.2). The fibroblasts were cultured in Dulbecco's modified Eagle's medium supplemented with 10% fetal bovine serum (FBS) in 35-mm dishes in a 5% CO_2 incubator. When cells became confluent, the culture medium was changed to 0.5% FBS-supplemented media. Fibroblasts were harvested from the dishes by treatment with trypsin-ethylenediaminetetraacetic acid (EDTA).

7.2.2 Penicillin-Streptomycin and Bottom Surface Treatment

Fibroblasts readily adhere to the surface of plastic culture dishes. We detached fibroblasts using trypsin-EDTA (Wako Pure Chemical Industry, Osaka, Japan) treatment (Tuan and Lo 2000) and then waited over 30 minutes to attempt to aspirate the fibroblasts. However, over time, detached cells readhere to the culture dish and cannot be aspirated. To avoid this problem, we treated the culture dish by painting the dish with a small amount of liquid PDMS (without the use of catalyst) for use in the following experiments. This method is also known as *siliconizing* (Gunnar and Bähr 2008); that is, coating a surface with silicon. The other method was to pour PDMS (using a catalyst) and cover the dish with a thin, solid PDMS layer. In the case of nontreated containers, less than half of the fibroblasts could be aspirated. On the other hand, the cells in the PDMS-coated dish were all easily aspirated.

7.2.3 Cell Suction System

In the acquisition process of a single cell, first the rotary pump (ISMATech Inc., Wertheim-Mondfeld, Germany) was connected to the dock side of the

PDMS chip via a Teflon tube (outer diameter 0.5 mm, inner diameter 0.3 mm). The main route starting from the dock side port (outlet port) to the glass microtube was on the same line. Therefore, flow speed and flow direction in the microchannel, as well as the speed on the tip of the glass microtube, were handled by this pump. During the experiments, we realized that small-diameter tubes decrease the possibility of creating cell stacks on the intersection point of the inlet port and the Teflon tube. Hence, the glass microtube and the cell delivery channel were connected using another Teflon tube (outer diameter 0.3 mm, inner diameter 0.2 mm). We used a glass microtube (0.30 mm outer diameter, 0.18 mm inner diameter) as a suction mouth for the oocyte cells. A glass microtube can easily vacuum single cells without inflicting any damage. In addition, it has a noncomplex fabrication procedure that makes it easy to apply for common procedures. For the fibroblast, the glass microtube was heated to decrease its diameter (inner diameter ~50 µm). The tip of the glass microtube was processed by a microforge (MF-830, Narishige Inc., Tokyo, Japan) and polishing machine (EG-44, Narishige Inc.).

7.2.4 Manufacture of the Microfluidic Chip

The microfluidic chip employed in this research has been designed to perform two main functions: aligning aspirated cells in the docking area and transferring them to the next module. We designed two different types of microfluidic chips that have two- and three-layer structures. A two-layer microfluidic chip has two molds, the main mold carrying the fluidic channel and the valves. The molds of the second fluidic chip are the main mold, valves (second mold), and air chamber (third mold), which were patterned on a silicon wafer with different heights using SU8-based photolithography, which has been described elsewhere (Zhang, Tan, and Gong, 2001). In the main mold, channels for delivering cells were 200 µm wide and 150 µm deep, dimensions sufficient to contain an oocyte. The main mold has a "Y"-shaped character and is completed with a snake-like dock, as shown in Figure 7.3.

After preparation of the mold, the PDMS device and the valves were fabricated using a classic multilayer soft lithography technique. Firstly, a thin layer of PDMS (thickness: ~300 µm, the first layer) was spin-coated on the main mold and then cured for less than 20 minutes at 100°C in an oven. The same method was repeated for the second layer, which also contained the valve. Incorrect placement of the second layer (thickness: ~250 µm), containing a thin membrane, may obstruct flow permanently. The first and second layers were carefully aligned together. The valve layer was completed by adding a PDMS slab containing an air chamber (depth: 500 µm). Then, the combined PDMS layers were treated by air plasma using an expanded plasma cleaner for 1 minute together with a glass slide rinsed in ethanol. The glass slide was placed on the prosthesis and pressure was applied until they were firmly bound to each other. Finally, the microfluidic chip was sealed with PDMS and cured a second time.

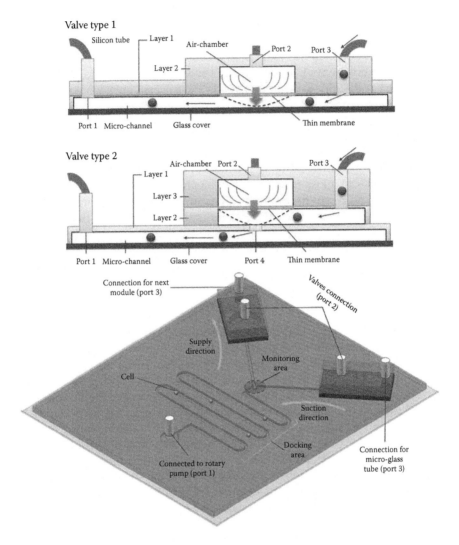

FIGURE 7.3
Port 1 is connected to a rotary pump that controls flow speed and direction in the fluidic channel. A thin PDMS membrane is actuated with Port 2 connected to a syringe pump. When the air chamber is filled with air, it closes the gate (Port 4) for the fluidic channel and stops cell flow from the loading inlet (Port 3). The "Y"-character channel controls supply suction and supply directions by switching valves.

7.2.5 Valve Control Principle

Within the PDMS chip, the valve region is closed by applying air pressure to the air chamber and obstructing the microchannel (Figure 7.4). The air pressure control valves for open and close actions are activated by a syringe pump (KDS270, Kd Scientific, Holliston, MA, USA). The syringe pump links

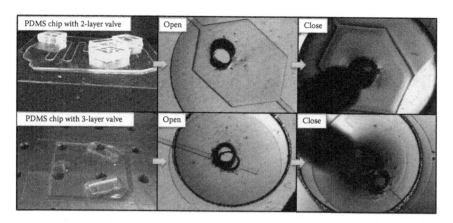

FIGURE 7.4

PDMS microfluidic chips and valve actuation. Figure shows valve deformation by applying air pressure.

two valves so that one becomes closed if the other becomes open. In addition, the flow behavior of the "Y"-shaped channel can be observed by the use of color pigments when the pump actuates. The control of the current direction in the microchannel is handled by the rotary motion of a high-precision rotary pump (ISMATech). Although the fabrication process of a three-layer microfluidic chip is more difficult than that for a two-layer chip, it has a better performance, in particular for response time. Table 7.1 shows a comparison of both valve designs.

7.2.6 Vision Systems

Two camera systems were assigned to monitor two important sections of the entire mechanism. The first camera (compact optical setup with Point grey Dragonfly camera, Point Grey Research, Richmond, BC, Canada) was placed on the cell container in order to detect the position of the oocyte or donor cells in the container. The second camera was boarded on the microfluidic chip with the purpose of actuating valves and changing flow direction.

The compact vision system provides good image quality, allowing data on the oocyte cell and donor cell to be extracted from the acquired images (Uvet et al. 2008). In this second version, we changed the optical setup and designed a task specific system that has a 1.5-mm monitoring area and light source on the same side as the complementary metal-oxide-semiconductor (CMOS) sensor. The specifications are given in Table 7.2.

The camera can be placed and aligned on a chip with the aid of xyz microstages. As shown in Figure 7.5, the new system is small and can be easily combined with the microfluidic chips. This makes it possible to observe the cell container and microfluidic chip simultaneously in a short distance. Otherwise, we would have to use two commercial microscopes, which

TABLE 7.1

Comparison of Two- and Three-Layer Valves

	Two-Layer Chip	Three-Layer Chip
Main fluidic channel	1st Layer	1st Layer
Valve position	1st Layer	2nd Layer
Air chamber	2nd Layer	3rd Layer
PDMS membrane	1st Layer	2nd Layer
Vertical movement between layers	No	Yes
Valve closing level	Low	High
Response speed	Slow	Fast

TABLE 7.2

The Compact Vision System Specifications

Design wavelength	587.6 nm
Focal length (objective lens)	7.5 mm
Effective aperture	1.85 mm
f-Number	4.1
NA	0.123
Refractive index (water)	1.3334
Depth of focus	25.8 μm
Magnification	4.7

Source: © 2009 IEEE.

requires a large workspace and the use of a long Teflon tube to connect the glass microtube to the inlet port of the PDMS chip.

In this study, the modulation transfer function (MTF) was also used as a measurement parameter of optical quality (Ray 2002; Smith 2000). MTF graphs show modulation of image contrast at different spatial frequencies. Diffraction limits the contrast in every optical system. Diffraction limited modulation transfer functions are given in MTF graphs with dashed curves for the purpose of comparison with perfect lens case. In this MTF analysis, defocusing, which causes blurry image, is set as 0.00. MTF performance was tested under a 587.6 nm wavelength. Four different MTF graphs plot the percentage of transferred contrast according to the distance from the center of the objective plane (center of the image). The MTF results at given radiuses are shown in Figure 7.6. The modulation (also known as *contrast*) is expressed in terms of a percentage (1.0 = 100%).

7.2.7 Cell Detection/Tracking and Control

The detection/tracking and control algorithm was mainly programmed for single-cell applications. Its execution steps can be described as follows:

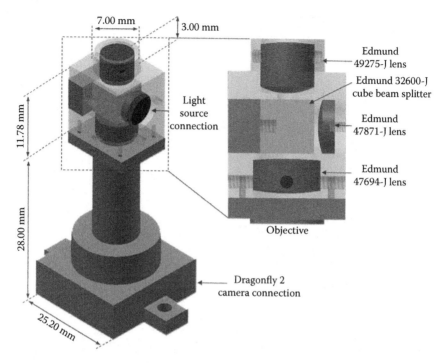

FIGURE 7.5
Compact vision system.

- Start the first camera and detect the position of single cells in the cell container.

- Align the glass microtube to the cell position and begin suction (ISMATech rotary pump).

- Toggle to the second camera and count the number of cells that pass the cross section in the PDMS chip.

- If the desired number of cells passes the cross point, switch valves and let the cells flow to the next module.

- Switch valves and cameras if a second group of cells is required.

A background subtraction algorithm was employed throughout the detection phase in order to eliminate redundant artifacts and to surpass optics-based aberrations. The background subtraction method was essentially applied to moving regions, and the object positions were automatically found after input images were compared with a background image. In this way, it is also possible to detect and track multiple objects. After the edge is identified, the algorithm makes a circular approximation to the edge of the object and draws a circle around it, which is taken as the diameter of the object.

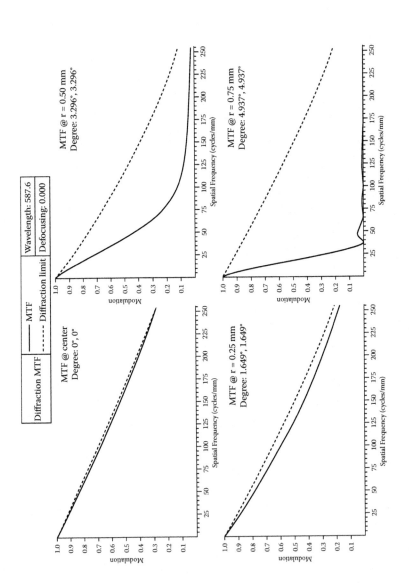

FIGURE 7.6
The graphs show the performance from the center of the image toward the corner (farthest from the center). MTF starts to slope down as moving away from the center, because sharpness is usually best in the center. The dashed curve represents the diffraction-limited results at f 4.1. The solid curves represent MTF. © 2009 IEEE.

It is important to note that the relative size of each pixel in a digital image is very important. To determine accurate diameter, the ratio between a single-cell image reconstructed on an image sensor and corresponding total pixel number must be calculated. The pixel ratio for each cell was calibrated by Olympus Ronchi Ruling glass (Olympus, Toyko, Japan) (100 lp/mm). A donor cell of ~15 µm corresponds to about 30 pixels. In addition, we consider the boundary of any moving region as an edge of the object, because cells always come into the observation area one by one. Once the background is fixed, any moving object is filtered according to its size and dimensions and labeled as a donor or oocyte. Thirty pixels are considered as a minimum detection size and an object below 30 pixels is omitted. We essentially applied the same idea to the two camera systems, but cells are only floating in the container viewed by the microscopic camera. In the case of the compact vision system, however, the program was plagued by some environmental problems such as bubbles and other unwanted objects, which appear similar to the fibroblast or the oocyte.

Becaus the oocytes are approximately ten times larger than the fibroblasts, requiring a deep channel depth (150 µm), the fibroblasts can easily go out of focus range and hence the image becomes blurry. Furthermore, the donor cell is very transparent under visible light. Even though its shape is nearly circular, because of the light conditions, in most cases it is complicated to extract its features from the background (Figure 7.7). After entering the microchannel, according to light dispersion over the donor cell, high-density parts become darker, whereas light areas frequently converge to the background color. Though the system could often capture the edges of the donor

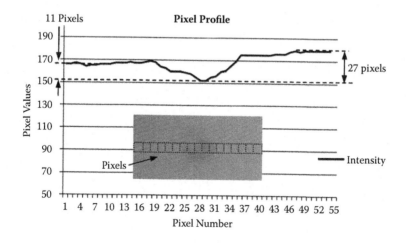

FIGURE 7.7
Pixel intensity changes according to pixel number to extract donor cells from the background. Minimum intensity change is used as default threshold value. © 2009 IEEE.

cell through consecutive frames, in some cases the system could not locate the edges of the fibroblast.

7.3 Experimental Results

7.3.1 Oocyte and Fibroblast Suction

After a number of treatments, explained in the previous section, oocytes and fibroblasts were dispersed in a random manner in different containers (Figure 7.8). Before dispersion, the required flow speed must be defined in order to stabilize cell detection. In the case of fibroblasts, the ideal flow speed is determined by changing the rotary pump speed as in Table 7.3.

After determining the optimum speed, we programmed an initial desired number of cells for suction. The program automatically starts searching for cells in the container if there is no cell on the monitoring area (Figure 7.9a). As soon as the program detects a cell or a cell group, it takes the position of the cells, draws circles around each detected cell, and displays their positional information (see Figure 7.8). The suction mouth of the glass microtube aligns with the nearest cell on the bottom surface, which is numbered 0, and then the rotary pump starts to flow. The required absorption time from the tip of the glass microtube to node A on the microchip is shown in Figure 7.10. According to the absorption time, the pump adjusts its speed automatically by decreasing the speed to the optimum detection level (see Table 7.3).

Once the suction of cell 0 is completed, the suction mouth returns to the original starting point, takes off from the surface to a safe height, and carries on suction of the medium without cells. After 6 seconds (an experimentally

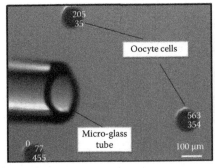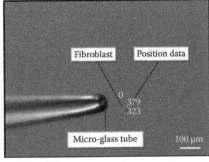

FIGURE 7.8
©2009 IEEE, Fibroblast and oocyte suction from a container. The tip size of the glass tube for the fibroblast is approximately 50 μm and for the oocyte it is approximately 180 μm. The detection algorithm locates the cells and aligns the glass microtube with them.

TABLE 7.3

Fibroblast Cell Detection Ratios for Different
Flow Speeds

Flow speed (in microchannel)	0.39 µL/min
Number of cells	55
Number of detected cells/ratio	55/100%
Flow speed (in microchannel)	0.50 µL/min
Number of cells	53
Number of detected cells/ratio	48/90.6%
Flow speed (in microchannel)	0.60 µL/min
Number of cells	46
Number of detected cells/ratio	34/74%
Flow speed (in microchannel)	0.65 µL/min
Number of cells	50
Number of detected cells/ratio	22/44%
Flow speed (in microchannel)	0.80 µL/min
Number of cells	50
Number of detected cells/ratio	0/0%

© 2009 IEEE.

calculated delay used in order to put a specific distance between each cell)
the suction mouth returns to the bottom surface and moves to the next cell,
numbered 1.

This procedure is repeated until the last cell is vacuumed from the screen
view. If the program reaches the total number of desired cells, it stops searching, moves to a safe height, and continues with the suction, even if there are
still some cells on the screen. The aspirated cells are batched in the docking area with a specific distance. The time interval between two connected
cells is given in Figure 7.9b for suction mode and supply mode. Although the
approximate absorption time for one cell to reach node A was found based
on the speed of the rotary pump and tube dimensions, the experimental
elapsed time values were different (Figure 7.11). The delay occurred due to
the drag resistance of cells as they move through the continuous fluid flow
in the Teflon tube.

7.3.2 Direction Control

Once aspiration of the desired number of cells is completed, the camera system on the cell container is toggled to the compact vision system placed on
the cross section of the "Y"-character microchannels (see Figure 7.11). The
task of the compact system is to ensure that the collected cells are gathered at
the dock and transported to the next module, by switching the valves. When
a new cell shows up in the upper right-hand corner, the program detects cells

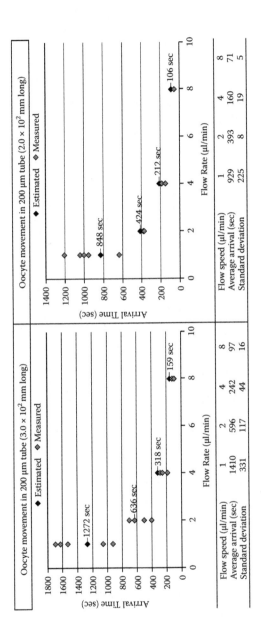

FIGURE 7.9
The cell suction system. (a) The glass microtube bent 45 degrees approaches approximately ~150 μm from an oocyte and vacuums it. (b) After dispersion, the time lag between two consecutive cells at points A and B. © 2009 IEEE.

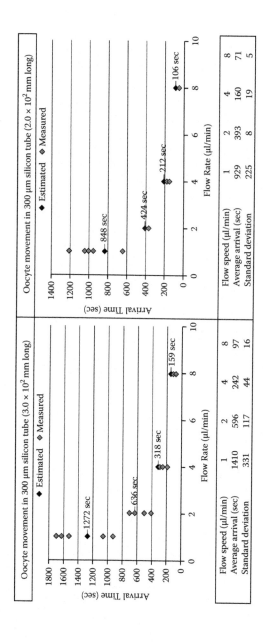

FIGURE 7.10

Approximate absorption time for one cell from the cell container to the microchip. (Flow liquid: TMB 199 liquid + 10% FBS; Oocytes: after removal of zona pellucida.)

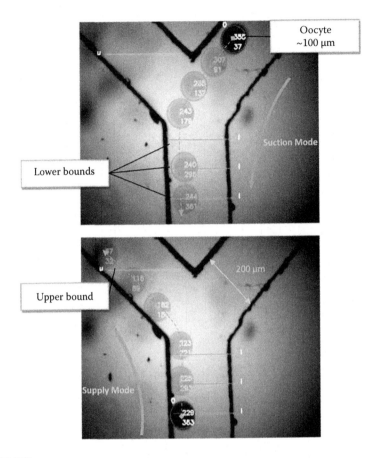

FIGURE 7.11
Experimental result for tracking and controlling an oocyte in the microfluidic chip. The images were taken by the compact vision system. Dashed lines with transparent oocyte figures for both images show trajectories in suction and supply modes. © 2009 IEEE.

and starts tracking. To avoid environmental failure in the PDMS chip and to maintain efficiency, four control parameters were added to the cell detection/ tracking and control program. These parameters are shown on the screen as sequential lines. The first three lines (green) confirm that a detected cell safely passes to the dock side. The second line, on the upper left-hand side (blue), counts the number of cells transferred. In the beginning, three green and one blue parameter toggle as false. As soon as the center of the detected circular area of the cell passes a single line, it toggles to true. After it passes three green lines in order, the program counts this as one cell and waits for the second cell. When the desired total number of cells is reached, cells in the dock are transported to the next module. Each time a single cell passes the blue line, this is recorded for final confirmation. To start cell transfer to the next module, the system runs as follows:

- The rotary pump connected to the end of the "Y"-shaped channel stops the flow.
- The syringe pump applies pressure to the right pneumatic valve (infusion) while releasing the left valves (withdraw). In the experiments, the time elapsed during valve switching was measured at approximately 3 seconds.
- The main flow direction is reversed.
- The rotary pump starts running again and transfers cells in the batch to the microchannel on the left.

7.4 Discussion and Conclusion

The system presented here allows individual cells to be aspirated from a container and transferred to other modules. The components, composed of pumps and micromanipulators, were connected to a computer that automatically controlled all functions carried out in the microfluidic device.

The pneumatic pressure valves were successfully applied on the fluidic chip. We demonstrated a potential application of this system, the automation of nuclear transplantation. We also demonstrated a potential application of this system, the automation of nuclear transplantation by singly transporting fibroblasts and oocytes. Cell coupling for nuclear transplantation can be automated by microfluidic devices. The detection method developed for this study is a simple and robust technique well suited for microfluidic systems. Experimental results showed that the synchronized camera modules together with this algorithm were able to handle the pumps and micromanipulators simultaneously. Data analyzed from the images were used to control the motion of the particles in the channels. The performance of the algorithm was tested with different parameters. It is capable of detecting different cell sizes, which also shows that the proposed system can be utilized as a support system with various on-chip single-cell analysis methods.

This device is by no means a final system for nuclear transplantation. Its efficiency may be increased by including automated cell fusion functions within networks of microchannels. Future research will focus on improving the algorithm and control, with the goal of executing simultaneous donor and oocyte manipulation in different fluidic chips before fusing them in a microfluidic chip.

References

Andrea, A. and Klavs, F. 2008. Microfluidic based single cell microinjection. *Lab on a Chip*, 8: 1258–1261.

Arai, T., Tanikawa, T., Arai, F., Satoh, O., Asouh, H., and Takahashi, S. 2007. Automated embryonic cell manipulation using micro robotics technology. Paper read at the International Conference on Intelligent Robots and Systems Workshop, October, San Diego, CA, October 29–November 2, 2007.

Cookson, S., Ostroff, N., Pang, W.L., Volfson, D., and Hasty, J. 2005. Monitoring dynamics of single-cell gene expression over multiple cell cycles. *Molecular System Biology*, 1: 2005–0024.

Cui, Y., Wei, Q., Park, H., and Lieber, C.M. 2001. Nanowire nanosensors for highly sensitive and selective detection of biological and chemical species. *Science*, 293(5533): 1289–1292.

Elfwing, A., LeMarc, Y., Baranyi, J., and Ballagi, A. 2004. Observing growth and division of large numbers of individual bacteria by image analysis. *Applied and Environmental Microbiology*, 70(2): 675–678.

Gunnar, P.H.D. and Bähr, M. 2008. Synthesis of cell-penetrating peptides and their application in neurobiology. *Methods in Molecular Biology*, 399: 181–186.

He, M., Edgar, J.S., and Jeffries, G.D.M. 2005. Selective encapsulation of single cells and subcellular organelles into picoliter- and femtoliter-volume droplets. *Analytical Chemistry*, 77(6): 1539–1544.

Huang, W.H., Aia, F., Wanga, Z.L., and Cheng, I-K. 2008. Recent advances in single-cell analysis using capillary electrophoresis and microfluidic devices. *Journal of Chromatography B*, 866(1–2): 104–122.

Jager, E.W.H., Inganäs, O., and Lundström, I. 2000. Microrobots for micrometer-size objects in aqueous media: potential tools for single-cell manipulation. *Science*, 288(5475): 2335–2338.

Lee, Y.C., Parviz, B.A., Chiou, J.A., and Chen, S. 2003. Packaging for microelectromechanical and nanoelectromechanical systems. *IEEE Transactions on Advanced Packaging*, 26(3): 217–226.

MacDonald, M.P., Spalding, G.C., and Dholakia, K. 2003. Microfluidic sorting in an optical lattice. *Nature*, 426: 421–424.

Ramesham, R. and Ghaffarian, R. 2000. Challenges in interconnection and packaging of microelectromechanical systems (MEMS). Paper read at the 50th Electronic, Components and Technology Conference, Las Vegas, NV, May 21–24, 2000.

Ray, S.F. 2002. *Applied Photographic Optics*, 3rd ed. Woburn, MA: Focal Press.

Schönholzer, F., Hahn, D., Zarda, B., and Zeyera, J. 2002. Automated image analysis and in situ hybridization as tools to study bacterial populations in food resources, gut and cast of *Lubricus terrestris*. *Journal of Microbiological Methods*, 48(1): 53–68.

Schwarz, M.A. and Hauser, P.C. 2001. Recent developments in detection methods for microfabricated analytical devices. *Lab on a Chip*, 1: 1–6.

Skelley, A.M., Kirak, O., and Suh, H. 2009. Microfluidic control of cell pairing and fusion. *Nature Methods*, 6: 147–152.

Smith, W.J. 2000. *Modern Optical Engineering: the Design of Optical Systems*, 3rd ed. New York: McGraw-Hill.

Toriello, N.M., Douglas, E.S., Thaitrong, N., Hsiao, S.C., Francis, M.B., Bertozzi, C.R. and ____ 2008. Integrated microfluidic bioprocessor for single-cell gene expression analysis. *PNAS*, 105(51): 20173–20178.

Tuan, R.S. and Lo, C.W. 2000. *Methods in Molecular Biology. Developmental Biology Protocols*, Vol III. New York: Humana Press.

Unger, A., Chou, H.P., and Thorsen, T., Scherer, A., and Quake, S.R. 2000. Monolithic microfabricated valves and pumps by multilayer soft lithography. *Science*, 288(5463): 113–116.

Uvet, H., Arai, T., Mae, Y., Takubo, T., and Yamada, M. 2008. Miniaturized vision system for microfluidic devices. *Advanced Robotics*, 22(11): 1207–1223.

Vilkner, T.T., Janasek, D., and Manz, A. 2004. Micro total analysis systems. Recent developments. *Analytical Chemistry*, 76(12): 3373–3386.

Walker, G.M., Zeringu, H.C., and Beebe, D.J. 2004. Microenvironment design considerations for cellular scale studies. *Lab on a Chip*, 4: 91–97.

Wu, H., Wheeler, A., and Zare, R.N. 2004. Chemical cytometry on a picoliter-scale integrated microfluidic chip. *PNAS*, 101(35): 12809–12813.

Yia, C., Lia, C.-W., Shenglin, J., and Yang, M. 2006. Microfluidics technology for manipulation and analysis of biological cells. *Analytica Chimica Acta*, 560(1–2): 1–23.

Zhang, J., Tan, K.L., and Gong, H.Q. 2001. Characterization of the polymerization of SU-8 photoresist and its applications in micro-electro-mechanical systems (MEMS). *Polymer Testing*, 20(6): 693–701.

8

Biomechanical Characterization of Human Red Blood Cells with Optical Tweezers

Youhua Tan and Dong Sun
City University of Hong Kong
Hong Kong, China

Wenhao Huang
University of Science and Technology of China
Hefei, China

CONTENTS

8.1 Introduction 148
8.2 Cell Mechanical Modeling 150
8.3 Cell Manipulation with Optical Tweezers 153
    8.3.1 Optical Tweezer System 153
    8.3.2 Experimental Materials Preparation 155
    8.3.3 Force Calibration 155
    8.3.4 Robotic Manipulation of Microbeads 156
    8.3.5 Optical Stretching of Human RBCs 157
8.4 Results and Discussion 158
8.5 Summary 161
References 161

Abstract

Human red blood cells (RBCs) are essential for transportation of oxygen and carbon dioxide for human bodies. The mechanical properties of cells are crucial to the exercise of normal cellular functions. Abnormity of cell mechanics may cause disorders. In this chapter, the biomechanical properties of human RBCs in hypotonic conditions are investigated using robotic manipulation technology with optical tweezers to understand the correlation between cell mechanics and osmotic environments. Optical traps serve as end-effectors to manipulate microbeads attached to the cell surface. The cell is stretched by progressively increasing the distance between the bead and the binding site, where the induced deformation responses are recorded for analysis. To extract the mechanical properties from the obtained force–deformation relationship, a cell mechanical model is developed from our previous work. This model is based on membrane theory and adopts a hyperelastic material to represent the deformation behavior of RBC membranes. By fitting the modeling results to the experimental data, the area compressibility modulus and elastic shear modulus are characterized as 0.29 ± 0.05 N/m and 6.5 ± 1.0 µN/m, respectively, which are less than the reported results of natural RBCs in isotonic conditions. This study indicates that hypotonic stress has a significant effect on the biomechanical properties of human RBCs, providing insight into the pathology of some human diseases and disease therapy.

8.1 Introduction

Human red blood cells (RBCs) are responsible for transportation of oxygen and carbon dioxide, which are crucial for maintaining normal physiological functions of human bodies. It is well known that RBCs have the ability to withstand large passive deformation when traversing narrow capillaries during microcirculation. An RBC mainly includes a liquid drop (hemoglobin) and a biomembrane, in which a lipid bilayer membrane is attached to a two-dimensional cytoskeletal network through some transmembrane proteins (Mohandas and Gallagher 2008). Compared to the biomembrane, the resistance of the inner fluid to stress is small and negligible. The deformability of human RBCs is thus dominated by the mechanical properties of biomembranes.

Cell mechanics is essential in maintenance and regulation of the physiological functions of biological cells. Abnormity of cell mechanics, especially biomechanical properties, may reflect microstructural alterations of the cytoskeleton and may lead to some disorders. Therefore, cell mechanics of human RBCs has received considerable attention in recent years. Accumulating evidence has reported that alterations of the mechanical properties of RBCs may be associated with the onset and progression of some diseases. For example, mechanical properties of oxygenated RBCs in sickle cell disease are significantly different from those of healthy RBCs (Nash, Johnson, and Meiselman 1984). RBCs parasitized by malaria virus, namely, *Plasmodium falciparum*, become rigid and poorly deformable and show abnormal circulatory behavior (Glenister et al. 2002; Shelby et al. 2003; Suwanarusk et al. 2004). The shear modulus of these infected RBCs was found to increase up to tenfold during parasite development (Suresh et al. 2005). Additionally, the cell mechanics of RBCs is related to some other disorders, such as diabetes mellitus (Tsukada et al. 2001), sepsis (Baskurt, Gelmont, and Meiseliman 1998), and chronic renal failure (Meier et al. 1991).

The cell mechanics of RBCs has been extensively investigated. It has been reported that several factors may regulate the cell properties of RBCs, such as chemical or drug treatment by thyroxine (Baskurt et al. 1990), nitric oxide (Bor-Kucukatay et al. 2003), and lanthanum (Alexy et al. 2007) and the effect of pH (Kuzman et al. 2000), temperature (Mills et al. 2007), and cell age (Sutera et al. 1985). An important physiological condition, osmotic stress has been found to have great influence on the biomechanical properties of some other types of cells; for example, articular chondrocytes (Guilak, Erickson, and Ting-Beall 2002), human neutrophils (Ting-Beall, Needham, and Hochmuth 1993), and Madin-Darby canine kidney cells (Steltenkamp et al. 2006). However, little attention has been paid to its effect on human RBCs.

To investigate the influence of osmotic stress on the mechanical properties of RBCs, robotic manipulation technology with optical tweezers is utilized to study the cell mechanics of human RBCs in hypotonic solutions. Increasing demands for both high precision and high throughput in cell manipulation highlights the need for automated processing with robotics technology. Benefiting from great advances such as visual servoing (Feddema and Simon 1998; Huang et al. 2009a, 2009b), microforce sensing and control (Wejinya, Shen, and Xi 2008; Xie et al. 2009), motion control (Sun and Mills 2002), microfabrication techniques (Zhang et al. 2004), and image processing (Li, Zong, and Bi 2001), robotic manipulation of biological objects has been achieved (Huang et al. 2009a, 2009b; Xie et al. 2009). In parallel, optical tweezer technology is known for its ability to impose force and deformation on a microscaled object on the order of piconewtons (pN, 10^{-12} N) and nanometers (nm, 10^{-9} m), respectively, in noncontact and noninvasive manners. Combining these two advanced techniques, biological cells can be manipulated with high precision and good controllability.

In this chapter, a cell mechanical model is developed from our previous work (Tan, Sun, and Huang 2010; Tan et al. 2008, 2009, 2010a, 2010b) to model the deformation behavior of human RBCs in optically induced cell stretching. Equilibrium equations are adopted to represent the force balance of the biomembrane; a hyperelastic constitutive material, namely, Evans–Skalak material, is utilized to describe the material characteristics of RBC membranes. According to the mechanical model, the relationship between the stretching force and the induced deformation can be established. To investigate the osmotic effect on the mechanical properties of human RBCs, robotic manipulation technology with optical tweezers is used to stretch human RBCs in hypotonic conditions. RBCs are stretched to different levels of deformation at various trapping forces. By fitting the modeling results to the experimental data, the area compressibility modulus and the shear elastic modulus of RBCs are obtained, which are less than the reported results of the natural RBCs in isotonic conditions. This indicates the significant effect of osmotic stress on the mechanical properties of human RBCs but also can be used to shed light on the therapy and pathology of some human diseases.

8.2 Cell Mechanical Modeling

In our previous work (Tan, Sun, and Huang 2010; Tan et al. 2008), we proposed a theoretical model to interpret the deformation response of biological cells in microinjection. This model was based on membrane theory and unitized a hyperelastic material to describe the deformation behavior of cell membranes. In this chapter, according to the practical conditions of RBCs stretching experiments by optical tweezers, the mechanical model is modified and extended to extract the mechanical properties of RBC membranes.

The experimental conditions of RBCs stretching meet the prerequisite and restriction of the mechanical model developed in our previous work. First, human RBCs in hypotonic solutions appear to be spherical or spheroidic; that is, rotationally symmetric. Second, RBC biomembranes are usually treated as incompressible homogeneous isotropic materials (Henon et al. 1999; Mills et al. 2004). Third, during the deformation process of RBCs, their internal volumes are generally considered to stay constant; that is, cytoplasm is incompressible (Dao, Lim, and Suresh 2003; Mills et al. 2007).

According to the shell theory of Landau and Lifshitz (1986), the contribution of the bending rigidity can be neglected due to the small thickness of biomembrane. Then, the deformation behavior of RBCs in optical stretching is mainly determined by membrane theory. Quasistatic equilibrium equations are used to describe the force balance in the meridian tangential and normal directions of the cell membrane, which are expressed by (Feng and Yang 1973; Tan, Sun, and Huang 2010; Tan et al. 2008, 2009):

$$\frac{\partial T_1}{\partial \lambda_1} \lambda_1' + \frac{\partial T_1}{\partial \lambda_2} \lambda_2' = \frac{\rho'}{\rho}(T_2 - T_1) \tag{8.1}$$

$$K_1 T_1 + K_2 T_2 = P \tag{8.2}$$

where T_1 and T_2, λ_1 and λ_2, and K_1 and K_2 are the principal tensions, stretch ratios, and curvatures, respectively. The indices 1 and 2 refer to the corresponding component in the meridian and circumferential directions of the deformed membrane, respectively. P is the external pressure acting on the membrane in the normal direction. ρ and η are the coordinates after deformation as shown in Figure 8.1. The prime denotes the derivative with respect to the angle ψ.

The principal tensions T_1 and T_2 are calculated according to the strain energy function of the chosen membrane material. Because the constitutive material proposed by Evans and Skalak (1980; ES material) is usually used to represent the deformation behavior of RBC membranes, it is adopted here to

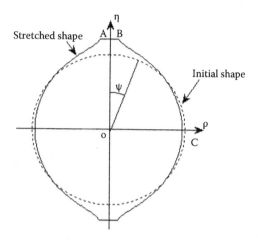

FIGURE 8.1
Coordinates definition before and after optical stretching. Image courtesy of Y. Tan, used with permission from IEEE (Tan et al. 2009).

model the stretching deformation. T_1 and T_2 can be derived from the strain energy function as follows:

$$\begin{cases} T_1 = k(\lambda_1\lambda_2 - 1) + \mu \dfrac{\lambda_1^2 - \lambda_2^2}{2(\lambda_1\lambda_2)^2} \\[4mm] T_2 = k(\lambda_1\lambda_2 - 1) + \mu \dfrac{\lambda_2^2 - \lambda_1^2}{2(\lambda_1\lambda_2)^2} \end{cases} \tag{8.3}$$

where k and μ are the area compressibility modulus and shear modulus, respectively.

There are two contact areas between an RBC and its exterior. One is between the bead and the RBC, and the other is between the glass surface and the other side of the cell. Because it is difficult to define the interactions in the contact areas, we simplify this problem by assuming that the interactions in both the contact areas are similar. This approximation is consistent with the treatment method reported previously (Mills et al. 2007). As shown in Figure 8.1, due to dual symmetry, only a quarter of the deformed cell shape is needed for analysis. According to the experimental conditions in cell stretching, appropriate boundary conditions are used, which are given as follows:

At point A: $\psi = 0$, $\lambda_1 = \lambda_2 = \lambda_0$;

At point B: $\psi = \psi_B$, $\rho_B = r_{contact}$;

At point C: $\psi = \pi/2$, $\rho' = 0$.

where $r_{contact}$ is the contact radius between the cell and the bead.

To solve the equilibrium Equations (8.1) and (8.2), the volume conservation constraint is imposed (Dao, Lim, and Suresh 2003; Mills et al. 2004; Tan, Sun, and Huang 2010; Tan et al. 2008, 2009, 2010a, 2010b). Moreover, the contact radius between beads and RBCs must be known prior by image processing. In the coordinates defined in Figure 8.1, K_1, K_2, ρ, and η can all be expressed as a function of λ_1 and λ_2, respectively (see more details in Tan et al. 2008). With the five equations, that is, Equations (8.1)–(8.3) and the volume conservation constraint, five unknowns λ_1, λ_2, T_1, T_2, and P can be solved. The deformed cell shapes are then determined as shown in Figure 8.2. The axial deformation d (along the stretching direction) is thus obtained. In parallel, the stretching force is acquired from the force balance in the equatorial plane. Therefore, the force and the induced deformation can be expressed as follows:

$$F = T_{1C} 2\pi\rho_C - P\pi\rho_C^2 \tag{8.4}$$

$$d = 2r_0 - 2\eta_B \tag{8.5}$$

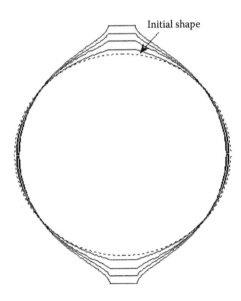

FIGURE 8.2
Calculated deformed cell shapes after optical stretching.

As stated above, the force–deformation relationship is determined when the area compressibility modulus k and the shear modulus μ are given in Equation (8.3). Different mechanical properties lead to different force–deformation curves. By minimizing the deviation between the modeling results and the experimental data, the biomechanical properties of RBCs can be characterized.

8.3 Cell Manipulation with Optical Tweezers

To study the cell mechanics of human RBCs, experiments of robotic cell manipulation with optical tweezers were conducted. Human RBCs are stretched at different levels of trapping forces. Through force calibrations and image processing, the relationship between the stretching forces and the induced deformations is established, from which the mechanical properties of RBCs can be characterized based on the cell mechanical model.

8.3.1 Optical Tweezer System

Figure 8.3 shows a schematic diagram of our optical tweezer system, which mainly consists of a single laser trap. The 808-nm diode laser source has a maximum power of 2.0 W. The laser beam is reflected by a dichroic mirror into a 40× objective and focused on the observation plane. To minimize the possible optical damage to living cells, the laser beam is focused on the attached polystyrene beads instead of RBCs. The biological sample is placed on a two-dimensional motorized stage that is driven by two DC motors with a positioning accuracy of 50 nm (PI M-111.1DG, Physik Instrumente Co., Shanghai, China). The cell manipulation process is guided by visual feedback provided by a CCD camera, from which the positions of cell and beads are obtained as well as the cell deformation. All of the mechanical components were supported on an antivibration table.

The mixture of RBCs and beads was contained in a home-built chamber, which was assembled with microscopic slides and coverslips conglutinated by super glue. All slides and coverslips were cleaned using ethanol. The coverslips were glued to the slide with super glue and sealed at the corners with nail polish. In cell stretching experiments, the surfaces of the chamber were bare glass. Once adhesion between cells and beads was confirmed, the diluted mixture was injected into the chamber from an open end, which was then sealed with a coverslip. The chamber was then reversed for about 10 minutes to let the cells settle down and adhere. Most RBCs were attached to the sidewall surface of the chamber, and unattached cells sank to the slide after inverting the chamber back to its original position. Then the chamber was ready for robotic manipulation experiments. It should be noted that all

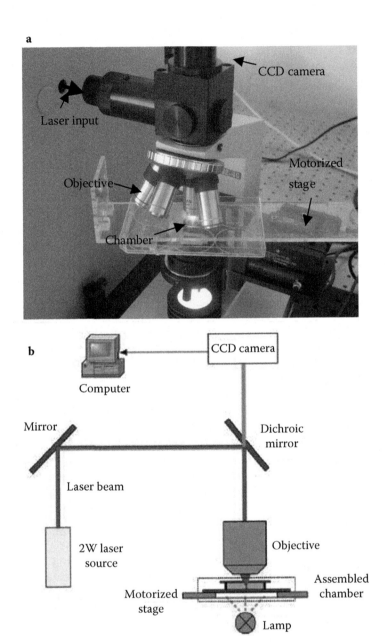

FIGURE 8.3
Robotic optical tweezer system: (a) experimental setup of optical tweezer system and (b) schematic diagram of optical tweezer system.

of the glass surfaces of the chamber were treated with 100 mg/mL bovine serum albumin (BSA, Sigma, St. Louis, MO, USA) to prevent the beads from sticking for microbead manipulation experiments (Tan et al. 2009, 2010b).

8.3.2 Experimental Materials Preparation

Fresh blood was drawn from healthy donors by fingertip prick. A small portion of blood was suspended in phosphate-buffered saline (PBS, Sigma) and then washed three times by centrifugation. A dense RBC sample was obtained after discarding the top layer of blood after rinsing. In parallel, streptavidin-coated polystyrene beads with a radius of 1.5 µm (Bangs Laboratories, Fishers, IN) were centrifuged three times in 0.1 mg/mL PBS-BSA solution. The washed beads were incubated with 1 mg/mL biotin-conjugated concanavalin A (Con A, Sigma) at 4°C for 40 minutes. The beads were then rinsed three more times in 0.1 mg/mL PBS-BSA and stored in 0.1 mg/mL PBS-BSA solution with Ca^{2+} and Mn^{2+}. The prepared polystyrene beads were added to the RBC suspension and incubated at 25°C for one hour to allow the adhesion between beads and RBCs. Once the adhesion was confirmed under an optical microscope, the mixture was diluted in 0.7% hypotonic sodium chloride buffer to allow RBCs to become swollen.

8.3.3 Force Calibration

To acquire the optical trapping force at a certain laser power, it is necessary to perform force calibration experiments because the trapping force cannot be measured directly. The usual viscous drag force calibration method was used here (Henon et al. 1999; Mills et al. 2004; Tan et al. 2010a). A polystyrene bead was trapped at the same separation distance h as that used in cell stretching experiments. As the chamber was driven to move via the motorized stage, the fluid flow exerted a viscous drag force on the trapped bead. When the flow velocity increased up to a critical value beyond which the bead just escaped the laser trap, the bead achieved equilibrium; that is, the trapping force equaled the viscous drag force. According to Stokes' law, the viscous drag force is expressed as (Svoboda and Block 1994)

$$F = \frac{6\pi R \eta_0 v_0}{1 - 9/16(R/h) + 1/8(R/h)^3 - 45/256(R/h)^4 - 1/16(R/h)^5} \quad (8.6)$$

where R is the radius of the trapped bead, η_0 is the fluid viscosity ($\eta_0 = 1.01 \times 10^{-3}$ Pa.s at 25°C), v_0 is the critical velocity, and h is the separation distance of the bead below the coverslip surface. Throughout calibration and cell stretching experiments, h was kept at 5 µm.

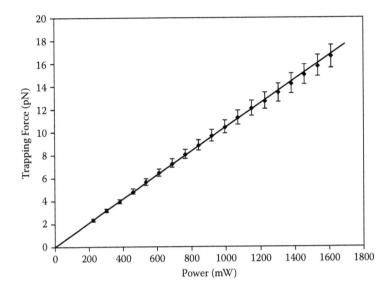

FIGURE 8.4
Optical force calibration versus various laser powers by trapping a polystyrene bead with radius of 1.5 μm at the separation depth $h = 5$ μm from the coverslip.

The force calibration results are shown in Figure 8.4 over a range of laser power. At each level of laser power, five separate measurements were conducted and the results were averaged. All data can be fitted by a straight line, which is consistent with the results reported by Svoboda and Block (1994) and Mills et al. (2004).

8.3.4 Robotic Manipulation of Microbeads

Robotic manipulation of biological cells has been reported in mechanical contacts (Huang et al. 2009a, 2009b; Li, Zong, and Bi 2001; Sun and Mills 2002; Wejinya, Shen, and Xi 2008; Xie et al. 2009). In many noninvasive cell manipulation applications (Arai et al. 2001; Gu, Kuriakose, and Gan 2007), cells were held and manipulated by laser traps directly. In this study, microbeads were attached to the cell surface, serving as handles to stretch the RBCs. The laser beam was focused on the attached bead instead of the cell to minimize the potential optical damage. Microbeads were manipulated by optical traps directly in RBC stretching experiments. Here, we first demonstrate the efficiency of bead manipulation by optical tweezers. Figure 8.5 illustrates the manipulation process. When the moving velocity of the motorized stage is lower than the critical value calculated from Equation (8.6), the trap holds the bead tightly, as shown in Figures 8.5a–c. As the velocity increases beyond this critical value, the bead escapes the trap, as shown in see Figure 8.5d. During cell manipulation, the centroids of microbeads can be obtained through image processing. Because

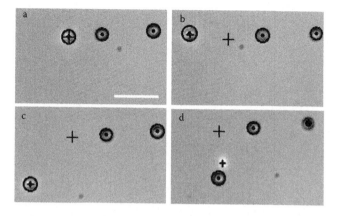

FIGURE 8.5
Robotic manipulation process of microbeads by optical tweezers: the large cross denotes the initial position of the manipulated bead, while the small cross denotes the position of the optical trap. The black circle and dot indicate the contour and the center of the microbeads, respectively. Scale bar is 10 μm. Reprinted with permission from IEEE (Tan et al. 2009).

the position of the trap is fixed, bead escape is detected when the centroid of the bead deviates from the trap position with a certain distance.

8.3.5 Optical Stretching of Human RBCs

Because our optical tweezer system consists of a single laser trap, a small portion of an RBC was required to be anchored to the side wall of the chamber while the attached bead on the opposite side was grasped by an optical trap, as shown in Figure 8.6 (Mills et al. 2007). As the chamber was driven to

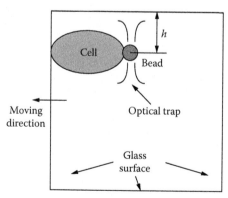

FIGURE 8.6
A schematic graph of cell stretching experiments, where one side of an RBC is fixed onto the glass surface and the other side is held by a laser trap. Reprinted with permission from IEEE (Tan et al. 2009).

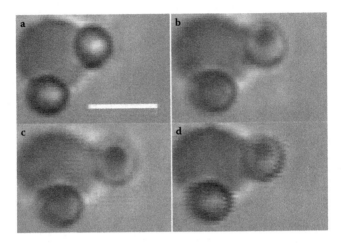

FIGURE 8.7
Stretching process of a swollen RBC: (a) before stretching, (b) during stretching, (c) stretched to the maximum deformation, and (d) the bead escapes the laser trap. Scale bar is 5 μm. Reprinted with permission from IEEE (Tan et al. 2009).

move by the motorized stage, the anchored side of the cell was moved with the stage. Because the trapped bead was kept fixed in the optical trap, the RBC was stretched until the trapped bead escaped from the trap. Note that the moving direction of the stage was determined along the line passing through the bead's centroid and the binding site of the cell. Figure 8.7 shows the cell stretching process.

For each stretching experiment, RBCs were stretched to different levels of deformation over a range of laser powers, which were recorded by the CCD camera for image analysis. The image at the moment when the trap could not hold the bead any longer was captured for cell deformation estimation. The trapping force can be acquired from the calibrated relationship between trapping force and laser power. Figure 8.8 shows the stretched cell shapes under a series of trapping forces. To obtain the deformations of RBCs, the digital image was processed by a home-built program to detect the edges of the stretched RBCs as shown in Figure 8.9. Then the axial deformation was measured.

8.4 Results and Discussion

Cell deformation was measured at each laser power. Then the relationship between the stretching force and the induced axial deformation was established for cell stretching experiments, which is shown in Figure 8.10. For each data point, ten separate tests were conducted and the obtained results were

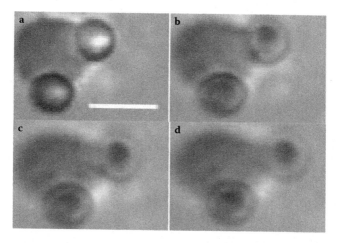

FIGURE 8.8
Deformed cell shapes of a swollen RBC at different levels of stretching forces: (a) 0 pN, (b) 8 pN, (c) 12 pN, and (d) 17.5 pN. Scale bar is 5 μm. Reprinted with permission from IEEE (Tan et al. 2009).

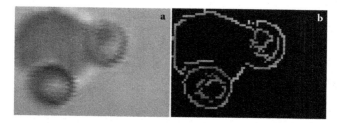

FIGURE 8.9
Image analysis for cell deformation estimation: (a) original image and (b) processed image. Reprinted with permission from IEEE (Tan et al. 2009).

averaged. It was found that RBCs tend to become stiff after repetitive stretching. To eliminate the influence of stretching-induced cell stiffening, we used the results from the first stretch for each cell for analysis. The error bar in Figure 8.10 represents the standard deviation of the measured cell deformation. According to Equations (8.4) and (8.5), the modeling relation between force and deformation can be obtained once the mechanical properties of RBCs are prescribed. The contact radius between the beads and RBCs $r_{connect}$ was measured as 0.8 μm. It was found that the experimental data agreed well with the modeling results when the area compressibility modulus and shear modulus were given as $k = 0.29 \pm 0.95$ N/m and $\mu = 6.5 \pm 1.0$ μN/m. The mechanical properties were determined through an identification procedure as reported in Tan, Sun, and Huang (2010). When the deviation between the experiments and the cell modeling was minimized, the most appropriate values of k and μ were obtained. The acquired mechanical properties of swollen RBCs are consistent with the reported values; for example, the area

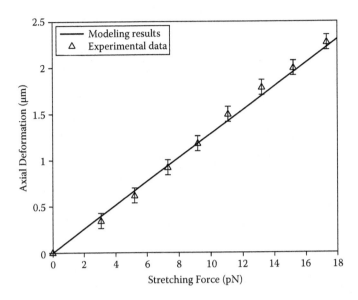

FIGURE 8.10
Comparison of experimental data and modeling results. Reprinted with permission from IEEE (Tan et al. 2009).

compressibility modulus of RBCs in hypotonic conditions is on the order of 0.2–0.45 N/m (Evans, Waugh, and Melnik 1976), and the elastic shear modulus is in the range of 2.5–10 μN/m (Dao, Lim, and Suresh 2003; Henon et al. 1999; Mills et al. 2004) but less than the elastic shear modulus of natural RBCs in isotonic conditions, which is reported to be 13 μN/m (Dao, Lim, and Suresh 2003). The results indicate that cell softening in hypotonic conditions may be related to the significant effect of osmotic stress on RBCs. Under hypotonic conditions, the osmotic pressure causes water influx from the exterior of the cell, which leads to the inflation of cytosol and the cytoskeleton. The decrease of cell stiffness is attributed to the fact that the phospholipids bilayer membrane swells faster than the cytoskeleton (Steltenkamp et al. 2006). As a consequence, the volume inflation leads to either rupture of cytoskeleton or its detachment from the lipid membrane. Moreover, the osmosis-induced increase of cell deformability has some potential biomedical significance and can provide a reasonable explanation for the observations reported previously. RBCs from sickle cell anemia patients appear to be much stiffer and less deformable than healthy RBCs (Nash, Johnson, and Meiselman 1984). It has been observed that treatment using hypotonic saline solution can reverse the sickling of the sickled RBCs, which may be beneficial in emergency therapy for painful sickle cell crises (Guy, Gavrilis, and Rothenberg 1973; McManus, Churchwell, and Strange 1995). This phenomenon can be explained by the outcome of this study in that the hypotonic solution makes the sickled RBCs much softer and more deformable, which may be beneficial in the alleviation of sickle cell disease. However, excessively hypotonic conditions will swell RBCs to an extreme extent and may cause hemolysis (Braasch 1971).

Additionally, the results show that the relation between the stretching force and the axial deformation is quasilinear, which is consistent with the results reported in Henon et al. (1999) and Mills et al. (2004). This finding indicates that when the stretching force is low enough (less than 18 pN), the swollen RBC behaves like a linear elastic spring, which reflects the intrinsic membrane deformation characteristics in this force range and sheds light on the study of the microstructures of RBC biomembranes.

8.5 Summary

In this chapter, mechanical characterization of human RBCs was successfully achieved through robotic manipulation with optical tweezers. A cell mechanical model was developed based on membrane theory, in which Evans-Skalak material was utilized to represent the deformation behavior of RBC biomembranes. To investigate the influence of osmotic stress on the mechanical properties of human RBCs, robotic manipulation technology with optical tweezers was used to stretch RBCs in hypotonic conditions. The linear relationship between the stretching force and the axial deformation was obtained in experiments. Comparing the experimental data to the modeling results, the mechanical properties of RBCs, for example, the area compressibility modulus and the elastic shear modulus, were characterized, which were lower than the counterpart RBCs in isotonic conditions. This preliminary study not only helps in understanding the significant effect of osmotic stress on human RBCs but provides insight into the pathology of some human diseases and disease therapy.

References

Alexy, T. Nemeth, N., Wenby, R.B., Bauersachs, R.M., Baskurt, O.K., and Meiselman, H.J. 2007. Effect of lanthanum on red blood cell deformability. *Biorheology*, 44(5–6): 361–373.

Arai, F., Ichikawa, A., Ogawa, M., Fukuda, T., Horio, K., and Itoigawa, K. 2001. High-speed separation system of randomly suspended single living cells by laser trap and dielectrophoresis. *Electrophoresis*, 22(2): 283–288.

Baskurt, O.K., Gelmont, D., and Meiseliman, H.J. 1998. Red blood cell deformability in sepsis. *American Journal of Respiratory and Critical Care Medicine*, 157(2):
421–427.

Baskurt, O.K., Levi, E., Temizer, A., Ozer, D., Caqlayan, S., Dikmenoqlu, N., and
Andac, S.O. 1990. In vitro effects of thyroxine on the mechanical properties of
erythrocytes. *Life Sciences*, 46(20): 1471–1477.

Bor-Kucukatay, M., Wenby, R.B., Meiselman, H.J., and Baskurt, O.K. 2003. Effects of
nitric oxide on red blood cell deformability. *American Journal of Physiology-Heart
and Circulatory Physiology*, 284(5): H1577–H1584.

Braasch, D. 1971. Red cell deformability and capillary blood flow. *Physiological Review*,
51(4): 679–701.

Dao, M., Lim, C.T., and Suresh, S. 2003. Mechanics of the human red blood cell
deformed by optical tweezers. *Journal of the Mechanics and Physics of Solids*,
51(11): 2259–2280.

Evans, E.A. and Skalak, R. 1980. *Mechanics and Thermodynamics of Biomembranes*. Boca
Raton, FL: CRC Press.

Evans, E.A., Waugh, R., and Melnik, L. 1976. Elastic area compressibility modulus of
red cell membrane. *Biophysical Journal*, 16(6): 585–595.

Feddema, J.T. and Simon, R.W. 1998. Visual servoing and CAD-driven microassem-
bly. *IEEE Robotics & Automation Magazine*, 5(4): 18–24.

Feng, W.W. and Yang, W.H. 1973. On the contact problem of an inflated spherical
nonlinear membrane. *Journal of Applied Mechanics*, 40: 209–214.

Fornal, M., Korbut, R.A., Lekka, M., Pyka-Fosciak, G., Wizner, B., Stycenz, J., and
Grodzicki, T. 2008. Rheological properties of erythrocytes in patients with high
risk of cardiovascular disease. *Clinical Hemorheology and Microcirculation*, 39(1–
4): 213–219.

Glenister, F.K., Coppel, R.L., Cowman, A.F., Mohandas, N., and Cooke, B.M.
2002. Contribution of parasite proteins to altered mechanical properties of
malaria-infected red blood cells. *Blood*, 99(3): 1060–1063.

Gu, M., Kuriakose, S., and Gan, X.S. 2007. A single beam near-field laser trap for
optical stretching, folding and rotation of erythrocytes. *Optics Express*, 15(3):
1369–1375.

Guilak, F., Erickson, G.R., and Ting-Beall, H.P. 2002. The effects of osmotic stress on
the viscoelastic and physical properties of articular chondrocytes. *Biophysical
Journal*, 82(2): 720–727.

Guy, R.B., Gavrilis, P.K., and Rothenberg, S.P. 1973. In vitro and in vivo effect of hypotonic saline on the sickling phenomenon. *The American Journal of the Medical
Sciences*, 266(4): 267–277.

Henon, S., Lenormand, G., Richert, A., and Gallet, F. 1999. A new determination of
the shear modulus of the human erythrocyte membrane using optical tweezers.
Biophysical Journal, 76(2): 1145–1151.

Huang, H.B., Sun, D., Mills, J.K., and Cheng, S.H. 2009a. Robotic cell injection system
with vision and force control: Towards automatic batch biomanipulation. *IEEE
Transactions on Robotics*, 25(3): 727–737.

Huang, H.B., Sun, D., Mills, J.K., and Li, W.J. 2009b. Visual-based impedance control
of out-of-plane cell injection systems. *IEEE Transactions on Automation Science
and Engineering*, 6(3): 565–571.

Kuzman, D., Znidarcic, T., Gros, M., Vrhovec, S., Svetina, S., and Zeks, B. 2000. Effect of pH
on red blood cell deformability. *European Journal of Physiology*, 440(7): R193–R194.

Landau, L.D. and Lifshitz, E.M. 1986. *Theory of Elasticity*. New York: Pergamon.

Lee, S.S., Kim, N.J., Sun, K., Dobbe, J.G., Hardeman, M.R., Antaki, J.F., Ahn, K.H., and Lee, S.J. 2006. Association between arterial stiffness and the deformability of red blood cells (RBCs). *Clinical Hemorheology and Microcirculation*, 34(4): 475–481.

Li, X.D., Zong, G., and Bi, S. 2001. Development of global vision system for biological automatic micromanipulation system. Paper read at the IEEE International Conference on Robotics and Automation, Seoul, Korea, May 21–26, 2001.

McManus, M.L., Churchwell, K.B., and Strange, K. 1995. Regulation of cell volume in health and disease. *The New England Journal of Medicine*, 333(9): 1260–1267.

Meier, W., Paulitschke, M., Lerche, D., Schmidt, G., and Zoellner, K. 1991. Action of rHuEpo on mechanical membrane properties of red blood cells in children with end-stage renal disease. *Nephrology Dialysis Transplantation*, 6(2): 110–116.

Mills, J.P., Diez-Silva, M., Quinn, D.J., Dao, M., Lang, M.J., Tan, K.S., Lim, C.T., Milon, G., David, P.H., Mercereau-Puijalon, O., Bonnefoy, S., and Suresh, S. 2007. Effect of plasmodial RESA protein on deformability of human red blood cells harboring *Plasmodium falciparum*. *Proceedings of the National Academy of Sciences of the United States of America*, 104(22): 9213–9217.

Mills, J.P., Qie, L., Dao, M., Lim, C.T., and Suresh, S. 2004. Nonlinear elastic and viscoelastic deformation of the human red blood cell with optical tweezers. *Molecular and Cellular Biomechanics*, 1(3): 169–180.

Mohandas, N. and Gallagher, P.G. 2008. Red cell membrane: Past, present, and future. *Blood*, 112(10): 3939–3948.

Nash, G.B., Johnson, C.S., and Meiselman, H.J. 1984. Mechanical properties of oxygenated red blood cells in sickle cell (HbSS) disease. *Blood*, 63(1): 73–82.

Shelby, J.P., White, J., Ganasan, K., Rathod, P.K., and Chlu, D.T. 2003. A microfluidic model for single-cell capillary obstruction by *Plasmodium falciparum*–infected erythrocytes. *Proceedings of the National Academy of Sciences of the United States of America*, 100(25): 14618–14622.

Steltenkamp, S., Rommel, C., Wegener, J., and Janshoff, A. 2006. Membrane stiffness of animal cells challenged by osmotic stress. *Small*, 2(8–9): 1016–1020.

Sun, D. and Mills, J.K. 2002. Manipulating rigid payloads with multiple robots using compliant grippers. *IEEE/ASME Transactions on Mechatronics*, 7(1): 23–34.

Suresh, S., Spatz, J., Mills, J.P., Micoulet, A., Dao, M., Lim, C.T., Bell, M., and Seufferlein, T. 2005. Connections between single-cell biomechanics and human disease states: Gastrointestinal cancer and malaria. *Acta Biomaterialia*, 1(1): 15–30.

Sutera, S.P., Gardener, R.A., Boylan, C.W., Carroll, G.L., Chang, K.C., Marvel, J.S., Kilo, C., Gonen, B., and Williamson, J.R. 1985. Age-related changes in deformability of human erythrocytes. *Blood*, 65(2): 275–282.

Suwanarusk, R., Cooke, B.M., Dondorp, A.M., Silamut, K., Sattabongkot, J., White, N.J., and Udomsangpetch, R. 2004. The deformability of red blood cells parasitized by *Plasmodium falciparum and P. vivax*. *The Journal of Infectious Diseases*, 189(2): 190–194.

Svoboda, K. and Block, S.M. 1994. Biological applications of optical forces. *Annual Review of Biophysics and Biomolecular Structure*, 23: 247–285.

Tan, Y., Sun, D., and Huang, W. 2010. Mechanical modeling of red blood cells during optical stretching. *Journal of Biomechanical Engineering-Transactions of ASME*, 132(4): 044504.

Tan, Y., Sun, D., Huang, W.H., and Cheng, S.H. 2008. Mechanical modeling of biological cells in microinjection. *IEEE Transactions on NanoBioScience*, 7(4): 257–266.

Tan, Y., Sun, D., Huang, W., and Cheng, S.H. 2010a. Characterizing mechanical properties of biological cells by microinjection. *IEEE Transactions on NanoBioScience*, 9(3): 171–180.

Tan, Y., Sun, D., Huang, W., and Li, H. 2009. Mechanical characterization of human red blood cells by robotic manipulation with optical tweezers. Paper read at the IEEE International Conference on Robotics and Biomimetics, Guilin, China, December 19–23, 2009.

Tan, Y., Sun, D., Wang, J., and Huang, W. 2010b. Mechanical characterization of human red blood cells under different osmotic conditions by robotic manipulation with optical tweezers. *IEEE Transactions on Biomedical Engineering*, 57(7): 1816–1825.

Ting-Beall, H.P., Needham, D., and Hochmuth, R.M. 1993. Volume and osmotic properties of human neutrophils. *Blood*, 81(10): 2774–2780.

Tsukada, K., Sekizuka, E., Oshio, C., and Minamitani, H. 2001. Direct measurement of erythrocyte deformability in diabetes mellitus with a transparent microchannel capillary model and high-speed video camera system. *Microvascular Research*, 61(3): 231–239.

Wejinya, U.C., Shen, Y.T., and Xi, N. 2008. In situ micro-force sensing and quantitative elasticity evaluation of living Drosophila embryos at different stages. IEEE/ASME International Conference on Advanced Intelligent Mechatronics, Xi'an, China, July 25, 2008.

Xie, Y., Sun, D., Liu, C., Cheng, S.H., and Liu, Y.H. 2009. A force control based cell injection approach in a bio-robotics system. Paper read at the IEEE International Conference on Robotics and Automation, Kobe, Japan, May 12–17, 2009, 3443–3448.

Zhang, X.J., Zappe, S., Bernstein, R.W., Sahin, O., Chen, C.-C., Fish, M., Scott, M.P., and Solgaard, O. 2004. Micromachined silicon force sensor based on diffractive optical encoders for characterization of microinjection. *Sensors and Actuators A: Physical*, 114(2): 197–203.

9

Nanorobotic Manipulation for a Single Biological Cell

Toshio Fukuda and Masahiro Nakajima
Nagoya University
Nagoya, Japan

Mohd Ridzuan Ahmad
Universiti Teknologi Malaysi
Skudai Johor, Malaysia

CONTENTS

9.1 Background of Nanorobotic Manipulations 166
9.2 Single-Cell Analysis and Nanosurgery System 167
9.3 Principles of Stiffness Measurements for a Single Cell 169
    9.3.1 Stiffness Measurement of a Single Cell Based on Nanoindentation Technique 169
    9.3.2 Stiffness Measurement Using Different Indenter Tip Shapes. 171
    9.3.3 Stiffness Measurement Using Nanoprobes 173
        9.3.3.1 Measurement of Single-Cell Stiffness Using a Soft Nanoprobe 174
        9.3.3.2 Measurement of Single-Cell Stiffness Using Hard Nanoprobes 175
9.4 Nanorobotic Manipulations inside Various Kinds of Microscopes ... 176
    9.4.1 Nanorobotic Manipulation System inside Electron Microscopes 176
    9.4.2 Observations of Biological Samples by E-SEM 177
9.5 Stiffness Measurements of Single Cells Using Conventional AFM Cantilevers 179
    9.5.1 Stiffness Measurement of Single Yeast Cells Depends on Cell Sizes 179
    9.5.2 Stiffness Measurement of Single Yeast Cells Depends on Growth Phases 181
9.6 Stiffness Measurements of Single Cells Using Nanoprobes 182
    9.6.1 Fabrication of Nanoprobes 182
    9.6.2 Calibration of Soft Nanoprobes 183

9.6.3   Stiffness Measurement of Single Yeast Cells by Nanoprobes . 184
9.7   Summary 185
Acknowledgments 186
References 186

Abstract

Nanorobotic nanomanipulation inside electron microscopes is presented
in this chapter. We constructed an environmental scanning electron
microscope (E-SEM) nanomanipulation system to observe and manipulate biological samples in nanoscale resolution with water-containing
condition. The system can be used for various applications in the direct
observation and manipulation of biological samples with nondrying,
nondyeing, noncoating treatments, with a 7-degrees of freedom nanomanipulator with a sharp pyramidal end-effector and a cooling stage;
that is, a temperature controller. We demonstrated in situ measurements
of mechanical properties of individual *W303* wild-type yeast cells using
several types of nanoprobes. Compression experiments to penetrate the
cell walls of single cells of different cell sizes (about 3–6 µm diameter)
and growth phases (early log, mid-log, late log, and saturation) were
conducted. The advantage of the integrated E-SEM nanomanipulation
system relies on its capability to perform in situ local direct observation
and manipulation of biological samples and its ability to control environmental conditions.

9.1 Background of Nanorobotic Manipulations

The possibility of controlling the structure of matter atom by atom, which
is now called *nanotechnology*, was first discussed seriously by Richard
Feynman in 1959 (Feynman 1960). Nanotechnology has an important role
in combinations of the top-down and bottom-up approaches to construct
highly-integrated devices as shown in Figure 9.1. Wide-scale controlled
devices from the atomic scale to meter scale will be realized in the near
future.

Presently, nanomanipulation can be applied to the scientific exploration of
mesoscopic phenomena and the construction of prototype nanodevices. It is
a fundamental technology for property characterization of nanomaterials,
nanostructures, and nanomechanisms; for the fabrication of nanoscale building blocks; and for the assembly of nanodevices. Nanoelectromechanical
systems (NEMS) are expected to realize highly integrated, miniaturized,
and multifunctional devices for various applications (Craighead 2000). To
realize such a high precision system, direct usage of bottom-up fabricated
nanostructures is effective.

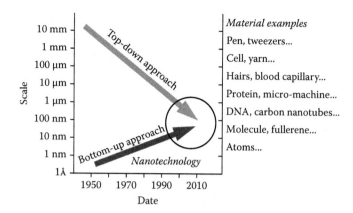

FIGURE 9.1
Schematic diagram of nanotechnology approaches (top-down and bottom-up).

Recently, the evaluation of bio-samples has received much attention for nano-bio applications in nanobiotechnology (Leary, Liu, and Apuzzo 2006; Staples et al. 2006). Single-cell analysis has received a lot of attention for its potential to reveal unknown biological aspects of individual cells. Nanomanipulation techniques are a promising way to develop nano-bio applications on the single-cell level for drug delivery, nanotherapy, nanosurgery, and so on.

9.2 Single-Cell Analysis and Nanosurgery System

Microbiology has traditionally been concerned with and focused on studies at the population level (10^5–10^7 cells; Sedgwick et al. 2008). On the other hand, single-cell analysis contributes to important research on the existence of cellular heterogeneity within individual cells. This technique is important for next-generation analysis methods in biological and medical fields.

Cellular heterogeneity is widespread in bacteria and increasingly apparent in eukaryotic cells (Ferrell and Machleder 1998). Heterogeneity at the single-cell level is typically masked and is therefore unlikely to be acknowledged in conventional studies of microbial populations, which rely on data averaged across thousands or millions of cells. Bulk-scale measurements made on a heterogeneous population of cells provide only average values for the population and are not capable of determining the contributions of individual cells.

The types of individual differences contributing to heterogeneity within a microbial population can be divided into at least four general classes: genetic differences, biochemical differences, physiological differences, and behavioral differences (Avery 2006).

The sizes of biological cells are distributed mainly around the 100 to 1 μm range. Their components, proteins, DNA, etc., are micrometer to nanometer sizes (Wilson and Hunt 2002). Hence, the micronanomechatronics and micronanorobotics contribute to investigating and imitating single-cell properties.

We proposed a single-cell nanosurgery system to realize single-cell diagnosis, extraction, cutting, injection, and embedded micronanodevices. A conceptual schematic is shown in Figure 9.2. Our approaches are based on nanomanipulation technologies using nanotools. As described in the following sections, we developed an environmental SEM (E-SEM) nanorobotic manipulation system to manipulate and control local environments for biological samples at the nanoscale. With this system we have realized the direct observation and manipulation of water-containing biological samples under nanometer high-resolution imaging. Based on the proposed system, the novel local stiffness evaluation, local electrical characterization, local cutting, local injection, and local extraction of biological organisms are presented by micronanoprobes based on the E-SEM nanorobotic manipulation system for a future single-cell diagnosis and surgery system.

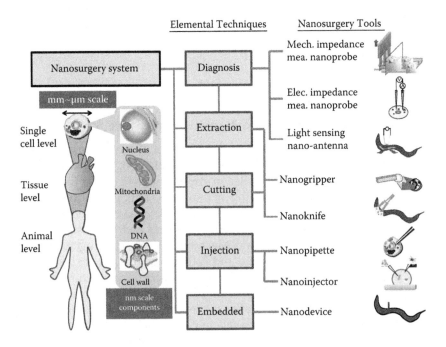

FIGURE 9.2
Schematic of the nanoindentation process.

9.3 Principles of Stiffness Measurements for a Single Cell

9.3.1 Stiffness Measurement of a Single Cell Based on Nanoindentation Technique

A schematic of a nanoindentation process for a single cell is shown in Figure 9.3. An atomic force microscope (AFM) cantilever with a standard or modified tip is mounted on the nanomanipulator stage. The

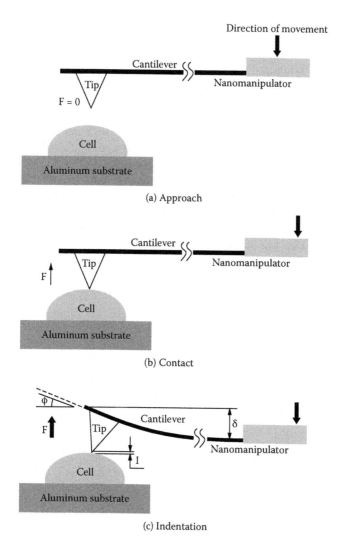

FIGURE 9.3
Schematic of nanoindentation process.

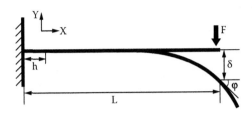

FIGURE 9.4
Schematic of beam deflection.

nanomanipulator is used to approach, contact, and indent the cantilever's tip on a single biological cell. Force is calculated from two parameters, that is, the cantilever's deflection angle, θ, and the cantilever's length, L, which can be obtained from the SEM images.

Figure 9.4 shows a schematic of the beam deflection. By using Macaulay's method (Stephen 2007), which is also known as the *double integration method,* the deflection of the beam can be represented in two relationships; that is, the length deflection, δ, and the angular deflection, φ.

Macaulay's method consists of three steps; that is, derivation of the bending moment, $M(x)$, which acts internally at every point in the interval between $x = 0$ and $x = L$; integration of $M(x)$ to obtain the beam slope; and second integration to get the elastic curve, $v(x)$. In integrating $M(x)$, integration of two constants will emerge; that is, C_1 and C_2. In order to evaluate these constants, appropriate boundary conditions of the beam will be used to determine their values. Finally, the value of $x = L$ is substituted into each equation to find the deflection and slope at the tip of the cantilever.

Equilibrium equation for the sum of moments around point h,

$$\sum M_h = -F(L-x) - M = 0 \tag{9.1}$$

Solving the moment equation for M gives

$$M = Fx - FL \tag{9.2}$$

The moment–curvature relationship can be expressed as

$$EI\frac{d^2v}{dx^2} = M = Fx - FL \tag{9.3}$$

Therefore, the general equations for the slope and deflection of the cantilever are

$$\frac{dv}{dx} = -\frac{FL^2}{2EI} = \varphi \ (angular\ deflection\ in\ radians) \tag{9.4}$$

$$v = -\frac{FL^3}{3EI} = \delta\,(length\ deflection) \tag{9.5}$$

The negative sign indicates the direction of the force. Now, we have the standard equations for the beam deflection under a condition as shown in Figure 9.4. Back to our discussion regarding the visual-based approach for force measurement of the AFM cantilever, the deflection of the AFM cantilever has to be expressed in angular deflection and not in length deflection.

By using basic mathematical manipulation from Equations (9.4) and (9.5), we arrive at the final equation of the cantilever deflection with respect to the angular deflection,

$$\delta = \frac{2}{3}\varphi L \tag{9.6}$$

where δ, φ, and L are the cantilever deflection, the angular deflection in radians, and the total length of the cantilever. The values of φ and L are determined from analysis of the SEM images. Finally, by using Equation (9.6), modification of the Hooke's law can be written as

$$F = k\delta = k\left(\frac{2}{3}\varphi L\right) \tag{9.7}$$

Evaluation of Equation (9.7) was conducted experimentally by comparing the result of δ obtained from a direct displacement measurement.

In our experiment, we obtain δ from the SEM image obtained from Equation (9.6). Because the base of the AFM cantilever was in fixed condition, the value of δ can be obtained directly from the length displacement of the cantilever's tip. Therefore, both parameters, δ and φ, can be determined from the high-magnification SEM image.

9.3.2 Stiffness Measurement Using Different Indenter Tip Shapes

Figure 9.5 shows a schematic of the indenter tip–sample contact for three different indenter tips; that is, cylindrical, conical, and spherical. The parameters I, h, r, θ, and R are indentation depth, sample height, radius of the cylindrical tip, and radii of the spherical tip for conical and spherical, respectively.

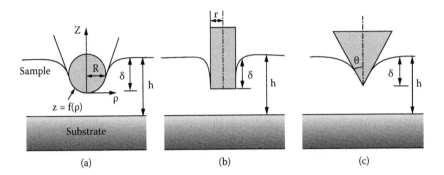

FIGURE 9.5
Schematics of the tip–sample contact for (a) spherical, (b) cylindrical, and (c) conical tips.

The Hertz model is used for the indentation based on a spherical tip and the Sneddon model is used for the indentation based on the cylindrical and conical tips. Therefore, the selection of the Hertz or Sneddon model depends on the shape of the indenter tip.

In 1882, Hertz published a classic paper that aroused considerable interest (Hertz 1882). The load–displacement relation based on a spherical tip from Hertzian analysis is

$$F_{spherical} = \frac{4}{3} \frac{E}{(1-v^2)} R^{1/2} I^{3/2} \tag{9.8}$$

where v is the Poisson's ratio of the sample.

In 1965, Sneddon published a paper on indentation of linear half spaces by rigid punches of arbitrary profile (Sneddon 1965). Although he showed the load–displacement relationship of several tip shapes, only the cylindrical and conical shapes are applied in our case. The load–displacement relations based on cylindrical and conical tips are

$$F_{cylindrical} = 2 \frac{E}{(1-v^2)} aI \tag{9.9}$$

$$F_{cone} = \frac{2}{\pi} \tan\theta \frac{E}{(1-v^2)} I^2. \tag{9.10}$$

The indenter is described by an arbitrary function, $z = f(\rho)$ that is rotated about the z axis to produce a solid of revolution. Nevertheless, Pharr, Oliver, and Brotzen (2002) have shown that Equations (9.8)–(9.10) are also valid for a nonrevolute indenter as well such as pyramidal tip.

9.3.3 Stiffness Measurement Using Nanoprobes

We designed two approaches for determining the stiffness of a single cell as shown in Figure 9.6.

The first approach is based on the buckling phenomenon of a nanoprobe. A schematic of this approach is shown in Figure 9.6a. It is, to the best of our knowledge, a novel technique in determining the stiffness of a cell (Ahmed et al., 2008a). In this technique, the nanoprobe and the cell can be modeled as two springs in series. In order to model the nanoprobe as a spring, firstly, the nanoprobe should be able to buckle linearly, and secondly, it should have a lower or equivalent spring constant as the cell. This technique prevents damage to the cell because the indentation is minimized from the buckling

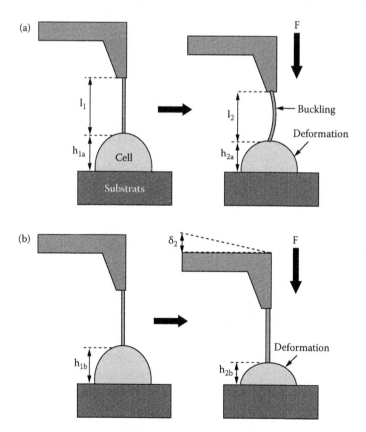

FIGURE 9.6
Schematic diagrams of nanoprobe indentation experiments indicate local single-cell stiffness measurement using (a) a soft nanoprobe and (b) a hard nanoprobe.

effect of the so-called soft nanoprobe, which avoids excessive indentation being applied to the cell.

The second approach for the measurement of cell stiffness is based on a hard nanoprobe, which relies on deformation of the cell in order to measure its stiffness. A schematic of this approach is shown in Figure 9.6b. By knowing the applied compression force and the deformation of the cell, the stiffness of the cell can be measured. In order to fabricate a hard nanoprobe, strong material that is hard to bend is needed. We used tungsten to construct a hard nanoprobe. To prevent excessive indentation force on the cell by the hard nanoprobe, this process has to be performed by avoiding any sudden pressure that can interrupt the chemical activities of the cell; for example, a mechanotransduction effect. The other preventive step is to use a lower cantilever spring constant.

The hard nanoprobe can also be used for single-cell surgery. In theory, all hard nanoprobes must be able to penetrate the cell; however, in practice, for yeast cells, only some nanoprobes can penetrate the cells, whereas others are only limited to cell stiffness measurement only. This is because to penetrate the cell, more compression force is needed. This excessive force may exceed the force limits of the nanoprobe, causing failure.

9.3.3.1 Measurement of Single-Cell Stiffness Using a Soft Nanoprobe

The spring constant of the cell, k_{cell}, can be calculated from the relationship of two springs in series as described in Equation (9.11).

$$k_{cell} = k_{needle} \left(\frac{\Delta_{total} - \Delta_{cell}}{\Delta_{cell}} \right) \qquad (9.11)$$

where k_{needle} is the spring constant of the soft nanoprobe, Δ_{total} is the total displacement of the nanoprobe and the cell, and Δ_{cell} is the deformation of the cell.

The Hertz and Sneddon models, which are based on the shape of the tips, that is, conical, spherical, and cylindrical, were used to estimate the Young's modulus of the cells. The equations are derived from the classic Hertz mechanics model for linear elastic material (Pharr, Oliver, and Brotzen 2002). Parameters E, v, α, R, a, and δ are the Young's modulus; the Poisson's ratio (v = 0.5 for soft biological materials; Lanero et al. 2006) of the elastic half space (cell's surface); the half opening angle of a conical tip; the radius of curvature of a spherical tip; the radius of a cylindrical tip; and the displacement of the cantilever, respectively. Values for α, R, and a were obtained from E-SEM images, and determination of the value of δ is obtained from Equation (9.6), respectively.

The following Equations (9.12)–(9.14) are used to estimate the stiffness of the cell from an indentation by an indenter, which has a body of revolution.

Si-Ti and W_2 nanoprobes are not a true body of revolution because the needles have a rectangular cross section. However, it has been shown that the error using models for a non-body of revolution is very small as explained in detail by Dao et al. (2001) and King (1987).

$$F_{cone} = \frac{2}{\pi} \tan \alpha \frac{E}{(1 - v^2)} \delta^2 \tag{9.12}$$

$$F_{spherical} = \frac{4}{3} \frac{E}{(1 - v^2)} R^{1/2} \delta^{3/2} \tag{9.13}$$

$$F_{cylindrical} = 2 \frac{E}{(1 - v^2)} a\delta \tag{9.14}$$

The models predict that the load depends on the indentation according to a power law related to the tip geometry (Lanero et al. 2006). In order to choose the correct tip geometry, an equation of the form $F = aI^b$ was fitted to force versus indentation curves using commercial fitting software, where the exponent b depends on the tip shape.

For buckling nanoprobe experiments, we obtained a value of b close to 2, characteristic of a conical tip. Interestingly, for a hard nanoprobe, a value close to 1 was obtained for b, from which the experimental data were then fitted using a cylindrical model. To calculate the applied force, F_{cone} in Equation (9.11), Hooke's law based on a cell spring constant, that is, $F = k_{cell} \Delta_{cell}$, was used.

The final equation of the Young's modulus of the cell obtained using a soft nanoprobe is expressed in Equation (9.15).

$$E_{cell} = \frac{(3.237)F_{cone}}{\delta^2} \tag{9.15}$$

9.3.3.2 Measurement of Single-Cell Stiffness Using Hard Nanoprobes

The estimation of the Young's modulus of a single cell by hard nanoprobes was also based on the Hertz–Sneddon continuum mechanics model.

The applied force, $F_{cylindrical}$, in Equation (9.14), was calculated using the following equation:

$$F = k\left(\frac{2}{3}\varphi L\right) \tag{9.16}$$

where k, φ, and L are the spring constant, the displacement angle in radians, and the length of the cantilever, respectively. It should be noted here, however, that the spring constant obtained from the manufacturer's specifications might not be accurate. Possible calibration methods can be performed to determine the exact spring constant of the cantilever prior to the application of the cantilever on the cell stiffness measurement such as a parallel beam approximation approach (Sader 1995), a scanning vibrometry method (Mendels et al. 2006), or a reference piezolever approach (Aksu and Turner 2007). Equation (9.10) was derived from Hooke's law; that is, $F = k\delta$, where δ is the displacement of the cantilever, which was obtained by using $\delta = \varphi(2/3)L$.

The final equation of the Young's modulus of the cell obtained using a hard nanoprobe is expressed in Equation (9.17):

$$E_{cell} = \frac{(2.930 \times 10^6)F_{cylindrical}}{\delta} \tag{9.17}$$

9.4 Nanorobotic Manipulations inside Various Kinds of Microscopes

Nanomanipulation has received much attention because it is an effective strategy for property characterization of individual nanoscale materials and the construction of nanoscale devices (Du, Cui, and Zhu 2006). A manipulation system and an observation system, in other words, a microscope, are necessary for nanomanipulations.

Figure 9.7 shows the strategies of two-dimensional and three-dimensional nanomanipulations under various kinds of microscopes. An optical microscope (OM) is one of the most common and basic microscopes. However, its resolution is limited to ~100 nm because of the diffraction limit of the optical wavelength (~400 to ~800 nm; Lewis et al. 2003). Hence, special techniques (using, for example, evanescent light or fluorescent light) are needed for the observation of nanometer scale objects (Hell 2007). To observe nanoscale objects, a resolution higher than nanoscale is required. Scanning probe microscopes (SPMs) and electron microscopes (EMs) are readily used for nanomanipulation techniques.

9.4.1 Nanorobotic Manipulation System inside Electron Microscopes

The sample chambers of conventional SEMs and transmission electron microscopes (TEMs) are set under a high vacuum (HV) to reduce the disturbance of the electron beam for observation (Fukuda, Arai, and Dong 2003).

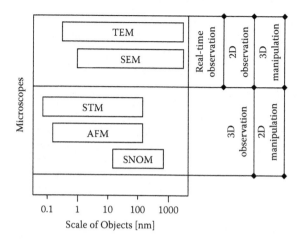

FIGURE 9.7
Elemental technologies of a nanosurgery system.

To observe water-containing samples—for example, bio-cells—appropriate drying and dyeing treatments are needed before observations. Hence, direct observations of water-containing samples are normally quite difficult using these electron microscopes. We have presented the assembly of carbon nanotubes (CNTs) based on a nanorobotic manipulation system inside an SEM and TEM, called a *hybrid nanorobotic manipulation system* (Nakajima, Arai, and Fukuda 2006). An overview of the constructed hybrid nanorobotic manipulation system is shown in Figure 9.8.

Recently, we have constructed nanorobotic manipulators inside an E-SEM (Ahmad et al. 2008a, 2008b, 2010). The E-SEM can realize direct observation of water-containing samples with nanometer high resolution by a specially built secondary electron detector, which is installed close to the sample. The evaporation of water is controlled by the sample temperature (~0 to ~40°C) and sample chamber pressure (10–2,600 Pa). An overview of the constructed E-SEM nanomanipulator is shown in Figure 9.9. It has been constructed with three units and 7 degrees of freedom (DOFs) in total. The temperature of sample is controlled by the cooling stage unit, as Unit3.

The unique characteristic of the E-SEM is the direct observation of the hydroscopic samples with no drying treatment. Generally, water is an important component to maintain biological cell life with chemical reactions. Nanomanipulation inside the E-SEM is considered to be an effective tool for a water-containing sample with nanometer resolution.

9.4.2 Observations of Biological Samples by E-SEM

Wild-type yeast cells were observed by the E-SEM. The samples were cultured with YPB medium for 24 hours in a 37°C chamber. The cultured cells

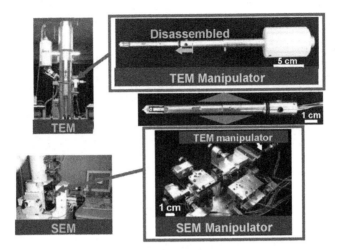

FIGURE 9.8
Photos of hybrid nanorobotic manipulation system inside a TEM and SEM.

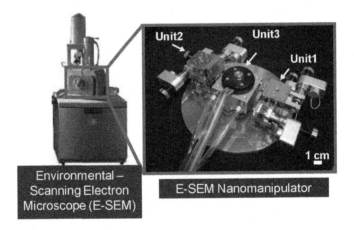

FIGURE 9.9
Photos of the nanorobotic manipulator inside an E-SEM.

were dispersed in pure water. Several microliters of the solution was dropped on an aluminum cooling stage with a micropipette.

Images of the yeast cells are shown with HV and E-SEM modes as shown in Figures 9.10a and 9.10b. The HV mode is operated with the conditions of room temperature (16.7°C) and ~2.0 × 10^{-3} Pa pressure. As shown in Figure 9.10a, almost all yeast cells show a concave and broken structure under HV mode. The E-SEM mode is operated with the conditions of 0.0°C using a cooling stage and ~650 Pa pressure. The accreted voltage was set at 15 kV. In the E-SEM mode, when decreasing the pressure from ~700 Pa, the water, which

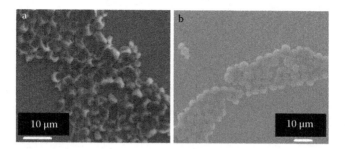

FIGURE 9.10
Electron microscopic images of yeast cells and culturing plate: (a) under HV mode and (b) under E-SEM mode.

is surrounding the cells, is gradually evaporated until showing up. From Figure 9.10b, the remaining water can be seen in the intercellular spaces of yeast cells as black contrast. Almost all of the yeast cells maintain their spherical shape in a water-containing condition with E-SEM operation.

To reveal the effect of observation with HV and E-SEM modes, the yeast cells were cultured again after observation. The plate was divided into three regions: cultured after water dispersion, SEM observation (HV), and E-SEM observation. The number of yeast cell colonies in the E-SEM mode were greater than in HV mode. From this experiment, the living cell rate using E-SEM mode was almost the same order as that under initial conditions of water dispersion.

9.5 Stiffness Measurements of Single Cells Using Conventional AFM Cantilevers

9.5.1 Stiffness Measurement of Single Yeast Cells Depends on Cell Sizes

The single-cell stiffness measurement is presented using an E-SEM nanorobotic manipulation system for yeast cells (Ahmad et al. 2008a, 2008b). A schematic of experimental setup is presented in Figure 9.11. The yeast cells were fixed on the temperature-controlled stage in perpendicular direction with an AFM cantilever. The position of the AFM cantilever was controlled by the nanomanipulator to apply the compression force on each cell. The E-SEM can provide real-time observations, that is, a cell being approached, touched, indented, and finally penetrated/burst by the AFM cantilever, can be seen clearly. The penetration of a single cell by the AFM cantilever was also measured from the occurrence of the cell bursting via real-time observation.

An E-SEM photo showing the penetration of single yeast cells is shown in Figure 9.12. The penetration forces clearly show a strong relationship between cell size and strength; the latter increases with an increase in cell

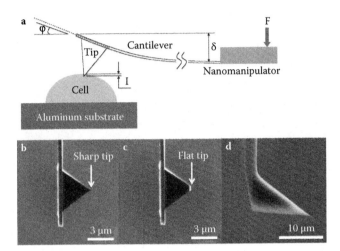

FIGURE 9.11
Schematic diagram of (a) an indentation experiment using (b) sharp and (c) flat AFM pyramidal cantilever tips under E-SEM mode. For the HV mode (d) a tetrahedral cantilever tip was used.

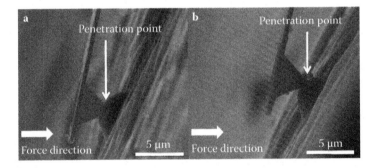

FIGURE 9.12
E-SEM photo during the penetration experiments of single yeast cells by an AFM cantilever tip: (a) sharp cantilever tip and (b) flat cantilever tip.

size as shown in Figure 9.13. The average penetration forces for 3, 4, 5, and 6 μm cell diameter ranges are 96 ± 2, 124 ± 10, 163 ± 1, and 234 ± 14 nN, respectively.

Yeast cell walls consist predominantly of glucan with (1,3)-β and (1,6)-β linkages and mannan covalently linked to protein (mannoprotein; Klis, Boorsma, and De Groot 2006; Lesage and Bussey 2006; Lipke and Ovalle 1998). Thus, it can be inferred that the β-glucans composition increases when the yeast cell size increases. The average Young's modulus obtained in this work, that is, 3.24 ± 0.09 MPa, is reasonable compared to reported local cell stiffness values of 0.73 MPa (Pelling et al. 2004) and 1.12 MPa (Lanero 2006),

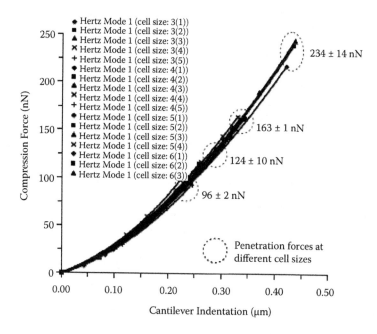

FIGURE 9.13
Penetration force using a sharp tip for different cell sizes. The curves are shown until the penetration points. Inner bracket () indicates the cell number for each cell size. Cell size is in micrometers.

because the E values obtained in this chapter represent not only the local elastic property of the cell but the whole cell stiffness.

9.5.2 Stiffness Measurement of Single Yeast Cells Depends on Growth Phases

All cells have a unique growth phase curve during their life cycle, which is normally divided into four phases: lag, log, saturation, and death phases. In the present study we did not investigate the death phase. These phases can be easily identified from the optical density (OD) absorbance–time curve. The lag phase is located at the initial lower horizontal line where the cells adapt themselves to growth conditions and the cells mature and divide slowly. The log phase can be seen from an exponential line where the cells have started to divide and grow exponentially. The actual growth rate depends upon the growth conditions. The saturation phase resembles a final upper horizontal line where the growth rate slows and ceases mainly due to lack of nutrients in the medium. During the death phase, all of the nutrients are exhausted and the cells die (Tortora, Funke, and Case 2003). It is believed that the mechanics of normal cells have different properties in each of the phases. In this section, the mechanical properties of *W303* yeast

TABLE 9.1

Penetrate Forces of the Single Cells at
Different Cell Growth Phases

Cell Growth Phase	Penetrate Forces (nN)
Early Log	161 ± 25 (n-8)
Mid Log	216 ± 15 (n-9)
Late Log	255 ± 21 (n-8)
Saturation	408 ± 41 (n-8)

cells at four different growth phases (early, mid, late log, and saturation) are discussed (Ahmad et al. 2008b).

The compression experiments were done from early log phase to saturation phase. Penetration force was analyzed for each phase as shown in Table 9.1. As expected, the force needed to penetrate a single cell increased from the early log to the saturation phase (161 ± 25, 216 ± 15, 255 ± 21, and 408 ± 41 nN), whereas the elastic properties of the cells appeared constant for all of the phases obtained; that is, 3.28 ± 0.17, 3.34 ± 0.14, 3.24 ± 0.11, and 3.38 ± 0.11 MPa.

These mechanical properties of the *W303* yeast cells at different growth phases are in agreement with reported increments of average surface modulus of *Saccharomyces cerevisiae* cell walls as 11.1 ± 0.6 N/m (log phase) and 12.9 ± 0.7 N/m (saturation phase) with no significant increase in the elastic modulus of the cell; that is, 112 ± 6 MPa (log phase) and 107 ± 6 MPa (saturation phase; Smith et al. 2000). Their values for elastic modulus are quite high is reasonable because they measured the whole elastic properties of the cell by compressing a single cell between two big flat indenters compared to local cell indentation in our case.

9.6 Stiffness Measurements of Single Cells Using Nanoprobes

9.6.1 Fabrication of Nanoprobes

Four kinds of nanoprobes were fabricated using a focused ion beam (FIB) process at the tip of AFM cantilevers as shown in Figure 9.14. Standard platinum-coated tetrahedral cantilever tips with a spring constant of 2 N/m were used in the fabrication of Si, Si-Ti, and tungsten nanoprobes. For the tungsten nanoprobe, a standard sharp pyramidal cantilever tip with a 0.09 N/m spring constant was used. The soft Si nanoprobe was fabricated by etching (Figure 9.14a). The first type of hard nanoprobe, that is, an Si-Ti nanoprobe, was fabricated by coating the former Si nanoprobe with Ti material by sputtering (Figure 9.14b). The second type of hard nanoprobe was fabricated by first flattening the apex of the sharp pyramidal cantilever tip by using FIB etching (Figure 9.14c). Another type of tungsten hard nanoprobe was fabricated by first flattening the apex of the sharp tetrahedral cantilever tip using

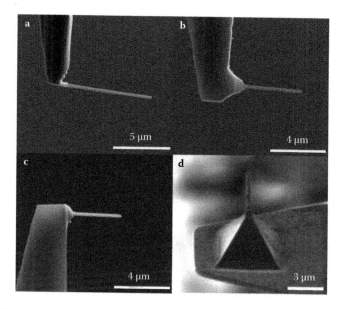

FIGURE 9.14
Actual images of (a) Si, (b) Si-Ti, (c) and (d) tungsten nanoprobes.

FIB etching, followed by tungsten deposition of a large area using FIB deposition, and finally trimmed to produce the nanoprobe structure using FIB etching (Figure 9.14d).

9.6.2 Calibration of Soft Nanoprobes

The Young's modulus and spring constant of the soft Si nanoprobe, E_{needle} and k_{needle}, were calibrated using a nanomanipulation technique. The soft nanoprobe was slowly pressed against another cantilever tip to experimentally determine the spring constant (0.110 N/m). The indentation was carried out until the nanoprobe begun to buckle. Then, the buckled nanoprobe was slowly retracted until the nanoprobe returned to a straight condition as shown in Figure 9.15. The value of E_{needle} was determined from the Euler buckling equation as shown in Equation (9.18), where ℓ_{buckle} is the length of the soft nanoprobe during the buckling condition.

$$E_{softnanoneedle} = \frac{7.68F_n \ell_{buckle}^2}{\pi^2 wb^3} \tag{9.18}$$

where F_n is the buckling force applied to the nanoprobe; E_{needle} is the Young's modulus of the nanoprobe; I is the second moment of area; K is the nanoprobe effective length factor, whose value depends on the conditions of the end support of the nanoprobe; and ℓ is the length of the nanoprobe. The

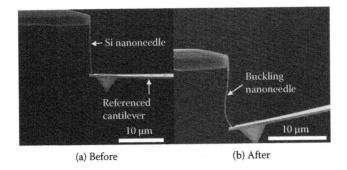

FIGURE 9.15
Calibration of the Si nanoprobe (a) before buckling and (b) after buckling.

value of the length of the soft nanoprobe was corrected with $K = 0.8$ for a structure that has one fixed end and the other end pinned (Timoshenko and Gere 1961). I is a property of a shape that is used to predict its resistance to buckling. A soft nanoprobe that has a rectangular cross section has the value of $I = (wb^3)/12$, where w and b are the width and height of the rectangular cross section. The values for w and b, which were obtained from an image analysis, were 165 and 170 nm, respectively.

9.6.3 Stiffness Measurement of Single Yeast Cells by Nanoprobes

The whole stiffness response of a single cell, that is, the deformation of the entire cell upon the applied load from a single point indentation, to the best of our knowledge, has not been previously reported. The difficulty in obtaining such data is due to the stiff indenter, which may penetrate or burst the cell. Our soft nanoprobe can be used to prevent cell penetration by its ability to buckle during indentation. The mechanism of cell deformation is stated as follows: upon indentation of the soft nanoprobe on the cell, local deformation occurs below the tip of the nanoprobe. Further indentation induces the whole cell to deform in addition to the local cell deformation. The ability to produce a large local point indentation could provide more information regarding the mechanical property of the organelles inside the cell. The global stiffness measurement of single cells from single point indentation was performed using an Si nanoprobe as shown in Figure 9.16. The measurement was performed using a standard indentation procedure. The Si nanoprobe started to buckle after the cell deformed about 0.5 µm. From this point, the buckling rate of the Si nanoprobe increased with increased indentation depth. The values of k_{cell} for approximately the same physical parameters of two yeast cells, that is, 0.92 ± 0.12 and 0.95 ± 0.36 N/m, show strongly similar mechanical properties.

The values that represent the whole cell spring constants are reasonable compared to the reported local spring constant of the *S. cerevisiae* yeast cell (0.06 ± 0.025 N/m). The values of whole E_{cell}; that is, 3.64 and 3.92 MPa, are

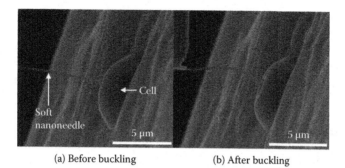

(a) Before buckling   (b) After buckling

FIGURE 9.16
Single-cell global stiffness measurement from a single point using an Si nanoprobe. Two images show the Si nanoprobe in (a) a straight condition and (b) buckling condition.

also rational because they represent the whole cell stiffness property compared to the reported local Young's modulus of the yeast cell; that is, 0.72 ± 0.06 MPa (Pelling et al. 2004). Our method shows improved data sensitivity compared to other global stiffness measurement methods that rely on compression of a single cell between one large indenter and a substrate. Data from this method may not represent the actual global cell stiffness because extra dissipation force may be included in the measurement as reported by Smith et al. (2000) for the global cell spring constant and Young's modulus of yeast cell as 11.1 N/m and 112 MPa.

9.7 Summary

In this chapter nanorobotic nanomanipulation inside electron microscopes was presented. An E-SEM nanomanipulation system was used to observe and manipulate biological samples in nanoscale resolution. The system can be used for various applications for the direct observation and manipulation of biological samples with nondrying, nondyeing, noncoating treatments, with a 7-DOF nanomanipulator with a sharp pyramidal end-effector and a cooling stage; that is, a temperature controller. We demonstrated in situ measurements of mechanical properties of individual *W303* wild-type yeast cells using several types of nanoprobes. Compression experiments to penetrate the cell walls of single cells of different cell sizes (about 3–6 μm diameter) and growth phases (early log, mid log, late log, and saturation) were conducted. Data clearly show an increment in penetration force; that is, 96 ± 2, 124 ± 10, 163 ± 1, and 234 ± 14 nN for 3, 4, 5, and 6 μm cell diameters, respectively. This was further confirmed from quantitative estimation of average cell rigidity through the Hertz model. The penetration forces at different cell growth phases also show the increment pattern from log (early, mid, and late) to saturation phases; that is, 161 ± 25, 216 ± 15, 255 ± 21, and 408 ± 41 nN, respectively.

The advantage of the integrated E-SEM nanomanipulation system relies on its capability to perform in situ local direct observation and manipulation of biological samples and its ability to control environmental conditions.

Acknowledgments

We thank Professors Michio Homma, Seiji Kojima, and Masaru Kojima at Nagoya University for discussion of biological aspects and Professor Toshifumi Inada at Nagoya University for providing us with the wild-type yeast strain W303 cells for the experiments. This work was partially supported by a Grant-in-Aid for Scientific Research from the Ministry of Education, Culture, Sports, Science and Technology of Japan and COE for Education and Research of Micro-Nano Mechatronics, Global COE Program of Nagoya University.

References

Ahmad, M.R., Nakajima, M., Kojima, S., Homma, M., and Fukuda, T. 2008a. In situ single cell mechanics characterization of yeast cells using nanoprobes inside environmental SEM, IEEE Transactions on Nanotechnology, Vol. 7, pp. 607–616.

Ahmad, M.R., Nakajima, M., Kojima, S., Homma, M., and Fukuda, T. 2008b. The effects of cell sizes, environmental conditions and growth phases on the strength of individual *w303* yeast cells inside ESEM. *IEEE Transactions on Nanobioscience*, 7: 185–193.

Ahmad, M.R., Nakajima, M., Kojima, S., Homma, M., and Fukuda, T. 2010. Nanoindentation methods to measure viscoelastic properties of single cells using sharp, flat, and buckling tips inside ESEM. *IEEE Transactions on Nanobioscience*, 9(1): 12–23.

Aksu, S.B. and Turner, J.A. 2007. Calibration of atomic force microscope cantilevers using piezolevers. *Review of Scientific Instruments*, 78: 1–8.

Avery, S.V. 2006. Microbial cell individuality and the underlying sources of heterogeneity. *Nature Reviews: Microbiology*, 4: 577–587.

Craighead, H.G. 2000. Nanoelectromechanical systems. *Science*, 290: 1532–1535.

Dao, M., Chollacoop, N., Van Vliet, K.J., Venkatesh, T.A., and Suresh, S. 2001. Computational modelling of the forward and reverse problems in instrumented sharp indentation. *Acta Materialia*, 49: 3899–3918.

Du, E., Cui, H., and Zhu, Z. 2006. Review of nanomanipulators for nanomanufacturing. *International Journal of Nanomanufacturing*, 1: 83–104.

Ferrell, J.E. and Machleder, E.M. 1998. The biochemical basis of an all-or-none cell fate switch in *Xenopus* oocytes. *Science*, 280: 895–898.

Feynman, R.P. 1960. There's plenty of room at the bottom. *Caltech's Engineering and Science*, 23: 22–36.

Fukuda, T., Arai, F., and Dong, L.X. 2003. Assembly of nanodevices with carbon nanotubes through nanorobotic manipulations. *Proceedings of the IEEE*, 91: 1803–1818.

Hell, S.W. 2007. Far-field optical nanoscopy. *Science*, 316: 1153–1158.

Hertz, H. 1882. On the contact of elastic solids. *Journal für die Reine und Angewandte Mathematik*, 92: 196–171.

King, R.B. 1987. Elastic analysis of some punch problems for a layered medium. *International Journal of Solids and Structures*, 23: 1657–1664.

Klis, F.M., Boorsma, A., and De Groot, P.W.J. 2006. Cell wall construction in *Saccharomyces cerevisiae*. *Yeast*, 23: 185–202.

Lanero, T.S. 2006. Mechanical properties of single living cells encapsulated in poly-electrolyte matrixes. *Journal of Biotechnology*, 124: 723–731.

Lanero, T.S., Cavalleria, O., Krol, S., Rolandi, R., and Gliozzi, A. 2006. Mechanical properties of single living cells encapsulated in polyelectrolyte matrixes. *Journal of Biotechnology*, 124: 723–731.

Leary, S.P., Liu, C.Y., and Apuzzo, M.L.J. 2006. Toward the emergence of nanoneuro-surgery: Part III—Nanomedicine: Targeted nanotherapy, nanosurgery, and progress toward the realization of nanoneurosurgery. *Neurosurgery*, 58: 1009–1026.

Lesage, G. and Bussey, H. 2006. Cell wall assembly in *Saccharomyces cerevisiae*. *Microbiology and Molecular Biology Reviews*, 70: 317–343.

Lewis, A., Taha, H., Strinkovski, A., Manevitch, A., Khatchatouriants, A., Dekhter, R., and Ammann, E. 2003. Near-field optics: From subwavelength illumination to nanometric shadowing. *Nature Biotechnology*, 21: 1378 –1386.

Lipke, P.N. and Ovalle, R. 1998. Cell wall architecture in yeast: new structure and new challenges. *Journal of Bacteriology*, 180: 3735–3740.

Mendels, D.-A., Lowe, M., Cuenat, A., Cain, M.G., Vallejo, E., Ellis, D., and Mendels, F. 2006. Dynamic properties of AFM cantilevers and the calibration of their spring constants. *Journal of Micromechanics and Microengineering*, 16: 1720–1733.

Nakajima, M., Arai, F., and Fukuda, T. 2006. In situ measurement of Young's modulus of carbon nanotube inside TEM through hybrid nanorobotic manipulation system. *IEEE Transactions on Nanotechnology*, 5(3): 243–248.

Pelling, A.E., Sehati, S., Gralla, E.B., Valentine, J.S., and Gimzewski, J.K. 2004. Local nanomechanical motion of the cell wall of *Saccharomyces cerevisiae*. *Science*, 305: 1147–1150.

Pharr, G.M., Oliver, W.C., and Brotzen, F.R. 2002. On the generality of the relationship among contact stiffness, contact area, and elastic modulus during indentation. *Journal of Materials Research*, 7: 619–617.

Sader, J.E. 1995. Parallel beam approximation for V-shaped atomic force, microscope cantilevers. *Review of Scientific Instruments*, 66: 4583–4587.

Sedgwick, H., Caron, F., Monaghan, P.B., Kolch, W., and Cooper, J.M. 2008. Lab-on-a-chip technologies for proteomic analysis from isolated cells. *Journal of the Royal Society Interface*, 5: S123–S130.

Smith, A.E., Zhang, Z., Thomas, C.R., Moxham, K.E., and Middelberg, A.P.J. 2000. The mechanical properties of *Saccharomyces cerevisiae*. *Proceedings of the National Academy of Sciences*, 97: 9871–9874.

Sneddon, I.N. 1965. The relation between load and penetration in the axisymmetric Boussinesq problem for a punch of arbitrary profile. *International Journal of Engineering Science*, 3: 47–57.

Staples, M., Daniel, K., Sima, M.J., and Langer, R. 2006. Applications of micro- and nano-electromechanical devices to drug delivery. *Pharnaceutical Research*, 23: 847–863.

Stephen, N.G. 2007. Macaulay's method for a Timoshenko beam. *International Journal of Mechanical Engineering Education*, 35: 285–292.

Timoshenko, S.P. and Gere, J.M. 1961. *Theory of Elastic Stability* (2nd ed.). New York: McGraw-Hill.

Tortora, G.J., Funke, B.R., and Case, C.L. 2003. *Microbiology: An Introduction* (8th ed.). San Francisco, CA: Benjamin Cummings.

Wilson, J. and Hunt, T. 2002. *Molecular Biology of the Cell*. New York: Garland Publishing.

10

Measurement of Brain Activity Using Optical and Electrical Methods

Atsushi Saito, Alexsandr Ianov, and Yoshiyuki Sankai
University of Tsukuba
Tsukuba, Japan

CONTENTS

10.1 Introduction 190
10.2 Methods to Measure Brain Activities 191
    10.2.1 Brain Wave Bioelectric Signal Measurement 191
    10.2.2 Measurement of Blood Information of the Brain 192
10.3 Device Development 194
    10.3.1 Hybrid Sensor Probe 194
    10.3.2 Signal Processing and Control Board 195
10.4 Experiment 196
    10.4.1 Operation Verification of the Hybrid Sensor Probe 196
    10.4.2 Optical Data Collection Experiment 197
    10.4.3 Assistive Device Control Experiment 198
10.5 Result 199
    10.5.1 Verification of Operation of the Hybrid Sensor Probe 199
    10.5.2 Optical Data Collection Experiment 199
    10.5.3 Assistive Device Control Experiment 200
10.6 Discussion 201
10.7 Conclusion 203
References 203

Abstract

There are patients who cannot produce bioelectric signals such as patients with advanced stages of amyotrophic lateral sclerosis or those who have suffered severe spinal cord injury. These patients are unable to use bioelectrical signal-based assistive devices such as the robot suit HAL. This chapter proposes a noninvasive brain activity scanning method for collecting the patient's movement intentions by developing a hybrid sensor that can measure both optical and bioelectrical signals of the same spot simultaneously and evaluate it. The developed sensor consists of holography laser modules and electrodes. The holography laser modules contain an emitter and receiver. In order to evaluate the hybrid sensor, three kinds of experiments were carried out: (1) operation verification of the hybrid sensor probe in which the pulse waves and the alpha wave were measured with the hybrid sensor probe; (2) an optical data collection experiment in which the optical output was found to be high when the participant was in relaxation state; on the other hand, while the participant was executing mental tasks such as algebraic calculations the optical output lowered; and (3) an assistive device control experiment in which the participant tried to move the upper limb assistive device 10 times. The upper limb movement was recorded 24 times during this period. However, 7 times (out of 24) upper limb movement corresponded to the participant's intention was recorded 5 s before or after the switch was pressed. We developed and evaluated a hybrid sensor that can collect both kinds of optical and bioelectrical signals from the same spot on the scalp in order to measure brain activity by using optical and bioelectrical data.

10.1 Introduction

It is difficult for patients suffering from advanced stages of amyotrophic lateral sclerosis (ALS) and severe spinal cord injuries to transmit bioelectrical signals from the brain to peripheral nerves. They cannot use assistive devices such as the robot suit HAL that are controlled using bioelectric signals (Hayashi et al. 2005; Kawamoto and Sankai 2005; Lee and Sankai 2003; Nakai et al. 2001; Okamura, Tanaka, and Sankai 1999; Suzuki et al. 2007) measured at the peripheral nerves. Residual functions such as voice or eye movements can be used with assistive devices, but these methods place great strain on patients. A brain–computer interface (BCI) that collects the patient's movement intentions and controls devices makes it easier for patients to use assistive devices in this manner.

In order to realize a user-friendly BCI, it is necessary to measure brain activity noninvasively. There are several methods for scanning brain activities. Functional magnetic resonance imaging (fMRI), positron emission tomography (PET), and magnetoencephalography (MEG) are methods that measure brain activity accurately. However, these methods require very large and expensive equipment. Their readings also contain a delay, due to the fact that they are based solely on blood flow. It is not possible to maintain a comfortable lifestyle and use these devices for long periods of time.

On the other hand, there are methods using portable devices, such as electroencephalograms (EEGs) and functional near-infrared spectroscopy (fNIRS). EEG is a method that measures brain activity using electrical brain waves that propagate through the scalp (Sanei and Chambers 2007). Brain waves can be measured using a small, portable device, so an EEG is suitable for daily use. EEG signals are, however, susceptible to noise. Bioelectrical signals originating from eye movements, facial muscular movement, and external power sources such as electronic devices are common noise sources. Furthermore, due to the fact that the electrical signals produced by the brain have to travel through the skull and cerebrospinal fluid, it is difficult to determine the origin of the signal.

fNIRS is a method that measures brain blood circulation information by using near-infrared spectroscopy (NIRS). Differences in blood flow volume reflect neural activities because higher neural activities require higher oxygen concentration and, therefore, higher blood circulation. By using noninvasive optical probes, it is possible to measure cortical neural activities around a brain (Koizumi et al. 2003; Koizumi et al. 2005). Combining bioelectrical activity data collected by brain electrodes with blood circulation data collected by optical probes, it is possible to measure brain activity and infer the area of the brain that is active with a higher degree of precision than with the methods currently available.

The objective of this chapter is to develop a hybrid sensor probe that can measure both optical and bioelectrical signals from the same spot simultaneously.

10.2 Methods to Measure Brain Activities

This section explains the methods used to measure brain activities.

10.2.1 Brain Wave Bioelectric Signal Measurement

EEG is the process of measuring electrical potential generated by several firing neurons simultaneously. These electrical signals propagate through the brain, skull, cerebrospinal fluid, and scalp. A common method for measuring brain waves is measuring voltage by placing noninvasive low-impedance electrodes on the patient's scalp.

Some common passive brain waves include the following:

- Delta: 3 Hz and lower (deep sleep, when awake pathological)
- Theta: 3.5–7.5 Hz (creativity, falling asleep)
- Alpha: 8–13 Hz (relaxation, closed eyes)
- Beta: 14–30 Hz and higher (concentration, logical and analytical thinking)

- Gamma: greater than 30 Hz (simultaneous processes)

It is important to note that voltages drop with the fourth power of the radius, so neural activities from deep sources are more difficult to register than activities from neurons near the skull (Johnson and Guy 1972).

In addition, the bioelectrical signals in the head reflect activation of the head musculature, eye movements, interference from nearby electric devices, and changing conductivity in the electrodes due to the subject's movements or physicochemical reactions at the electrode sites. All of these activities that are not directly related to the current cognitive processing of the subject are considered noise.

Bioelectrical signals were analyzed by using common signal processing techniques.

10.2.2 Measurement of Blood Information of the Brain

In order to measure blood information of the brain using optical data, Lambert–Beer's law was used.

According to Lambert–Beer's law, there is a logarithm relationship between the incident light beams I_{in} and the transmitted light beam I_{out}, absorption coefficient ε, the distance the light travels d, and concentration of the solution C.

$$I_{out} = I_{in}10^{-\varepsilon Cd} \tag{10.1}$$

The light absorbance *Abs* for liquids is defined as:

$$Abs = -\log_{10}\left(\frac{I_{in}}{I_{out}}\right) = \varepsilon Cd \tag{10.2}$$

Lambert–Beer's law, however, usually does not apply for very high concentrations or if the material is highly scattering. When light is applied to blood it is attenuated by both absorption and scattering phenomena. Furthermore, when light is used on the head, the light emitter and receiver are not facing each other. Therefore, a modified version of Lambert–Beer's law is necessary. The modified Lambert–Beer's law is as follows:

$$Abs = \varepsilon C \langle d \rangle + S \tag{10.3}$$

<d> is the average length of the path followed by the light and *S* is a component affected by scattering.

When a light beam is applied to a living organism, its intensity also varies according to the organic tissues under the target region and blood flow.

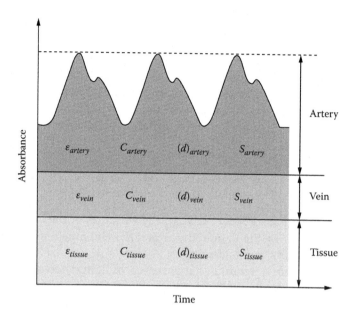

FIGURE 10.1
Variation of light absorbance with time. The components affecting light passing through a living body are classified into three components: organic tissues, veins, and arteries.

The components affecting light passing through a living body are classified into three components: organic tissues, veins, and arteries, as shown in Figure 10.1. In this case, absorbance is expressed as formula (10.4):

$$Abs = \varepsilon_{tissue} C_{tissue} \left\langle d_{tissue} \right\rangle + S_{tissue} + \varepsilon_{vessel} C_{vessel} \left\langle d_{vessel} \right\rangle + S_{vessel} + \varepsilon_{artery} C_{artery} \left\langle d_{artery} \right\rangle + S_{artery}$$

$$(10.4)$$

ε_{tissue}, ε_{vessel}, and ε_{artery} are the absorption coefficients of tissues, vessels, and arteries. C_{tissue}, C_{vessel}, and C_{artery} are the concentration variations of tissues, vessels, and arteries. $<d_{tissue}>$, $<d_{vessel}>$, and $<d_{artery}>$ are the average lengths of the light paths in tissues, vessels, and arteries. S_{tissue}, S_{vessel}, and S_{artery} are the scatter of tissues, veins, and arteries.

If we consider the intensity and wavelength of the incisive light constant and if we also consider that the variation caused by scattering can be ignored, we can evaluate the impact of each component in formulas (10.4).

Organic tissues are static elements; therefore, the concentration, light path, and absorption rate are constant.

Venous blood flow has a constant flow rate. Therefore, the shape of the veins is constant and the light path does not change. But because blood under a beam of light is always changing and because the blood does not have a uniform concentration, the fluid concentration and absorption rate are not constant.

Arterial blood flow is periodical. Therefore, there are changes in pressure, which are responsible for changes in the shape of the arteries. This variation of shape changes the light path. Similar to venous blood, the presence of blood flow means that the concentration and absorption rate are variable.

If S_{tissue}, S_{vein}, and S_{artery} are constant, variation of absorbance is expressed as formula (10.5):

$$\Delta Abs = \varepsilon_{artery} C_{artery} \left\langle \Delta d_{artery} \right\rangle + K \tag{10.5}$$

ΔAbs is variation of absorbance. $<\Delta d_{artery}>$ is variation of the average length of the path followed by the light in the artery. K is the constant including the effect of tissues, veins, and scattering.

Therefore, it is safe to assume that variation of light detected by the light receiver is a direct result of the variation in blood flow and concentration.

10.3 Device Development

10.3.1 Hybrid Sensor Probe

The objective is to develop a sensor that can capture both optical and bioelectrical data simultaneously by using a single sensor probe. A hybrid sensor probe consists of the following components.

- Optical elements
- Electrode
- Amplifier

Optical elements include a light emitter, a light receiver, and a light-guiding transparent acrylic bar. Holography laser modules were used as light sources for the optical sensors. The laser module has a laser diode and photodiodes and is able to keep the size of the sensor small. Common near-infrared imaging devices usually collect the light using optical fibers and the optical signals are converted into electric signals on the external control board. The hybrid sensor probe converts optical signals into electrical signals. Therefore, an optical fiber is not necessary, and handling of the hybrid sensor probe is easy. The light is emitted to the scalp through the light-guiding bar. The light-guiding bar is also used to push hair aside.

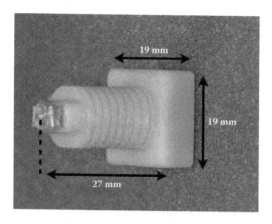

FIGURE 10.2
The hybrid sensor probe developed. Dimensions: 19 mm × 19 mm × 27 mm; weight 4.5 g.

The material chosen for the electrode was silver chloride. Silver chloride was chosen because of its low price and good performance. It has very low impedance and can be acquired for relatively low prices. A buffer circuit was added to the electrode because the electrical current drained from the scalp by the electrode may not be enough to overcome the relative high impedance from the cable. The electrode was located in the end of the hybrid sensor probe. The light-guiding bar was located in the center of the electrode.

An amplifier converted small current signals from the photodiodes output into voltage signals. It also worked to buffer the signals measured on the electrode to decrease output impedance.

Figure 10.2 shows the hybrid sensor probe developed. Its dimensions were 19 mm × 19 mm × 27 mm and its weight was 4.5 g. It was attached directly to a standard EEG cap.

10.3.2 Signal Processing and Control Board

In order to process signals measured by the hybrid sensor probes, a signal processing and control board was developed. The board consisted of signal processing circuits, laser driver circuits, and a microcontroller.

Analog signal processing circuits amplified and filtered the signals measured at the hybrid sensor probes. It was able to change the gain and cutoff frequency using the microcontroller.

Laser drive circuits stabilized the power of the laser diode and controlled the light emission. The timing of the light emission was controlled by the microcontroller.

The microcontroller worked to control the signal processing circuits and the laser drive circuits, to convert analog signals into digital signals, and to communicate with the other devices. The board had a USB port and some digital I/O ports to allow communication with an external device such as a computer or actuators. The microcontroller chosen was powerful enough to execute simple calculations and basic digital processing techniques. More advanced software technologies such as neural networks and genetic algorithms require an external PC. The controller analog sampling rate was set to 1 kHz and A/D conversion resolution was set to 12 bit.

10.4 Experiment

In order to evaluate the hybrid sensor, three experiments were carried out. The first one was to verify the operation of the hybrid sensor probes. The second experiment was to collect optical data using the hybrid sensor probes. The third was to control the assistive device using the hybrid sensor probes.

10.4.1 Operation Verification of the Hybrid Sensor Probe

The purpose of this experiment was to verify the operation of the hybrid sensor probes. In this experiment, two hybrid sensor probes and a reference electrode were used. One sensor acted as an emitter and the other acted as a receiver. The optical sensor emitted a laser wavelength of 805 nm. This wavelength has high permeability on human skin. Furthermore, as shown in Figure 10.3, 805 nm is the isosbestic point of oxyhemoglobin and deoxyhemoglobin. Hence, it suffers little influence from oxygen saturation.

In order to measure brain blood information, it is necessary to reach the light emitted by the probe to the cortex. The distance from the scalp to the cortex is 15–20 mm. The depth to which light infiltrates depends on the distance between the emitter and the receiver. If a brain is active, the influence

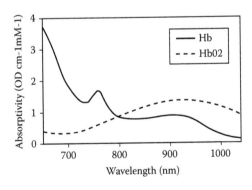

FIGURE 10.3
Hemoglobin absorptivity versus wavelength: 805 nm is the isosbestic point of oxyhemoglobin and deoxyhemoglobin. This wavelength has high permeability on human skin and is well absorbed by hemoglobin. © 2009 IEEE.

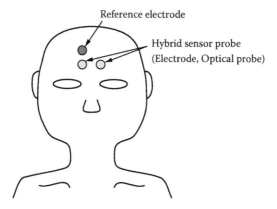

FIGURE 10.4
Position of the hybrid sensor probes and a reference electrode attached to the participant's forehead. © 2009 IEEE.

that light receives from a brain is greater than the influence from other tissues such as skull and skin. Considering the effect of the distance between the emitter and the receiver, a distance greater than 20 mm is enough to measure brain blood information (Kato 2004). Therefore, the distance between the emitter and the receiver was set to 20 mm.

The hybrid sensors and a reference electrode were connected to the signal processing and control board. The board was connected to the PC through a USB port. The board communicated with the PC using a baud rate of 460800 via a serial communication method. The signals measured by the hybrid sensors were saved on the PC.

The probes and the electrode were placed on the participant's forehead, as shown in Figure 10.4. The participant was healthy 25-year-old male. The participant was seated in a relaxed sitting position. First, to verify the optical part of the hybrid sensor probe, the returning pulse wave was measured on the forehead. Second, to verify the electrode of the hybrid sensor probe, alpha waves were measured. When the subject's eyes were closed, the alpha waves increased. The voltage between the reference electrode and the electrode on the hybrid sensor probe was measured. We computed the short-time Fourier transform of the bioelectrical signals. The size of the window was 4096 points.

10.4.2 Optical Data Collection Experiment

In this experiment two hybrid sensors were used. One sensor acted as an emitter and the other acted as a receiver. The optical sensor emitted a wavelength laser of 805 nm. The setup was the same as in the last experiment.

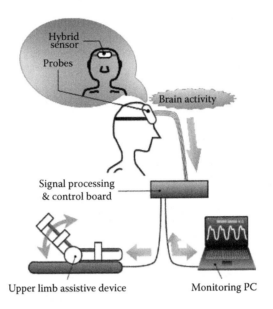

FIGURE 10.5
Experimental system setup for assistive device control experiment. The hybrid sensors and a reference electrode were connected to the signal processing and control board. The board was connected to the PC through a USB port. The board communicated with the PC using a baud rate of 460800 via a serial communication method. The signals measured by the hybrid sensors were saved on the PC. The sensors were placed on the participant's forehead.

The participant was a healthy 23-year-old male. The participant was seated in a relaxed sitting position with his eyes closed. He was asked to perform mental calculations.

10.4.3 Assistive Device Control Experiment

The purpose of this experiment was to control the upper limb assistive device, a part of the robot suit HAL, by using brain activity signals measured by the hybrid sensors. Figure 10.5 shows the experimental system setup for the assistive device control experiment. In this experiment, two hybrid sensor probes and a reference electrode were also used. The connection of the sensors, the board, and the PC were the same as in the last experiment. The board was connected to the upper limb assistive device through the digital I/O ports. A push switch was also connected to the board through a digital I/O port.

During a task that requires mental concentration such as mental arithmetic, blood flow volume of the prefrontal cortex is increased (Tanida et al. 2004). In this experiment, we used this phenomenon as the switch to control the assistive device. If blood flow volume was increased, the optical output measured by the hybrid sensor probe was decreased. Upon detection of a decrease in the optical output, the movement of the assistive device was changed into bend or extension. A single binary signal created by the controller after analyzing the signals from the optical sensor turned the actuator inside the device on and off. The control board was programmed to invert the state of the actuator. The state of the actuator was controlled every 0.8 sec. The control signal was inverted when the maximum of the signals measured by optical sensors during 0.8 s went below a threshold value. The threshold value was chosen by observing the data collected during the relaxation and metal calculation phase of the optical data collection experiment. A period of 0.8 s was chosen because that was the average heartbeat period of the participant. Ideally, each time the participant focused on a mental task the assistive device would turn on or off.

The participant and his task were the same as in the last experiment. He was given a push switch to use to press to signify when he started the mind task. The timing of the beginning of the mental calculations was determined by the participant.

10.5 Result

10.5.1 Verification of Operation of the Hybrid Sensor Probe

Figure 10.6 shows the variation of the optical output. The intensity changed periodically. Pulse waves rise up in the heart's contraction phase and fall in the diastole phase. The pulse wave has an inflection point in the diastole phase. The signals measured in this experiment had the same characteristics of the pulse waves.

Figure 10.7 shows a spectrogram of the EEG signals measured by the electrodes. The frequency band of alpha waves is 8–13 Hz. While the subject's eyes were closed, the signal intensity around 10 Hz was strong. At 18 s, the subject's eyes opened and the signal intensity around 10 Hz became weak. Therefore, alpha waves could be measured with the hybrid sensor probe.

10.5.2 Optical Data Collection Experiment

As shown in Figure 10.8, the optical output was found to be high when the participant was in relaxed state. On the other hand, while the participant was executing mental calculations such as algebra the optical output was lowered.

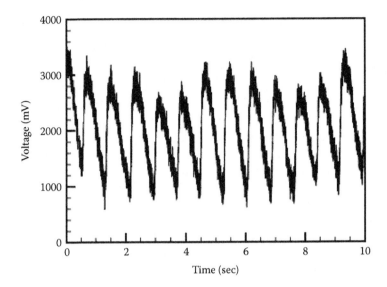

FIGURE 10.6
Optical data measured from the participant's forehead.

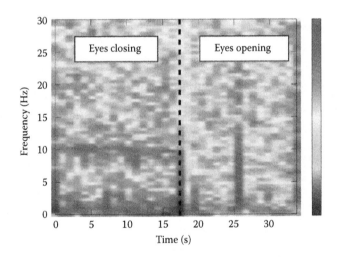

FIGURE 10.7
Spectrogram calculated from EEG signals measured by the electrodes.

10.5.3 Assistive Device Control Experiment

The participant tried to control the upper limb assistive device ten times, shown in Figure 10.9. Upper limb movement was recorded twenty-four times during this period; however, seven times (out of twenty-four), upper limb movement corresponding to the participant's intention was recorded 5 s before or after the switch was pressed.

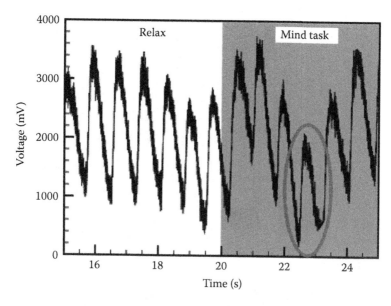

FIGURE 10.8

Results corresponding to data collection experiment. Data included brain blood circulation information measured using optical module of the hybrid sensor. The circle shows that the optical density was lowered when the participant switched from relaxed mode to mental task mode. © 2009 IEEE.

10.6 Discussion

In Figure 10.9 the uppermost graph shows data for the first 100 s, during which the participants tried to move the upper limb assistive device four times. However, the assistive device moved fifteen times, and the movement corresponded to the participant's intention twice by moving within 5 s before or after the button was pressed. Between 100 and 195 s the participant tried to move the upper limb assistive device six times, and the device moved nine times, during which the movement corresponded to the participant's intention five times by moving within 5 s before or after the button was pressed.

During the first few tries the chance of success was found to be low. But, after several trials, the probability of success increased considerably.

The reason for the low success rate in the initial stage of the experiment can be attributed to a lack of learning history. However, the human brain can adapt itself to unfamiliar conditions through repeated learning and can operate precisely. There were cases when the assistive device moved before the participant pressed the button. This may be attributed to the fact that because the participant was free to decide when to start the mental calculations, his brain was already prepared to start calculating.

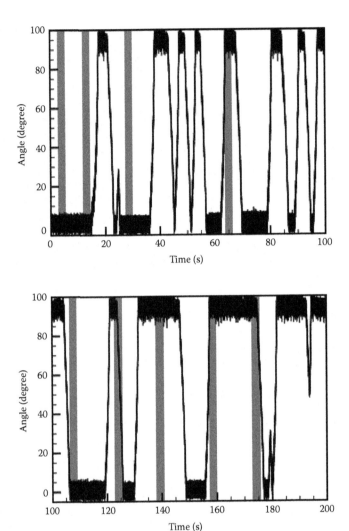

FIGURE 10.9
Graphs showing results of assistive device control experiments. Gray area represents the period of mind task performance, and the black line is the angle of the upper limb assistive device. The uppermost graph shows data from 0 to 100 s. The graph below shows the data corresponding to 100 to 195 s. © 2009 IEEE.

The user set the threshold value based on observations during the optical data collection experiment. There was no learning process executed by the controller. The optical data collection experiment and assistive device control experiment were executed at different times. The human body's biochemical state is dynamic; therefore, the threshold value varies according to different periods of the day. Implementing a dynamic threshold value by using learning algorithms can potentially increase the success rate of the experiment. It is important to notice that bioelectrical signals from the brain were not used. The use of bioelectrical signals could increase the accuracy of the test.

10.7 Conclusion

In this chapter, a hybrid sensor that can collect both bioelectrical and optical data from the same spot on the scalp was developed and evaluated in order to measure brain activity. Data analysis during and after the experiments showed that the bioelectrical data collected by the hybrid sensor were very similar to the data collected by an ordinary disposable electrode. Similarly, the optical data collected by the hybrid sensor were similar to the data collected using a standard functioning near-infrared imaging device.

Our next step is to use this new technology to accurately register the user's movement intentions and use these data to accurately control assistive devices.

References

Hayashi, T., Kawamoto, H., and Sankai, Y. 2005. Control method of RobotSuit HAL working as operator's muscle using biological and dynamical information. IEEE/ RSJ International Conference on Intelligent Robots and Systems, Edmonton, Canada, August 2–6, 2005.

Johnson, C. and Guy, A. 1972. Nonionizing electromagnetic wave effect in biological matherials and systems. *Proceedings of the IEEE*, 60(6): 692–718.

Kato, T. 2004. Principle and technique of NIRS-Imaging for human brain FORCE: Fast-oxygen response in capillary event. *International Congress Series*, 1270: 85–90.

Kawamoto, H. and Sankai, Y. 2005. Power assist method based on PhaseSequence and muscle force condition for HAL. *Advanced Robotics*, 19(7): 717–734.

Koizumi, H., Maki, A., Yamamoto, T., Sato, H., Yamamoto, Y. and Kawaguchi, H.. 2005. Non-invasive brain-function imaging by optical topography. *Trends in Analytical Chemistry*, 24(2): 147–156.

Koizumi, H., Yamamoto, T., Maki, A., Yamashita, Y., Sato, H., Kawaguchi, H. and Ichikawa, N. 2003. Optical topography: practical problems and new applications. *Applied Optics*, 42(16): 3054–3062.

Lee, S. and Sankai, Y. 2003. The natural frequency-based power assist control for lower body with HAL-3. International Conference on Systems, Man and Cybernetics, Washington, DC, October 5–8, 2003.

Nakai, T. Lee, S., Kawamoto, H. and Sanaki, Y. 2001. Development of powered assistive leg for walking aid using EMG and Linux. Asian Symposium on Industrial Automation and Robotics, Bangkok, May 17–18, 2001.

Okamura, J., Tanaka, H., and Sankai, Y. 1999. EMG-based prototype powered assistive system for walking aid. Asian Symposium on Industrial Automation and Robotics, Bangkok. May 6–7, 1999.

Sanei, S. and Chambers, J.A. 2007. *EEG Signal Processing*. New York: Wiley-Interscience.

Suzuki, K., Mito, G., Kawamoto, H., Hasegawa, Y. and Sankai, Y. 2007. Intention-based walking support for paraplegia patients with RobotSuit HAL. *Advanced Robotics*, 21(12): 1441–1469.

Tanida, M., Sakatanib, K., Takanoc, R. and Tagaic, K. 2004. Relation between asymmetry of prefrontal cortex activities and the autonomic nervous system during a mental arithmetic task: near infrared spectroscopy study. *Neuroscience Letters*, 369: 69–74.

11

Bowel Polyp Detection in Capsule Endoscopy Images with Color and Shape Features

Baopu Li and Max Q.-H. Meng
The Chinese University of Hong Kong
Hong Kong, China

CONTENTS

11.1 Introduction 206
11.2 Color and Shape Feature Analysis 209
    11.2.1 Color Feature 210
    11.2.2 Shape Feature 212
11.3 Experimental Results 213
11.4 Conclusions 216
Acknowledgment 216
References 216

Abstract

Capsule endoscopy (CE) has been widely applied in hospitals because it can be used to directly view the whole small intestine in the human body. However, a major drawback of this technology is the tedious review process of about 50,000 images produced in each examination. To relieve physicians and provide support for their decision making, computerized detection of disease is highly desired. In this chapter, we put forward a novel scheme for bowel polyp detection for CE images that integrates color and shape information, which are important visual clues for physicians. An illumination-invariant color feature built upon a chromaticity histogram is suggested. Combining it with Zernike moments that are scale, translation, and rotation invariant, we exploit the integrated information as color and shape features to discriminate polyp CE images from normal ones. By using a multilayer percetron neural network and support vector machine as classifiers, we perform experimental results on our collected CE data, illustrating encouraging performance of detection for polyp CE images.

11.1 Introduction

The gastrointestinal (GI) tract is a 30-foot-long structure composed of a pharynx, esophagus, stomach, small intestine, large intestine, and rectum. Diseases of the GI tract, such as stomach and intestinal cancer, pose a great threat to human's health. According to a publication in Hong Kong (Hospital Authority of Hong Kong 2006), GI tract–related cancers of the colon, stomach, and rectum are ranked as the third, fourth, and fifth causes of cancer deaths, respectively, accounting for 18% of the total cancer deaths in Hong Kong in 2003. Gastroscopy and colonoscopy are the most commonly used approaches for diagnosis of GI diseases. Although they can provide good images that reveal the status of the GI tract, neither can reach the small intestine. Moreover, these techniques require sedating the patient, are uncomfortable, and may include a risk of perforation. Furthermore, these operations require that doctors be very skillful, concentrated, and experienced to navigate the endoscope because the GI tract is very flexible. In 2000, a new kind of GI endoscopy, that is, capsule endoscopy (CE), was developed. This new endoscopy technology, developed by Given Imaging Corporation in Israel, has revolutionized the diagnosis methodology for the digestive tract because this small device can directly view the entire small intestine without pain, sedation, or air insufflation, which is a significant breakthrough.

As demonstrated in Figures 11.1 and 11.2, a CE, measuring 26 mm × 11 mm, is a pill-shaped device that consists of a short-focal-length complementary metal oxide semiconductor (CMOS) camera, light source, battery, and radio transmitter. A patient must fast for about 12 hours before ingesting the CE. After ingestion, this small device starts to work with the peristalsis of mucosa of the GI tract and takes images while moving forward along the digestive tract. Images recorded by the miniature camera are sent out wirelessly to a special recorder attached to the waist. Such a process continues for about 8 hours until CE battery life ends. Finally, all of the image data in the recorder are downloaded into a personal computer or a computer workstation, and physicians can view the images and analyze potential sources of different diseases in the GI tract with the help of specific software. The diagnosis process is time consuming due to the large amount of video, so the diagnosis is not a real-time process, paving a potential way for off-line postprocessing and computer-aided diagnosis. CE was approved by the U.S. Food and Drug Administration (FDA) in 2001, and it has been reported that this novel technology has provided great value in evaluating GI bleeding, Crohn's disease, ulcers, and other diseases of the digestive tract (Adeler and Gostout 2003). Moreover, over 800,000 patients have been diagnosed using CE technology (Given Imaging Ltd. 2009).

One major issue associated with CE is that it takes a long time for physicians to evaluate the large number of images produced. There are about 50,000 images per examination for one patient, and it costs an experienced

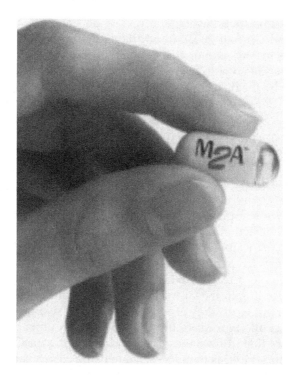

FIGURE 11.1
Capsule endoscopy.

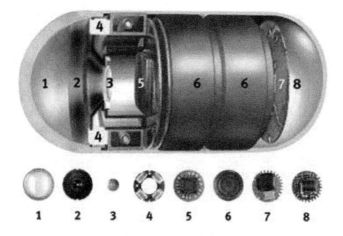

FIGURE 11.2
M2A capsule endoscopy: (1) optical dome, (2) lens holder, (3) lens, (4) illuminating sources, (5) CMOS imager, (6) battery, (7) transmitter, and (8) antenna.

clinician about 2 hours on average to review and analyze all of the video data (Adeler and Gostout 2003). In addition, abnormalities in the GI tract may be present in only one or two frames of the video, so they might be missed by physicians due to oversight. Moreover, some abnormalities cannot be detected by the naked eye due to their size, texture, and distribution. Furthermore, different clinicians may have different findings when viewing the same images. Such problems motivate researchers to design reliable and uniform assistive approaches to relieve physicians. However, such a goal is very challenging because true features associated with diseases are not exactly known or well defined. Moreover, different diseases have different symptoms in the digestive tract, and some diseases show great variations in color and shape.

Due to CE's wide application, many efforts have been made to develop computer-aided detection of CE images to decrease the burden on doctors. Bashar et al. (2008) proposed a method using color and texture to choose informative frames from the CE video. A novel scheme for choosing MPEG-7 visual descriptors as a feature extractor to recognize several diseases such as ulcers and bleeding in the GI tract was proposed in Coimbra and Cunha (2006). Based on this work, they proceeded to develop two approaches to segment the GI tract into four major topographic areas (Cunha et al. 2008), and the first software that utilizes these approaches aiming for CE examination was also introduced in this paper. A scheme using color distribution to discriminate stomach, intestine, and colon tissue in CE images was proposed by Berens, Mackiewicz, and Bell (2005). In Zabulis, Argyros, and Tsakiris (2008), the authors employed two cues, that is, lumen and illumination highlight, for navigation of active CE. Recently, Bejakovic et al. (2009) proposed making use of color, texture, and edge features to analyze Crohn's disease lesions from CE images. Szczypinski et al. (2009) suggested a novel model of deformable rings to interpret CE video, which allows a quick review of the whole video. We have investigated bleeding, ulcer, and tumor region detection for CE images in our previous works (Li and Meng 2009a, 2009b, 2009c, 2009d), which mainly concentrate on features that are suitable to describe bleeding, ulcers, and tumors in CE images.

Because polyps are common in the GI tract, we focus on polyp CE image recognition in this chapter. To achieve this goal, we advance a new scheme that exploits color and shape features. The proposed new feature integrates a chromaticity histogram with a Zernike moment shape descriptor to differentiate between a normal CE image and a polyp image. Experimental results from our present data validate this new scheme's ability to achieve performance for polyp CE image detection when using a multilayer perceptron neural network as the classifier.

The remainder of this chapter is organized as follows. The color and shape features for polyp detection are discussed in detail in the following section. In Section 11.3, experimental results are presented and discussed. Conclusions are drawn at the end of this chapter.

11.2 Color and Shape Feature Analysis

A polyp is an abnormal growth of tissue protruding from the mucous membrane. Polyps are commonly found in the intestine, stomach, and so on. Intestinal polyps grow out of the lining of the small and large bowels, and they come in a variety of shapes—round, droplets, and so on. They also exhibit different colors. Figure 11.3 shows a few normal CE images, and Figure 11.4 shows some CE images with different polyps that vary in color, size, and shape (refer to color originals in Li and Meng 2009e). From these illustrations, it can be noticed that polyps show some differences in color compared to normal CE images. Moreover, polyps demonstrate some specific shape features. These interesting properties motivated us to investigate the combination of color and shape features to discriminate normal CE images from polyp CE images. We proposed a novel color feature based on a histogram of the chromaticity channel in hue, saturation, intensity (HSI) color space and then integrated it with a traditional but powerful shape feature, that is, Zernike moments, for CE images.

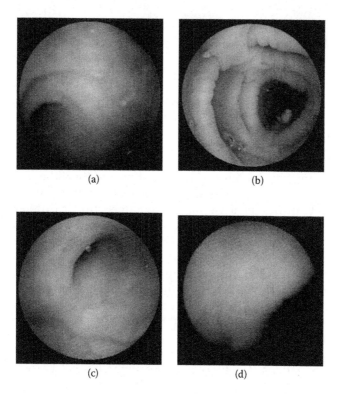

(a)   (b)

(c)   (d)

FIGURE 11.3
Representative normal intestinal CE images.

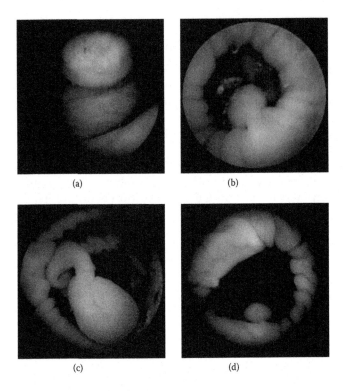

(a)   (b)

(c)   (d)

FIGURE 11.4
Representative intestinal CE images with polyps.

11.2.1 Color Feature

CE images usually suffer from illumination variation due to the specific imaging circumstances such as camera motion and the rather limited range of illumination in the digestive tract. Moreover, different images from different patients in the database may be obtained under different imaging conditions with a great deal of variation in lighting and so on. Therefore, it may be beneficial to consider illumination variations and geometric deformation effects on the colors of CE images because colors are different when objects are viewed under different angles and different lighting conditions.

There are many techniques to solve the problem of identifying the presence of an object under varying imaging conditions (Gevers and Stokman 2004; Gevers, Voortman, and Aldershoft 2005). One kind of algorithm estimates transformations and compensates for such effects. An alternative method is to obtain invariant features, namely, deriving features that are robust to different transformations. Benefits of the latter method is that it avoids expensive parameter estimations such as camera and light source calibration and so on. In this chapter, we adopt the latter strategy due to this advantage. Specifically, we take into account color invariance because CE images are color images.

Gevers, Weijer, and Stokman (2005) demonstrated that the following equations hold for hue and saturation in HSI color space:

$$h = \arctan \frac{\sqrt{3}(k_G - k_B)}{(k_R - k_G) + (k_R - k_B)} \tag{11.1}$$

$$s = 1 - \frac{\min\{k_R, k_G, k_B\}}{(k_R + k_G + k_B)} \tag{11.2}$$

where $k_c = \int_\lambda f_c(\lambda) r_b(\lambda) d\lambda \quad for \quad c = R, G, B$

is the constructed variable that depends only on sensors and surface, $f_c(\lambda)$ is the channel sensor response function, and $r(\lambda)$ is the surface reflectance function. They further verified that hue (H) and saturation (S) in HSI color space are invariant to viewing orientation, illumination direction, and illumination intensity. The HSI color space is devised to be used intuitively in manipulating color and to approximate the manner in which humans perceive and interpret color. In the human vision system, perception of an image is decomposed into luminance and chroma components, and HSI color space separates an image into intensity and chromaticity just as in human vision perception. Three properties of color, that is, hue, saturation, and intensity, are defined in order to differentiate the color components. HSI color space will facilitate our investigation of features for polyp image detection because we can study color features in chromaticity channels while investigating shape features in intensity channels. Moreover, the invariant property of HSI color space compared to other color models is attractive for employment as the basis for the color feature analysis.

Distribution of colors in an image provides useful cues for object recognition. Physicians also use color as a primary clue to conduct diagnosis for CE images (Li and Meng 2007). To represent color features, we resort to a two-dimensional (2D) histogram of HS channels in HSI color space because a histogram is robust to image scale changes, translation and rotation about the viewing axis, and partial occlusion (Swain and Ballard 1991). Because HS only represents the chromaticity information for a color image, we call this 2D histogram a *chromaticity histogram*. However, direct usage of a chromaticity histogram may be computationally intensive if full use of the histogram is made; for example, a quantization scheme of 180 bins in H and 50 bins in S. To overcome this shortcoming, we apply a discrete cosine transform (DCT) to compress the chromaticity histogram. Because the lower frequencies can represent most of the energy of an image, we truncate the higher frequency coefficients to reduce the number of features to characterize color features. Through experiments, we found that using only twenty-eight coefficients, which lie in the upper left corner of the DCT coefficients matrix, worked well for our purpose, as shown in Figure 11.5. Using these twenty-eight coefficients of the chromaticity histogram, we obtained color features for CE images that were invariant to illumination change. Furthermore, the color features obtained were also robust to scale, translation, and rotations.

The quantization scheme may affect the performance of such a color representation. However, because the emphasis of this chapter is not to find an optimal quantization scheme for detecting polyp CE images, this remains as one point for our future work. At present, we experimentally use the quantization scheme of forty bins in H and twenty bins in S, producing satisfactory detection results.

11.2.2 Shape Feature

As illustrated in Figure 11.4, the polyps in CE images also show different characteristics of shape. Shape is another primary low-level image feature exploited by clinicians. There are two main types of shape representation methods; namely, contour-based methods and region-based methods (Zhang

1	2	6	7	15	16	28					
3	5	8	14	17	27						
4	9	13	18	26							
10	12	19	25								
11	20	24									
21	23										
22											

FIGURE 11.5
Coefficients chosen from DCT.

and Lu 2003). Because it is very challenging to obtain an accurate and clear contour of polyps in CE images due to the complex background, in this chapter we turn to the region-based shape descriptor.

Taking into account the specific imaging circumstances required for CE images mentioned previously, we need a shape feature that is invariant to rotation, scale, and translation. Fortunately, Zernike moments satisfy these properties. A basis function for the Zernike moment is defined by (Teague 1980):

$$V_{nm}(x, y) = V_{nm}(\rho \cos \theta, \rho \sin \theta) = R_{nm}(\rho) \exp(jm\theta) \tag{11.3}$$

where

$$R_{nm}(\rho) = \sum_{s=0}^{n-\frac{|m|}{2}} (-1)^s \frac{(n-s)!}{s!(\frac{n+|m|}{2} - s)!(\frac{n-|m|}{2} - s)} \rho^{n-2s} \tag{11.4}$$

where ρ is the radius from (x,y) to the shape centroid, θ is the angle between ρ and the x-axis. n,m are integers that satisfy the condition $n-|m| = even$, $|m| \le n$. A Zernike moment can be then defined as:

$$A_{nm}(\rho) = \frac{n+1}{\pi} \sum_x \sum_y f(x, y) V_{nm}^*(x, y) \quad x^2 + y^2 \le 1 \tag{11.5}$$

where * represents complex conjugate. A_{nm} is a complex number and the magnitude of A_{nm} is rotation invariant. The unit disk can be centered on the center mass of an image, which enables both scale and translation invariance of the moments (Ye and Peng 2002). Zernike moment invariance can be constructed in an arbitrary order. In our implementation, we obtained different orders of Zernike moments, that is, tenth-order and fifth-order, directly on the I channel in HSI color space, thus obtaining the shape feature for each CE image.

11.3 Experimental Results

Gastroenterologists selected a data set composed of 300 representative polyp (150) and normal (150) CE images from two patients' video data. The original images were manually labeled to provide the ground truth. A CE image containing any polyp region is labeled as a positive sample; otherwise, it is labeled as a negative sample. In order to prevent overfitting of the classification results, we exploited threefold cross-validation for all of our classification experiments. To demonstrate the performance of the proposed features, we compare the proposed scheme with color wavelet covariance (CWC) features used in Karkanis et al. (2003) to detect tumors in traditional endoscopic images. CWC features are new techniques to represent color features that are built upon the covariance of second-order textural measures in the wavelet domain of color channels of images.

We also exploited a multilayer perceptron (MLP) neural network and support vector machines (SVM) to find a better classifier for our work. A three-layer MLP with two nonlinear outputs was employed in the experiments. The number of input nodes of the MLP depends on the number of input features, and the number of epochs for training the MLP was set to 5,000. Because the number of hidden nodes has a strong impact on the final classification results, several variations on the number of hidden layer neurons, ranging from five to fifty, with five-node increments, were carried out. For SVM implementation, we referred to the work of Chang and Lin (2001). The radial basis function was found to be the kernel function that yielded the best classification performance in our experiments. The highest classification accuracy of an SVM from seven different sets of the key parameters in an SVM, that is, the penalty parameter and the kernel parameter, was chosen as the classification performance.

Classification of CE images using MLP or SVM is measured by accuracy, specificity, and sensitivity, which are widely employed to evaluate the performance of classification. Some definitions are as follows:

$$\text{Accuracy} = \frac{\textit{Number of Correct Predictions}}{\textit{Number of Positives} + \textit{Number of Negatives}} \tag{11.6}$$

$$\text{Specificity} = \frac{\textit{Number of Correct Negative Predictions}}{\textit{Number of Negatives}} \tag{11.7}$$

$$\text{Sensitivity} = \frac{\textit{Number of Correct Positive Predictions}}{\textit{Number of Positives}} \tag{11.8}$$

We performed experiments using different orders of Zernike moments, that is, fifth- and tenth-order, and the number of these moments corresponds to twelve and thirty-six, respectively, so the number of whole features is forty and sixty-four, respectively. The average recognition results of the proposed features using MLP and SVM with fifth-order and tenth-order Zernike moments are shown in Tables 11.1 and 11.2, respectively. The classification results of CWC features are demonstrated in Table 11.3.

From these three tables, it can be noticed that the proposed color and shape feature shows much better performance for polyp recognition from CE images compared to the CWC method when choosing MLP or SVM as the classifier. This is expected because the proposed color and shape features hybrid color invariance with shape invariance. Moreover, the proposed feature with fifth-order Zernike moments and a chromaticity histogram shows an encouraging recognition accuracy of 94.20% when using MLP as the classifier, together with a promising specificity (93.33%) and sensitivity (95.07%). An unexpected result is that the performance of an SVM is inferior to that of an MLP for the proposed color and shape features. Such a result may be due to the fact that the parameters used in SVM experiments are not optimized.

TABLE 11.1

Classification Results of the Proposed Algorithm with Fifth-Order Zernike Moment and the Chromaticity Histogram (%)

	MLP	SVM
Accuracy	94.20	85.33
Specificity	93.33	80.67
Sensitivity	95.07	90.00

TABLE 11.2

Classification Results of the Proposed Algorithm with Tenth-Order Zernike Moment and the Chromaticity Histogram (%)

	MLP	SVM
Accuracy	93.47	89.00
Specificity	93.53	81.34
Sensitivity	93.42	96.67

TABLE 11.3

Classification Results of CWC Method (%)

	MLP	SVM
Accuracy	58.67	70.50
Specificity	63.67	63.67
Sensitivity	53.67	76.33

11.4 Conclusions

In this chapter we have presented a new scheme that uses color and shape features to detect intestinal polyps from CE images. The novel features combine the advantages of a chromaticity histogram and Zernike moments in HSI color space, leading to color invariance and shape invariance. Thus, the proposed feature shows greater discriminative ability for polyp detection in CE images compared to a CWC method. Experiments with our present CE images show that this method is promising for detection of polyp images. Future work will be directed to collecting more patients' data in order to test the robustness of the proposed scheme. Moreover, a suitable quantization approach for HS histograms is worth further investigation to achieve better performance.

Acknowledgment

This work was supported by SHIAE project #8115021 of the Shun Hing Institute of Advanced Engineering of The Chinese University of Hong Kong, awarded to Max Meng.

References

Adeler, D.G., and Gostout, C.J. 2003. Wireless capsule endoscopy. *Hospital Physician*, 39(5): 14–22.

Bashar, M.K., Mori, K., Suenaga, Y., Kitasaka, T., and Mekada, Y. 2008. Detecting informative frames from wireless capsule endoscopic video using color and texture features. Paper read at the 11th Medical Image Computing and Computer-Assisted Intervention, New York, September 6–10, 2002.

Bejakovic, S., Kumar, R., Dassopoulos, T., Mullin, G., and Hager, G. 2009. Analysis of Crohn's disease lesions in capsule endoscopy images. Paper read at the IEEE International Conference on Robotics and Automation, Kobe, Japan, May 12–17, 2009.

Berens, J., Mackiewicz, M., and Bell, D. 2005. Stomach, intestine and colon tissue discriminators for wireless capsule endoscopy images. *Proceedings of SPIE on Medical Imaging*, 5747: 283–290.

Chang, C.-C. and Lin, C.-J. 2001. LIBSVM: A library for support vector machines. Available at http://www.csie.ntu.edu.tw/cjlin/libsvm. Accessed August 18, 2010.

Coimbra, M.T. and Cunha, J.P.S. 2006. MPEG-7 visual descriptors—Contributions for automated feature extraction in capsule endoscopy. *IEEE Transactions on Circuits and Systems for Video Technology*, 16(5): 628–637.

Cunha, J.S., Coimbra, M., Campos, P., and Soares, J.M. 2008. Automated topographic segmentation and transit time estimation in endoscopic capsule exams. *IEEE Transactions on Medical Imaging*, 27(1): 19–27.

Gevers, T. and Stokman, H. 2004. Robust histogram construction from color invariants for object recognition. *IEEE Transactions on Pattern Analysis and Machine Intelligence*, 26(1): 113–118.

Gevers, T., Voortman, S., and Aldershoft, F. 2005. Color feature detection and classification by learning. *Proceedings of the IEEE International Conference on Image Processing*, 2: 714–717.

Gevers, T., Weijer, J.V.D., and Stokman, H. 2006. *Color Image Processing: Emerging Applications*. Boca Raton, FL: CRC Press.

Given Imaging Ltd. 2009. Corporate overview. Available at http://www.givenimaging.com. Accessed July 12, 2010.

Hospital Authority of Hong Kong. 2006. Highlights on cancer statistics 2003. *Hong Kong Cancer Registry*, 1–29.

Karkanis, S.A., Iakovidis, D.K., Maroulis, D.E., and Korras, D.A. 2003. Computer-aided tumor detection in endoscopic video using color wavelet features. *IEEE Transactions on Information Technology in Biomedicine*, 7(3): 141–152.

Li, B. and Meng, M.Q.-H. 2007. Analysis of wireless capsule endoscopy images using chromaticity moments. Paper read at the IEEE International Conference on Robotics and Biomimetics, Sanya,China, December 15–18, 2007.

Li, B. and Meng, M.Q.-H. 2009a. Computer aided detection of bleeding regions in capsule endoscopy images. *IEEE Transactions on Biomedical Engineering*, 56(4): 1032–1039.

Li, B. and Meng, M.Q.-H. 2009b. Computer-based detection of bleeding and ulcer in wireless capsule endoscopy images by chromaticity moments. *Computers in Biology and Medicine*, 39(2): 141–147.

Li, B. and Meng, M.Q.-H. 2009c. Small bowel tumor detection for wireless capsule endoscopy images using textural features and support vector machine. Paper read at the IEEE/RSJ International Conference on Intelligent Robots and Systems, St. Louis, MO. October 11–15, 2009.

Li, B. and Meng, M.Q.-H. 2009d. Texture analysis for ulcer detection in capsule endoscopy images. *Image and Vision Computing*, 27(9): 1336–1342.

Swain, M.S. and Ballard, D.H. 1991. Color indexing. *International Journal of Computer Vision*, 7(1): 11–32.

Szczypinski, P.M., Sriram, R.D., Sriram, P.V.J., and Reddy, D.N. 2009. A model of deformable rings for interpretation of wireless capsule endoscopic videos. *Medical Image Analysis*, 13(4): 312–324.

Teague, M.R. 1980. Image analysis via the general theory of moments. *Journal of the Optical Society of America*, 70(8): 920–930.

Ye, B. and Peng, J. 2002. Invariance analysis of improved Zernike moments. *Journal of Optics A: Pure and Applied Optics*, 4: 606–614.

Zabulis, X., Argyros, A.A., and Tsakiris, P.D. 2008. Lumen detection for capsule endoscopy. Paper read at the IEEE/RSJ International Conference on Intelligent Robots and Systems, Nice, France, September 22–26, 2008.

Zhang, D. and Lu, G. 2003. Evaluation of MPEG-7 shape descriptors against other shape descriptors. *Multimedia Systems*, 9: 15–30.

12

Classification of Hand Motion Using Surface EMG Signals

Xueyan Tang, Yunhui Liu, Congyi Lu, and Weilun Poon
Chinese University of Hong Kong
Hong Kong, China

CONTENTS

12.1 Introduction 220
12.2 System Configuration 222
    12.2.1 Multichannel sEMG Sensor Ring 222
    12.2.2 sEMG Signal Preprocessing 223
12.3 Classification of Hand Movements 223
    12.3.1 Automatic Relocation of sEMG Electrodes 223
    12.3.2 Feature Extraction from Multiple Channels 226
12.4 Identification of Movement Force and Speed 230
    12.4.1 STFT Method 231
    12.4.2 Features Based on STFT 231
    12.4.3 Experimental Results 232
12.5 Summary 233
References 237

Abstract

The human hand has multiple degrees of freedom (DOFs) to achieve high dexterity. Identifying the five-finger movements using surface electromyography (sEMG) is challenging. Moreover, the success rate of identifying the hand movements is sensitive to many aspects; for example, the sEMG electrode placements, variant movement forces, or movement speeds. In this chapter, a robust sEMG system for identifying the hand movements is developed. First, a multichannel sEMG sensor ring is designed, which is easy to wear on the human forearm even without knowledge of the exact location of the corresponding muscles. However, a new problem of using the multichannel sensor ring is followed and unsolved in the current research. The problem is how to relocate the sEMG electrodes with the same sequence as the last trial. This chapter introduces the concordance correlation coefficient to investigate the relationships of all channels, and autorelocation of the sEMG electrodes is possible. The process of the successful hand motion classification can be divided into collecting original sEMG signals, calculating features basd on original signals, and classifying motions based on features. If the calculated features are robust to some variances in the movement forces and speed, the motion classification results also have robustness. Thus, to make classification of the hand movements robust to some variances in the movement forces and speed, a new ratio measure of the multiple channels is defined as the feature, which is based on the results of the temporal square integral values of each channel signal. Finally, real-time classification of the hand movements is possible, using the statistical classifier based on Mahalanobis distance. In addition to classification of the hand movement types, knowing the movement force and the movement speed are important. In this chapter, the levels of the movement forces are described using spectral moments based on the short-time Fourier transform (STFT) results. The levels of the movement speeds, which are seldom studied in the current research, are also identified. Based on the results of STFT, the spectral flatness feature is firstly introduced for the sEMG signal to describe the different speeds of the hand movements.

12.1 Introduction

The surface electromyography (sEMG) signal is generated by the electrical activity of muscle fibers during a contraction and is noninvasively recorded by electrodes attached to the skin (Merletti and Parker 2004). Its application to control of artificial limbs or duplication of human movements using a remote mechanism is challenging. In the rehabilitation field, sEMG signals have been applied to control prosthetic legs (Jin et al. 2000) and prosthetic arms (Doringer and Hogan 1995; Ito et al. 1992; Saridis and Gootee 1982). Identification of human hand movements is relatively difficult, because the hand possesses more degrees of freedom (DOFs) than the legs and arms. Due to identification difficulties, the dexterity of some sEMG prosthetic hands in the market is far less than that of the human hand, achieving only a limited number of movements; that is, hand open and hand close. Many researchers focus on dexterity improvement of sEMG prosthetic hands (Farry, Walker, and Barabiuk 1996; Fukuda, Tsuji, and Kaneko 1997; Hudgins and Parker 1993; Kuribayashi, Okimura, and Taniguchi 1993), and discrimination of two to six patterns can be achieved. In this chapter the aim is to further increase the number of identified hand movements, and classification of seven hand movements is achieved.

The placement of sEMG electrodes is a critical issue for successful identification of hand movements. Most of the current research is based on the idea that the distribution of the corresponding muscles for hand movements is known. The classification success rates are dominantly determined by the placement of the sEMG electrodes. However, in many applications, for example, commercial products, most users lack knowledge of the muscle distribution, and thus there is a risk of classification failure due to misalignment of the sEMG electrodes. To solve this problem, in recent research, multichannel sensor rings have been designed (Y.-C. Du et al. 2010; Saponas et al. 2008). Since multichannel sensor rings envelop the whole or half circumference of the forearm, sensor rings can capture all signals from the extensor or flexor muscles of the forearm. In this chapter, the sEMG sensor is designed as a half wristband, and the user can easily wear the sensor ring on the wrist as if wearing a watch.

The features extracted from the raw sEMG signals are another critical issue for successful identification. For research in which sEMG electrodes are pasted exactly above the corresponding muscles, methods include the temporal features (Zecca et al. 2002) for noncomplex and low-speed movements and temporal–spectral features; for example, short-time Fourier transform (STFT) and short-time Thompson transform (STTT), which can provide more transient information for complex and high-speed movements (S. J. Du and Vuskovic 2004; Farry, Walker, and Barabiuk 1996; Hannaford and Lehman 1986). For a multichannel sensor ring, the methods of feature extraction include the ratios of the temporal and spectral features among the different channels (Saponas et al. 2008) and six temporal features directly used for the motion classifier (Y.-C. Du et al. 2010). This chapter further improves the feature extraction method for the multichannel sensor ring by increasing classification robustness to some variances of the movement forces and speed. A new ratio measure of the multiple channels is defined as the feature, which is based on the results of the temporal square integral values of each channel signal.

For a multichannel sensor ring, a new problem has arisen, which is how to recognize the same channel sequence as the last trial after the user arbitrarily wears the sensor ring. Currently, no studies have been conducted to solve this problem. This chapter is inspired by research using the cross-correlation coefficient to investigate the cross-talk among the different channels (Mogk and Keir 2003). The concordance correlation coefficient is introduced to study the relationship between multiple channels and check the feasibility of channel sequence recognition.

The speed of hand movements is also critical for movement description. Currently, there are few studies concentrated on this topic. In this chapter, the levels of the movement speeds are identified. Based on the results of STFT, the spectral flatness feature is firstly introduced for the sEMG signal to describe the different speeds of hand movements.

12.2 System Configuration

The sEMG-based sensing system is configured as shown in Figure 12.1. The potential user wears a small, lightweight sEMG sensor ring on the wrist. The sEMG sensor ring has six-channel electrodes, integrated with analog circuits, an A/D converter, and a wireless module. The sEMG signals, accumulated on the skin covering the wrist, are amplified, filtered, and converted digitally and then transferred to a computer via the wireless module. The computer processes the hand movements for identification.

12.2.1 Multichannel sEMG Sensor Ring

The sensor ring has six pairs of sEMG sensor electrodes, and each pair is for one channel, as shown in Figure 12.2. The six-channel sensor ring covers the overall posterior side of the forearm; that is, it includes all of the extensor muscles for the finger movements. Each sEMG electrode has a diameter of $\phi 10$ mm, and one channel is composed of two electrodes. Each pair of channels is placed 15 mm apart. Before wearing the sEMG electrodes, the forearm should be washed to ensure good conductivity between the skin surface and the electrodes.

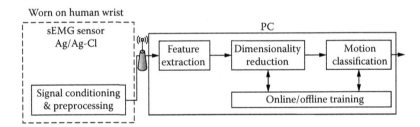

FIGURE 12.1
Configuration of the sEMG-based sensing system.

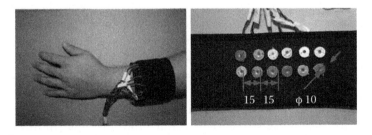

FIGURE 12.2
Multichannel sEMG sensor ring: (a) sensor ring on the forearm and (b) six-channel sEMG electrodes.

12.2.2 sEMG Signal Preprocessing

The amplitudes of the raw sEMG signals are miniature, at the scale from several microvolts to millivolts. Moreover, several types of noise are mixed with the useful sEMG signals; that is, low-frequency cross-talk, 50-Hz AC frequency, and high-frequency noises. Therefore, the differential amplifier and filters are designed to strengthen and clarify the useful signals. The sEMG signal is amplified to the scale of *V* by the differential amplifier. The high-pass (>20 Hz), notch (50 Hz), and low-pass (<500 Hz) filters eliminate the three types of noise mentioned above. The amplifier and filters are miniature sized and are integrated with the sEMG sensor ring to be worn on the human forearm. The advantage of integration of the sEMG sensor and the analog circuits is that there is no extra noise introduced during long-distance wire transfer.

After amplification and filtration, the analog voltages of the sEMG signal are converted digitally by a 10-bit A/D converter. The digital signals are transferred to the computer via wireless communication using standard radio frequency (RF) technology.

12.3 Classification of Hand Movements

This section addresses the classification of hand movements using the six-channel sensor ring. We defined seven types of hand movements, as shown in Figure 12.3.

12.3.1 Automatic Relocation of sEMG Electrodes

The advantages of using the multichannel sensor ring include convenience for the user and the low possibility of classification failure due to misalignment

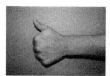 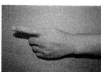 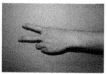 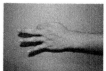

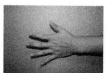 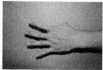 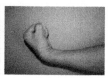

FIGURE 12.3
Seven classes of hand movements: (a) thumb, (b) index, (c) V sign, (d) OK gesture, (e) all fingers extended, (f) four fingers extended, and (g) grasp.

of the sEMG electrodes. However, especially for the whole sensor ring, some channels are redundant. The multichannel sensor ring always has redundant channels, and it is important to determine which channels are meaningful. To ensure that the extracted features are uniform, especially when the user arbitrarily wears the sensor ring, it is important to determine where the first-channel electrodes among the selected meaningful channels are located for every trial.

For multichannel sEMG sensors, the definition of the cross-correlation coefficient, also called the *Pearson's product-moment coefficient*, has been used to investigate cross-talk among the channels (Mogk and Keir 2003). However, the cross-correlation only measures the extent of the linear relationship between two variables. When two variables have a nonlinear relationship, the value of the cross-correlation coefficient is zero. Thus, the cross-correlation coefficient has the risk during evaluating the relationship of two variables. Here, the concordance coefficient is introduced in this chapter to evaluate the agreement of each two-channel sEMG signal. The concordance correlation coefficient, defined by Lin (1989), measures the agreement between two variables and has been widely used in studies on data reproducibility (Lin 1989) and image comparison analysis (Lange et al. 1999). In this chapter, we use the concordance coefficient to investigate the agreement between sEMG signals for each two-channel signal.

The concordance correlation coefficient of the N-length variables of x and y is defined as

$$\rho = \frac{2\sigma_{xy}}{\sigma_x^2 + \sigma_y^2 + \left(\mu_x - \mu_y\right)^2} \tag{12.1}$$

μ_x and μ_y are the mean of the two variables, and μ_y has the same formula as μ_x:

$$\mu_x = \frac{1}{N}\sum_{i=1}^{N} x_i \tag{12.2}$$

σ_x and σ_y are the variances of the two variables, and σ_y has the same formula as σ_x:

$$\sigma_x^2 = \frac{1}{N}\sum_{i=1}^{N}\left(x_i - \mu_x\right)^2 \tag{12.3}$$

σ_{xy} is the covariance of x and y:

$$\sigma_{xy} = \frac{1}{N} \sum_{i=1}^{N} (x_i - \mu_x)(y_i - \mu_y)$$

$$(12.4)$$

For the generalized formulation, it is assumed that there are a total of M pairs of sEMG electrodes in the multichannel sensor ring. The M-channel sEMG signals are represented by an $N \times M$ matrix of $X = \begin{bmatrix} X_1, & ..., & X_i, & ..., & X_M \end{bmatrix}$. Each column X_i of an N-length vector is the time-series sEMG signal of channel i. The concordance correlation coefficient of any two channels channel i and channel j is defined as

$$R_{X_i X_i} = \rho_{X_i X_j}, \qquad i = 1,...M-1, \qquad j = i+1,...M$$

$$(12.5)$$

For each hand movement, we can obtain a $1 \times \sum_{i=1}^{M-1} (M-i)$ vector R of the concordance correlation coefficients as

$$R = \begin{bmatrix} R_1, & ..., & R_i, & ..., & R_{M-1} \end{bmatrix}$$

$$(12.6)$$

where

$$R_1 = \begin{bmatrix} R_{x_1 x_2}, & R_{x_1 x_3}, & ..., & R_{x_1 x_M} \end{bmatrix},$$

$$R_i = \begin{bmatrix} R_{x_i x_{i+1}}, & R_{x_i x_{i+2}}, & ..., & R_{x_i x_M} \end{bmatrix},$$

$$R_{M-1} = \begin{bmatrix} R_{x_{M-1} x_M} \end{bmatrix}.$$

In our case, there are a total of six channels for the sEMG electrodes. Before the derivation of the concordance correlation coefficients, we explain why six channels for the sEMG electrodes are chosen. It is well known that most muscles responsible for hand movements are clustered on the posterior side of the forearm. The extensor digitorum is responsible for the movements of the index, middle, ring, and little fingers; the extensor pollicis longus and brevis control the thumb; the extensor indicis controls the index finger; and the extensor digiti minimi controls the little finger (Miller 2008). The muscles on the posterior of the forearm must be included in the area enveloped by the sensor ring. Six channels are enough to cover the circumstance of the posterior side. The six-channel sEMG signals of each hand movement are represented by an $N \times 6$ matrix of $X = \begin{bmatrix} X_1, & X_2, & X_3, & X_4, & X_5, & X_6 \end{bmatrix}$. For each hand movement, we can obtain a 1×15 vector R of the concordance correlation coefficients as

$$R = \begin{bmatrix} R_1, & R_2, & R_3, & R_4, & R_5 \end{bmatrix}$$

$$(12.7)$$

where

$$R_1 = \begin{bmatrix} R_{X_1 X_2}, & R_{X_1 X_3}, & R_{X_1 X_4}, & R_{X_1 X_5}, & R_{X_1 X_6} \end{bmatrix},$$

$$R_2 = \begin{bmatrix} R_{X_2 X_3}, & R_{X_2 X_4}, & R_{X_2 X_5}, & R_{X_2 X_6} \end{bmatrix},$$

$$R_3 = \begin{bmatrix} R_{X_3 X_4}, & R_{X_3 X_5}, & R_{X_3 X_6} \end{bmatrix},$$

$$R_4 = \begin{bmatrix} R_{X_4 X_5}, & R_{X_4 X_6} \end{bmatrix},$$

$$R_5 = \begin{bmatrix} R_{X_5 X_6} \end{bmatrix}.$$

The concordance correlation coefficients of three kinds of gestures were investigated, including thumb (Figure 12.3a), index (Figure 12.3b), and the OK configuration (Figure 12.3d). For each kind of gesture, thirty trials were sampled. In the first step, the same onset point of six-channel signals for each movement was found using the Bonato method (Staude et al. 2001). In the second step, 500-ms signals were selected. Finally, the concordance correlation coefficients were computed. In Figure 12.4, the results show that for each kind of hand movement, the concordance correlation coefficients of thirty trials have similar and stable distributions, which fall in the narrow bands with the maximum and minimum values as the boundaries.

Here we apply the results in Figure 12.4 to the generalized case in which the sEMG sensor ring has M channels ($M > 6$) for the electrodes. Before each use, the user only needs to perform these three gestures several times as calibration. For each hand movement, a

$$1 \times \sum_{i=1}^{M-1} (M - i)$$

vector can be obtained. From this vector, six continuous channels, of which concordance correlation coefficients are all located within the boundaries shown in Figure 12.4, can be selected. If, for each calibration, the concordance correlation coefficients of the same six continuous channels fall within the boundaries, it can be concluded that the channel at the beginning of these six channels is the first channel.

12.3.2 Feature Extraction from Multiple Channels

The spectral method of square integral feature defined in Equation (12.8) has been widely used as the calculated feature for motion classification.

$$E_i = \sum_{i=1}^{N} X_i^2(t) \tag{12.8}$$

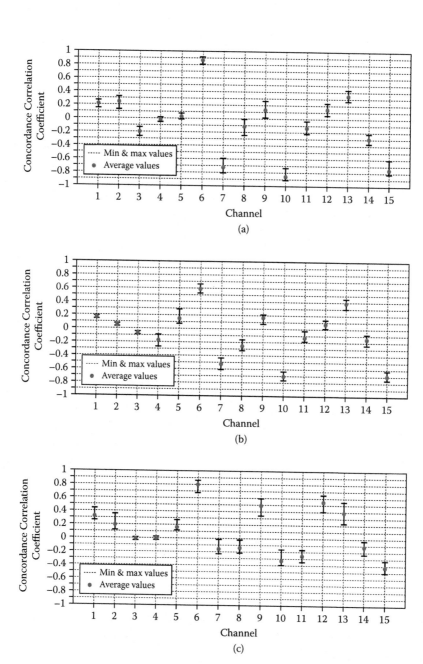

FIGURE 12.4

Concordance correlation coefficients for three gestures: (a) thumb, (b) index, and (c) OK gesture.

where i represents the ith channel, $X_i(t)$ is the time-series sEMG signal of the ith channel, and N is the data number of the time-series sEGM signal from one channel.

However, there is a limitation when using the spectral integral of the temporal sEMG signals as the feature. For the same type of the movement, the square integral values of the temporal signal vary with the movement force and movement speed. The changes in the feature's values can affect the classification results. The ideal case is that classification of the types of hand movements is not affected by some variances such as movement forces and speed. To make the classification result robust to these variances, the ratios of the square integral values of the multiple channels are defined as the feature. The ratio of the ith channel to first-channel signals is defined as

$$RE_{i1} = \frac{E_i}{E_1}, \qquad i = 2, ..., M \qquad (12.9)$$

All of the ratios of single-channel to first-channel signals are defined as

$$RE_1 = \begin{bmatrix} RE_{21}, & ..., & RE_{M1} \end{bmatrix} \qquad (12.10)$$

The ratio of the ith channel to the jth channel signal is represented as

$$RE_{ij}^* = \frac{E_i}{E_j}, \qquad i = 2, ..., M-1, \qquad j = i+1, ..., M \qquad (12.11)$$

Normalize RE_{ij}^* with reference to first-channel signal:

$$RE_{ij} = \frac{E_i/E_j}{E_j/E_1} = \frac{E_i \times E_1}{E_j^2} \qquad (12.12)$$

All of the ratios of the ith channel to jth channel signals with reference to the first-channel signal are represented as

$$RE_i = \begin{bmatrix} RE_{(i+1)i}, & ..., & RE_{Mi} \end{bmatrix}, \qquad i = 2, ..., M-1 \qquad (12.13)$$

Combining Equations (12.10) and (12.13), we can obtain the newly defined feature of channel ratio, a vector formulated as

$$RE = \begin{bmatrix} RE_1, & ..., & RE_i, & ..., & RE_{M-1} \end{bmatrix} \tag{12.14}$$

where M is the channel number. RE_1 is a $1 \times (M-1)$ vector, and RE_i is a $1 \times (M-i)$ vector. So RE is a row vector with $\sum_{i=1}^{M-1}(M-i)$ columns.

In our case, there is a total of six channels, and thus RE is a 1×15 vector of:

$$RE = \begin{bmatrix} RE_{21}, & ..., & RE_{61}, & RE_{32}, & ..., & RE_{62}, & RE_{43}, & ..., & RE_{63}, & RE_{54}, & RE_{64}, & RE_{65} \end{bmatrix}.$$

Using the above definition and the six-channel sensor ring shown in Figure 12.2, the seven types of hand movements determined as shown in Figure 12.3 can be distinguished. For each type of hand movement, thirty trials were sampled. First, the Bonato method was used to find the onset points, and 500-ms signals from the onset points were selected, as shown in Figure 12.5. Then, the feature measures defined in Equation (12.14) were calculated, and the results are shown in Figure 12.6.

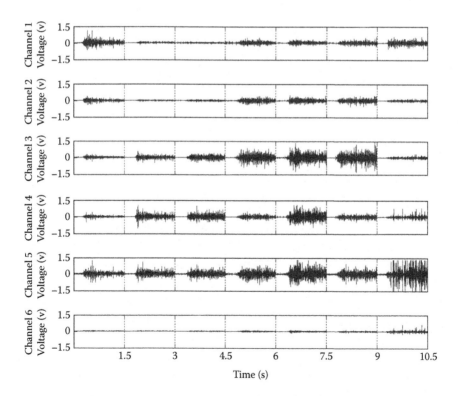

FIGURE 12.5
Six-channel raw sEMG signals for seven types of hand movements.

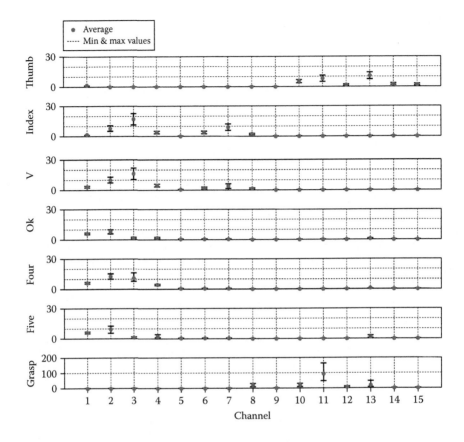

FIGURE 12.6
Channel ratio features of seven types of hand movements.

The features shown in Figure 12.6 are selected as the trained data sets and then clustered by the Mahalanobis distance theory. Another ten trials for each type of hand movement were sampled as the test data. The success rate was around 90%. The results show that the proposed feature measure is effective. In future work, we will improve the proposed feature measure to check the feasibility of applying the same trained data set to different users.

12.4 Identification of Movement Force and Speed

Force and speed are also important parameters for movement description. Currently, there is no effective method for identifying movement speed. Movement speed is related to the transient portion of the sEMG signals. Here, the STFT results are used to obtain the distribution of the sEMG signal in both time and frequency domains. Then, the spectral flatness feature is introduced and used to describe the speed. The description of the movement speed is also based on STFT results, and then the spectral moment is calculated as the feature.

12.4.1 STFT Method

The basic idea of STFT is to divide a signal into several segments in the time domain and apply discrete Fourier transform (DFT) to each time segment.

Given a finite-length time sequence $x(i), i \in [0, \quad ..., \quad L-1]$, the DFT of the time sequence $x(i)$ is

$$X[m] = X[mF] = \sum_{i=0}^{L-1} x[i] e^{(-j2\pi(mF)(iT_s))} \tag{12.15}$$

where T_s is the sampling frequency, and $F = 1/LT_s$ is the frequency sampling step size. STFT for each segmented window is the sum of these DFTs with respect to T_s and F,

$$P[k, \quad m] = P[kT_s, \quad mF] = \sum_{i=0}^{L-1} x[i] W[i-t] e^{(-j2\pi mi/L)} \tag{12.16}$$

where $W[i]$ is the window function. The sampling step size in the time domain is $T = kT_s$.

A critical issue for STFT is tradeoff between time and frequency resolution. This means that a spectrum computed from a relatively long time window will resolve detailed frequency features but change little if the center time of the window is shifted by a small amount. Conversely, a narrow window will have a high time resolution but show few details in the computed spectrum. Thus, the acceptable resolutions of time and frequency are lower bounded. Balance can be found from the time-bandwidth uncertainty principle or Heisenberg inequality,

$$\Delta t \times \Delta f \geq \frac{1}{4\pi} \tag{12.17}$$

12.4.2 Features Based on STFT

Based on the results of STFT, the nth spectral moment of the frequency distribution at time t is defined as

$$M_n(t) = \sum_{f=l_b}^{u_b} \left(f^n \hat{P}(t,f) \right)$$

(12.18)

where n is the order of the spectral moment, l_b and u_b are the lower and upper boundaries of the frequency, and $p(t,f)$ is the calculated spectrum from STFT.

Based on the results of STFT, the spectral flatness feature is introduced to describe the characteristics of the sEMG signal. Spectral flatness has been widely used in the field of audio for description of the spectral power distribution of the sound. Here we introduce this definition to the sEMG signal. The spectral flatness is defined as

$$SF(t) = \frac{\left[\prod_{f=l_b}^{u_b} \hat{P}^2(t,f) \right]^{\frac{1}{u_b - l_b + 1}}}{\frac{1}{u_b - l_b + 1} \sum_{f=l_b}^{u_b} \hat{P}^2(t,f)}$$

(12.19)

where l_b and u_b are the lower and upper boundaries of the frequency. $\hat{P}(t,f)$ is the calculated spectrum from STFT in Equation (12.16).

A high spectral flatness indicates that the spectrum has a similar amount of power in all spectral bands. A low spectral flatness indicates that the spectral power is concentrated within a relatively small number of bands.

12.4.3 Experimental Results

To test the levels of the forces and speeds, the movement is designed as ball grasping, shown in Figure 12.7. We chose the sEMG signal from a middle channel, where the signals have large amplitude. First, the raw sEMG signals were processed by STFT, and the results are shown in Figures 12.8 and 12.9. According to the Heisenberg inequality in Equation (12.17), the segmented window number in the time domain was chosen as fifty, with a window overlap of 30%, and 100 points were selected over the frequency range from 0 to 500 Hz.

Based on the STFT results, the spectral moment features were calculated, as shown in Figure 12.10. It can be seen that the spectral moment features of the higher force have larger amplitudes than the lower force. Thus, the force levels can be distinguished. Based on the STFT results, the spectral flatness features were calculated, as shown in Figure 12.11. The significant differences of the spectrum distribution at the different time points can be seen. The spectral flatness feature showed that the flatness changes at low speed were more significant than those at high speed. Thus, the speed classification can be differentiated based on the spectral flatness features.

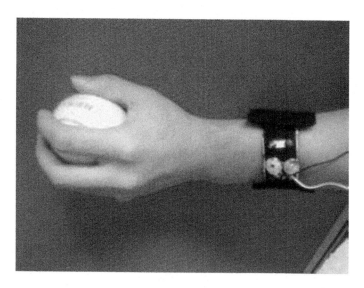

FIGURE 12.7
Ball grasping.

12.5 Summary

In this chapter, a robust sEMG sensor system was designed for identification of human hand movements. The sEMG sensor was designed as a multichannel ring. This chapter addresses the advantages of the multichannel sensor ring and also states the necessity of relocating the electrodes for each trial. Autorelocation of the electrodes is proposed using the concordance correlation coefficients for each two channels. The results show that the proposed method is effective. For classification of the movement types, to make the classification result robust to some variances such as the movement forces and speeds, a new feature measure based on multiple channels was proposed and applied to distinguish seven types of hand movements. The classification success rate was as high as 90% using the proposed feature measure of multiple channels and statistical Mahalanobis distance classifier. In future work, we will further improve the method of feature extraction and investigate the feasibility of using the same features for different users. Finally, in this chapter, identification of different movement speeds was achieved by introducing the spectral flatness feature to describe the spectral power distribution of sEMG signals. Different movement forces were also identified by the spectral moment feature based on the STFT results.

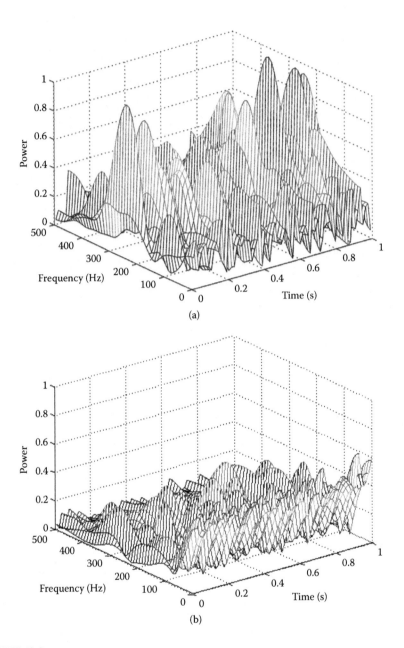

FIGURE 12.8
STFT results at different forces: (a) high force and (b) low force.

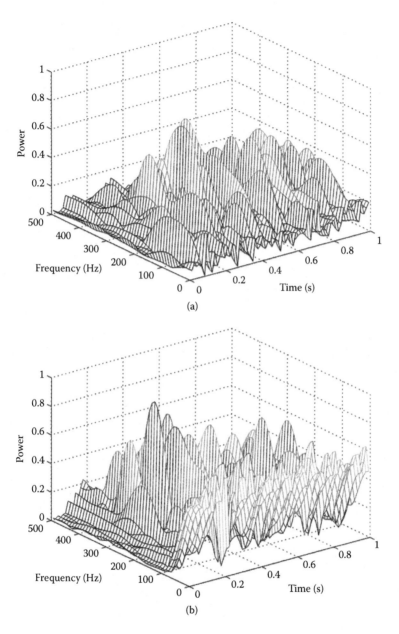

FIGURE 12.9
STFT results at different speeds: (a) low speed and (b) high speed.

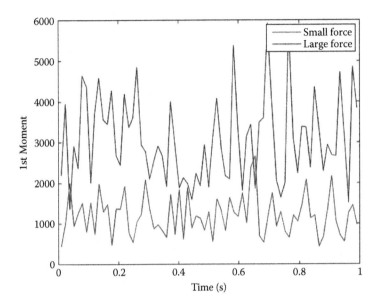

FIGURE 12.10
Spectral moment features based on STFT at different forces.

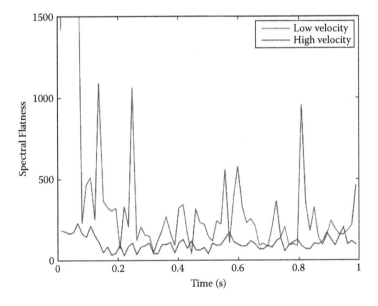

FIGURE 12.11
Spectral flatness features based on STFT at different speeds.

References

Doringer, J.A. and Hogan, N. 1995. Performance of above elbow body-powered prostheses in visually guided unconstrained motion tasks. *IEEE Transactions on Biomedical Engineering*, 42: 621–631.

Du, S.J. and Vuskovic, M. 2004. Temporal vs. spectral approach to feature extraction from prehensile EMG signals. Paper read at the IEEE International Conference on Information Reuse and Integration, Las Vegas, NV, November 2009.

Du, Y.-C., Lin, C.-H., Shyu, L.-Y. and Chen, T. 2010. Portable hand motion classifier for multi-channel surface electromyography recognition using grey relational analysis. *Expert Systems with Applications*, 37(6): 4283–4291.

Farry, K.A., Walker, I.D., and Barabiuk, R.G. 1996. Myoelectric teleoperation of a complex robotic hand. *IEEE Transactions on Robotics and Automation*, 12: 775–788.

Fukuda, O., Tsuji, T., and Kaneko, M. 1997. An EMG controlled robotics manipulator using neural networks. Paper read at the IEEE International Workshop on Robot and Human Communication, Sendai, Japan, October 1997.

Hannaford, B. and Lehman, S. 1986. Short time fourier analysis of the electromyogram: fast movements and constant contraction. *IEEE Transactions on Biomedical Engineering*, 33: 1773–1181.

Hudgins, B. and Parker, P. 1993. A new strategy for multifunction myoelectric control. *IEEE Transactions on Biomedical Engineering*, 40: 82–94.

Ito, K., Tsuji, T., Kato, A., and Ito, M. 1992. EMG pattern classification for a prosthetic forearm with three degrees of freedom. Paper read at the IEEE International Workshop on Robot and Human Communication, Toyko, Japan, September 1992.

Jin, D.W., Zhang, R.H., Zhang, J.C., Wang, R.C., and Gruver, W.A. 2000. An intelligent above-knee prosthesis with EMG-based terrain identification. Paper read at the IEEE International Conference on Systems, Man and Cybernetics, Nashville, TN, October 2002.

Kuribayashi, K., Okimura, K., and Taniguchi, T. 1993. A discrimination system using neural network for EMG-controller prostheses—Integral type of EMG signal processing. Paper read at the IEEE/RSJ International Conference on Intelligent Robots and Systems, Tokyo, Japan, July 1993.

Lange, N., Strother, S.C., Anderson, J.R., Nielsen, F.A., Holmes, A.P., Kolenda, T., Savoy, R., and Hansen, L.K. 1999. Plurality and resemblance in fMRI data analysis. *Neuroimage*, 10: 282–303.

Lin, I.-K. 1989. A concordance correlation coefficient to evaluate reproducibility. *Biometrics*, 45(1): 255–268.

Merletti, R. and Parker, P. 2004. *Electromyography: Physiology, Engineering and Noninvasive Applications.* Hoboken, NJ: Wiley.

Miller, C.J. 2008. Real-time feature extraction and classification of prehensile EMG signals. Master's thesis, San Diego State University.

Mogk, P.M. and Keir, J. 2003. Crosstalk in surface electromyography of the proximal forearm during gripping tasks. *Journal of Electromyography and Kinesiology*, 13: 63–71.

Saponas, T. S., Tan, D., Morris, D. and Balakrishnan, R. 2008. Demonstrating the feasibility of using forearm electromyography for muscle–computer interfaces. Paper read at the Conference on Human Factors in Computing Systems, Florence, Italy, April 2008.

Saridis, G.N. and Gootee, T.P. 1982. EMG pattern analysis and classification for a prosthetic arm. *IEEE Transactions on Biomedical Engineering*, 29: 403–412.

Staude, G., Flachenecker, C., Daumer, M., and Wolf, W. 2001. Onset detection in surface electromyographic signals: A systematic comparison of methods. *EURASIP Journal on Applied Signal Processing*, (1): 67–81.

Zecca, M., Micera, S., Carrozza, M.C., and Dario, P. 2002. Control of multifunctional prosthetic hands by processing the electromyographic signal. *Critical Review in Biomedical Engineering*, 30: 459–485.

13

Multifunctional Actuators Utilizing Magnetorheological Fluids for Assistive Knee Braces

H. T. Guo and W. H. Liao

The Chinese University of Hong Kong
Hong Kong, China

CONTENTS

13.1 Introduction 240
13.2 Design of Multifunctional Actuator 242
    13.2.1 Motor Design 243
    13.2.2 Clutch/Brake Design 246
13.3 Analysis of Multifunctional Actuator 249
13.4 Modeling of Multifunctional Actuator 251
13.5 Prototype Testing 254
13.6 Conclusion 258
Acknowledgments 260
References 260

Abstract

Knee braces are a kind of wearable lower extremity exoskeleton that can enhance people's strength and provide desired locomotion. It is possible to use knee braces to assist elderly or disabled people in improving their mobility to solve many daily life problems, like going up and down stairs and over obstacles. A well-designed actuator is the key component for assistive knee braces. In this design, magnetorheological (MR) fluids are integrated into a motor to work with multiple functions as a motor, clutch, and brake in order to meet the requirements of normal human walking. To design multifunctional actuators, several design considerations including configurations, mechanical and electromagnetic designs, and the influence of a permanent magnet on MR fluids are discussed. Finite element models of the actuator are built and analyzed. Modeling of the actuator in different functions is presented. A prototype of the actuator is fabricated and each function is tested. Torque tracking in brake function of the actuator is investigated. The results show that the developed multifunctional actuator is promising for assistive knee braces.

13.1 Introduction

With aging comes various types of physical deterioration, which often affects mobility. The muscular strength of older people may decrease and they may be unable to walk or lose their stability during walking. Without appropriate exercise and rehabilitation, their muscles will further deteriorate and they may become bedridden. It has been found that exercise training can increase strength and may improve motor activity in people with cerebral palsy (CP) without adverse effects (Damiano et al. 2000). It was also demonstrated that exercise increases the strength of affected major muscle groups in stroke survivors (Teixeira-Salmela et al. 1999). Therefore, an effective way to relieve these problems and enable older people to fulfill their activities of daily living is to provide a means for them to be able to continue walking.

Assistive knee braces are a species of wearable lower extremity exoskeletons. Such assistive equipment can enhance people's strength and provide desired locomotion and have advantages over wheelchairs, which are commonly used for patients with mobility disorders. For example, assistive knee braces could help the wearer walk on his or her own legs and therefore exercise the own lower body. Moreover, it is possible to use this kind of lower extremity exoskeleton to assist older or disabled people to improve their mobility in order to solve many daily life problems, such as going up and down stairs and over obstacles.

Some research groups have developed several wearable assistive knee braces for walking support. The Berkeley Lower Extremity Exoskeleton (BLEEX) was developed (Kazerooni and Steger 2006) to support a human's walking while carrying a heavy load on his or her back. The Hybrid Assistive Limb (HAL; Kawamoto and Sankai 2002) was developed to help people walk, climb stairs, and carry things around. The RoboKnee (Pratt et al. 2004) provides assistance in climbing stairs and bending the knees while carrying a heavy load. The Wearable Walking Helper (WWH; Nakamura, Saito, and Kosuge 2005) and Walking Power Assist Leg (WPAL; F. Chen et al. 2007) were designed to augment human power during walking based on human–robot interactions. Some companies, including Honda, have also developed assistive walking devices to support bodyweight and reduce the load on the wearer's legs while walking, climbing stairs, and in a semi-crouching position (Honda 2008).

All of the above assistive knee braces use powerful actuation devices to provide adequate supporting torque as well as smooth locomotion. To assist the wearer in various postures and prevent knee braces from exceeding the restricted motion, actuators that function as a brake/clutch combined with the ability to safely interlock are desirable. Power consumption by the actuation devices is another consideration in lengthening the working time of batteries after they are fully charged. Therefore, well-designed actuators would be the key component for assistive knee braces in terms of performance and safety.

Generally, actuation devices in assistive knee braces can be classified as active and semi-active actuators. The most widely used active actuators are electric DC motors in rotary or linear forms. In addition to electric motors, hydraulic and pneumatic actuators are other active actuators used in assistive knee braces and exoskeletons.

For active actuators, especially for electric DC motors, brake function requires a large amount of power to maintain any posture and might cause safety problems. Some researchers have adopted smart fluids in actuation mechanisms; for instance, a rehabilitative knee orthosis equipped with electrorheological (ER) fluids-based actuators (Nikitczuk, Weinberg, and Mavroidis 2005). An orthopedic active knee brace using a magnetorheological (MR) fluids-based shear damper was developed to make the knee brace have controllable resistance (Ahmadkhanlou, Zite, and Washington 2007). All of the knee braces developed using smart fluids provide controllable torque by passive and semi-active means while consuming little power. Furthermore, according to clinical gait analysis (CGA), the knee joint dissipates power during walking (Zoss and Kazerooni 2006). Hence, the knee joint dynamics could be closely matched by a controlled energy-dissipative device; for example, smart fluids-based actuators. However, in some situations, such as going upstairs or stepping over obstacles, such knee braces do not help in active ways.

To combine the advantages of active and semi-active actuation devices, like electric motors and smart fluids-based actuators, a hybrid assistive knee brace that integrates an MR actuator with an electric motor was developed (J. Z. Chen and Liao 2010). The MR actuator can function as a brake when adjustable torque is preferred and requires low power consumption or it can work as a clutch to transfer torque from the motor to the brace. With adaptive control, the actuation system worked well and could provide the desired torque with better safety and energy efficiency. However, the actuator seemed a bit bulky to be used on the human body and could not fulfill the tasks of bidirectional rotation. Therefore, designing a more compact, multifunctional actuator is desired for assistive knee braces.

The objective of this research is to develop a novel actuator with multiple functions such as motor, clutch, and brake for assistive knee braces. Utilizing MR fluids, the actuator provides torque safely as a motor and clutch and produces controllable torque with little power consumption for braking. Moreover, the braking torque control of the actuator could be easily implemented.

13.2 Design of Multifunctional Actuator

The actuator in this research is comprised of two main components, the motor and the clutch/brake, and each component is associated with corresponding coils. The motor and clutch/brake are filled with MR fluids.

The motor converts electric power into mechanical power to provide active torque. Utilizing MR fluids, the clutch/brake transfers the torque generated from the motor to the outside as a clutch or provides controllable semi-active torque as a brake. Multiple functions can be achieved by applying current on different coils. Figure 13.1 shows a schematic of the multifunctional actuator.

When current is applied to the outer coil of the motor, the induced electromagnetic field drives the rotor to rotate and then provide active torque. If current is applied to both outer and inner coils simultaneously, the MR fluids produce shear stress under the electromagnetic field induced from the inner coil. As a result, the clutch/brake transfers the torque from the motor to the outside as a clutch. When current is applied only to the inner coil, the actuator functions as a brake. By adjusting the current, the actuator produces controllable torque. In this situation, with no current applied on the outer coil, the rotor will not rotate because of the magnetic interaction force between the stator and permanent magnets. The advantage of this design is that it can deal with the tradeoff between the brake function and bidirectional rotation.

Figure 13.2 shows a person moving through a normal gait cycle and the location of each walking state (Wikenfeld and Herr 2003). According to the gait cycle shown, in the state of stance flexion and extension, the actuator works as brake; in the state of preswing and swing extension, the actuator works as a motor and clutch; in the state of swing flexion, the clutch is off.

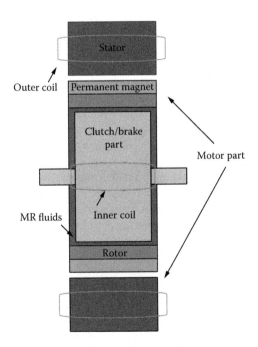

FIGURE 13.1
Schematic of the multifunctional actuator.

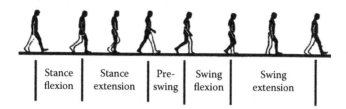

| Stance flexion | Stance extension | Pre-swing | Swing flexion | Swing extension |

FIGURE 13.2
Gait cycle and walking states for normal walking (Wikenfeld and Herr 2003).

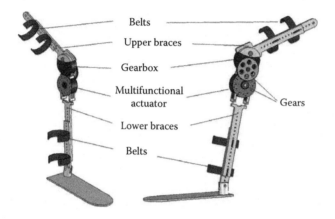

FIGURE 13.3
Configuration of the assistive knee brace with the actuator.

Thus, the multifunctional actuator developed meets any motion required of an assistive knee brace.

The configuration of the knee brace that utilizes the multifunctional actuator is shown in Figure 13.3, where the multifunctional actuator provides active and semi-active torque to help the wearer achieve better mobility.

13.2.1 Motor Design

The motor is designed based on conventional electric motors. Considering the advantages of simple construction and maintenance, as well as high efficiency and torque per volume, a brushless permanent magnet (BLPM) DC motor was modified for the motor.

Generally, BLPM DC motors are constructed in three basic physical configurations as shown in Figure 13.4, in the form of an interior rotor, exterior rotor, or axial rotor. The interior rotor configuration is an appropriate choice because high torque with low speed is needed. Such a configuration can be made with a large hole through the center of the rotor, which provides valuable space for other parts of the mechanism (Hendershot and Miller 1994).

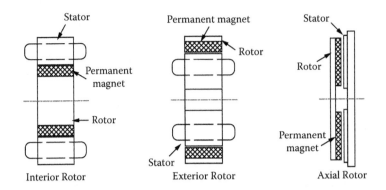

FIGURE 13.4
Three basic BLPM DC motor configurations.

To design a motor that produces sufficient torque while having good performance, several design factors should be considered. The number of stator slots and magnet poles is one of the considerations in motor design. The number of poles is inversely proportional to the maximum speed of rotation. By increasing the number of poles, the overall diameter can be reduced.

Cogging force is a kind of magnetic force between the stator and permanent magnets, which usually causes oscillation during rotation. For conventional motor design, many efforts have been made to reduce the cogging force. However, in this design, the magnetic force between the stator and permanent magnets has a special function. When there is no current applied on the stator coils, this magnetic interaction force holds the rotor still and plays an important role in the operation as a brake.

Increasing the cogging force improves the brake function but impairs the dynamic performance of motor function. Hence it is a trade-off to determine the suitable magnetic force between the stator and permanent magnets. In this design, fractional slots/poles were adopted to minimize the cogging force while maintaining an appropriate magnetic force between stator and permanent magnets.

In order to provide sufficient active torque, the motor needs to produce an electromagnetic torque as large as possible. There are some factors affecting the value of the torque, such as grade of the permanent magnet, permeability of the magnetic material, windings of the coil, and air gap. In the motor, magnetic flux passes between the stator and permanent magnets through the air gap. The output torque or the electromagnetic torque is proportional to the flux in it. The electromagnetic torque provided by the motor is calculated with the following equation:

$$T_M = C_T \Phi_M I_M \qquad (13.1)$$

where C_T is the torque constant relating to the windings, I is the current applied on the outer coils, Φ is the magnetic flux in the air gap, and the subscript M represents the motor part.

According to the Ampere's law, there is

$$HL = nI = F \tag{13.2}$$

where H is the magnetic field intensity, L is the length of the magnetic circuit, n is the turns of coil, and F is the magnetomotive force (MMF). Also,

$$\Phi = \int_A B \cdot da = BA \tag{13.3}$$

$$B = \mu H \tag{13.4}$$

where B is the magnetic flux density, A is the cross-sectional area, and μ is the magnetic permeability. Using the above equations in the motor, it can be derived that

$$F_M = nI_M = \sum_{i=1}^{j} \Phi_i \frac{l_i}{\mu_i A_i} = \Phi_M \left(\frac{g}{\mu A_g} + \sum_{i=1}^{k} \frac{l_i}{\mu_i A_i} \right) \tag{13.5}$$

where subscript i represents each component within the magnetic circuit and l is the length of the magnetic circuit in the motor that includes the air gap g. Because each component in the magnetic circuit is connected in serial, their magnetic fluxes are the same.

Therefore, considering Equations (13.1) and (13.5), in a steady state, decreasing the air gap would decrease the magnetic reluctance and increase the air gap flux and thus increase the output torque.

The windings of the outer coil are connected with three coils in the form of *wye*. Based on the desired specification and parameters obtained above, the maximum outer coil current or the demagnetizing line current can be calculated by the following equation:

$$I_{demag} = \left[\frac{1000}{4\pi \times 39.37} \right] \times \frac{2(L_{PM} + g_M)H_d}{z_M / 2p_M} \times a_M = 2.02 \times \frac{4p_M a_M (L_{PM} + g_M)H_d}{z_M} \tag{13.6}$$

where L_{PM} and H_d are the length and coercive force of the permanent magnets; z is the total number of conductors actually carrying current; p is the number of pole pairs; and *a* is the number of parallel paths in the winding. When the current is larger than this value, the permanent magnet will be demagnetized and thus impair the performance of the motor part.

In order to design a compact actuator used in assistive knee braces, the hall sensor commonly used in BLPM DC motors was removed. The indirect rotor position sensing can be obtained through back electromagnetic field (EMF) detection in an unexcited phase winding.

13.2.2 Clutch/Brake Design

The clutch/brake is placed inside the motor together with the MR fluids to produce the torque. Similar to designing the motor, there are several configurations of the clutch/brake. The clutch/brake of the actuator may be implemented in the form of an inner armature with slots and shoes. In this case, inner coils are wound on each shoe in the inner armature. An example of such a clutch/brake element is illustrated in Figure 13.5.

Alternatively, the clutch/brake can be implemented in the form of a plurality of input–output plates separated by nonmagnetic spacer rings forming gaps in between to carry the MR fluids. An example of such a clutch/brake is illustrated in Figure 13.6. In this configuration of the clutch/brake, the inner coil can be implemented in the form of an interior coil, exterior coil, or axial coil.

Based on the above discussion, three main configurations of a BLPM DC motor are possible for the motor. Because there are three different inner coil configurations for the clutch/brake, that is, in the form of input–output plates, the clutch/brake can be implemented in four forms. Therefore, there are various combinations of motor and clutch/brake available for the design of the multifunctional actuator. Table 13.1 shows the possible combinations.

Although all of the above configurations can be implemented in designing the multifunctional actuator, only a motor with an interior rotor configuration is discussed in this chapter. For the clutch/brake made in the form

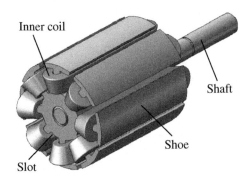

FIGURE 13.5
Clutch/brake in the form of an inner armature.

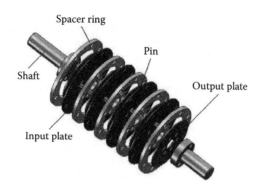

FIGURE 13.6
Clutch/brake in the form of input–output plates.

TABLE 13.1

Combinations of Motor and Clutch/Brake

		Motor		
		Interior Rotor	**Exterior Rotor**	**Axial Rotor**
Clutch / Brake	Inner armature	+	+	+
	Input–output plates (with interior coil)	+	+	+
	Input–output plates (with exterior coil)	+	+	+
	Input–output plates (with axial coil)	+	+	+

of an inner armature (Guo and Liao 2009), in order to produce the desired electromagnetic field, the length of the inner armature has to be increased so that the dimension of the smart actuator as well as the weight are increased accordingly. Though the multifunctional actuator is promising for assistive knee braces, the compactness is still an issue. Hence, the clutch/brake discussed in this chapter is in the form of input–output plates. Figure 13.7 shows a sectional view of the actuator.

The torque generated by the clutch/brake can be calculated as follows:

$$T_{CB} = \int_A \tau_{mr} r_{CB} dA_{CB} \tag{13.7}$$

where τ_{mr} is the yield shear stress of MR fluids, A is the overlapping surface, and r_{CB} is the radius of the clutch/brake.

The overlapping surface on the plates where the MR fluids are activated by applied magnetic field intensity can be calculated by

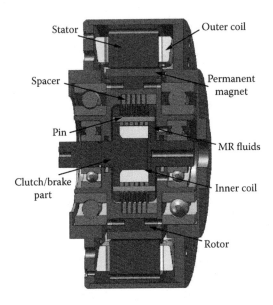

FIGURE 13.7
Configuration of the multifunctional actuator.

$$A_{CB} = 2n\pi \int_{r_i}^{r_o} r_{CB} dr_{CB} = 2n\pi(r_o^2 - r_i^2) \tag{13.8}$$

where n is number of the surfaces of the plates in contact with MR fluids, and r_i and r_o are radii of the input and output plates, respectively.

The characteristics of the MR fluids can be described using the Bingham plastic model (Phillips 1969), for which the shear stress τ is

$$\tau_{mr} = \tau_y + \eta\dot{\gamma} \tag{13.9}$$

where τ_y is the yield stress due to the applied magnetic field and can be obtained from the specifications of the MRF-132DG fluids as shown in Lord (2008); η is the off-field plastic viscosity of the MR fluids; and $\dot{\gamma}$ is the shear rate, which can be written as

$$\dot{\gamma} = \frac{\omega r_{CB}}{g_{CB}} \tag{13.10}$$

where ω is the angular velocity, and g_{CB} is the gap between each pair of an input and output plate (also the thickness of the MR fluids in between the pair).

Referring to Equations (13.7)–(13.10), the torque produced by the clutch/brake can be obtained as follows:

$$T_{CB} = n_{CB} \int_{r_i}^{r_o} (\tau_y + \eta\dot{\gamma}) r_{CB}(2\pi r_{CB}) dr_{CB} = \frac{2n_{CB}\pi\tau_y}{3}(r_o^3 - r_i^3) + \frac{n_{CB}\pi\omega\eta}{2g_{CB}}(r_o^4 - r_i^4)$$

(13.11)

If the angular velocity is slow when the torque caused by the fluid viscosity is negligible, the torque produced by the clutch/brake can be rewritten as

$$T_{CB} = n_{CB} \int_{r_i}^{r_o} \tau_y r_{CB}(2\pi r_{CB}) dr_{CB} = \frac{2n_{CB}\pi\tau_y}{3}(r_o^3 - r_i^3)$$

(13.12)

13.3 Analysis of Multifunctional Actuator

The actuator is modeled and analyzed using a finite element method (FEM). A three-dimensional model was built to analyze the influence of permanent magnets on MR fluids and the electromagnetic torque between the stator and the permanent magnets in the motor. A two-dimensional model was built to analyze the electromagnetic flux from the inner coil in MR fluids and the yield stress produced in the clutch/brake. Simulations were carried out using ANSYS (Canonsburg, PA, USA).

Figure 13.8 shows the contour plot of the magnetic flux density in the motor when no current is applied on the outer coil. The torque between the stator and permanent magnets can be calculated based on this flux density distribution. The result of the simulation was about 0.733 Nm. This magnetic interaction torque between the stator and permanent magnets can be used to hold the rotor static and plays a role in the operation as a brake.

Figure 13.9 shows the distribution of magnetic flux in the rotor. The magnetic flux from the permanent magnets does not enter the inside of the rotor. Therefore, the MR fluids will not be affected by the permanent magnets.

An FEM was also utilized to determine whether the magnetic flux in MR fluids is perpendicular to the input and output plates so that the maximum shear stress could be produced. It was illustrated that the maximum stress occurred when the direction of the magnetic field was perpendicular to the shear motion of the MR fluids (Kordonsky et al. 1990). The simulation result is shown in Figure 13.10. The direction of the magnetic flux in MR fluids was along the normal direction of the plates so that the maximum yield shear stress was obtained.

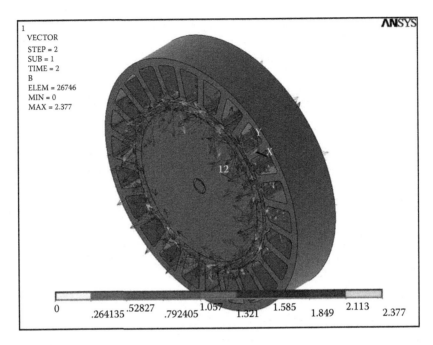

FIGURE 13.8
Contour plot of the magnetic flux density in the motor.

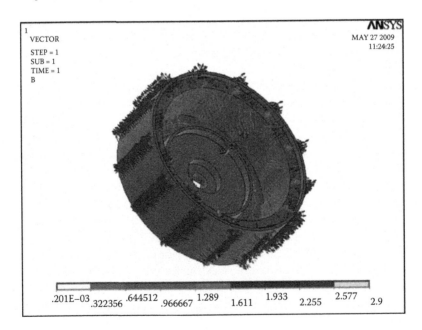

FIGURE 13.9
Magnetic flux distribution in the rotor.

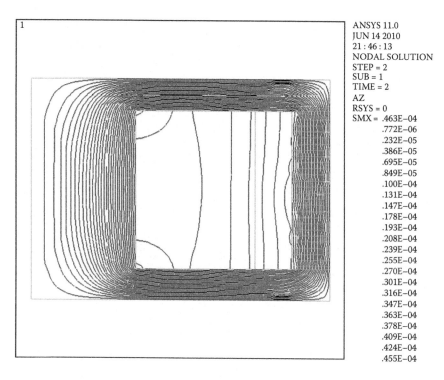

FIGURE 13.10
Magnetic flux distribution in the clutch/brake.

The torque generated from the clutch/brake was estimated using an FEM. Figure 13.11 shows the contour of electromagnetic flux density in the clutch/brake for an input current of 1.5 A. According to the properties of MRF-132DG and its relationship between the flux density and the yield shear stress, the output torque from the clutch/brake can be obtained as 0.23 Nm using Equation (13.12). It can be found that the output torque is proportional to the current applied on the inner coil. This indicates that the clutch torque transferred from the motor and the brake torque provided by the clutch/brake depend on the value of current applied to the inner coil. Therefore, the torque control of the multifunctional actuator in brake function would be straightforward.

13.4 Modeling of Multifunctional Actuator

Because the actuator has multiple functions, modeling of the actuator can be illustrated for different functions. For motor function, the model is similar to the conventional DC motor. Equations (13.13)–(13.16) are used for the dynamic model of the motor function:

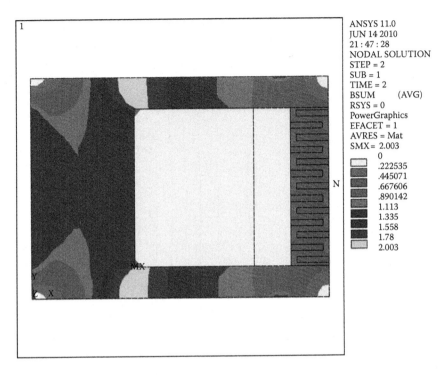

FIGURE 13.11
Contour of flux density in the clutch/brake.

$$V_M = R_M I_M + L_M \frac{dI_M}{dt} + E \qquad (13.13)$$

$$E = K_e \omega \qquad (13.14)$$

$$T_M = K_t I_M w \qquad (13.15)$$

$$T_M = J_M \frac{d\omega}{dt} + D\omega + T_L \qquad (13.16)$$

where V_M is the supply voltage on the outer coil, R_M is the resistance of the outer coil, I_M is the current, L_M is the inductance, E is the back-EMF, ω is the angular velocity, T_M is the motor torque, J_M is the moment of inertia, T_L is the load torque including the external load and the friction torque, D is the viscous damping coefficient, and K_e and K_t are EMF constant and torque constant, respectively. The model of the motor function then can be expressed in state–space form as follows:

$$\begin{cases} \dot{x} = Ax + Bu \\ y = Cx + Du \end{cases}$$

where

$$A = \begin{bmatrix} -\dfrac{D}{J_M} & \dfrac{K_i}{J_M} \\ -\dfrac{K_e}{L_M} & \dfrac{R_M}{L_M} \end{bmatrix}; B = \begin{bmatrix} -\dfrac{1}{J_M} & 0 \\ 0 & \dfrac{1}{L_M} \end{bmatrix}; C = \begin{bmatrix} 1 & 0 \end{bmatrix}; D = \begin{bmatrix} 0 \\ 0 \end{bmatrix}$$

$$x = \begin{bmatrix} \omega \\ I_M \end{bmatrix}; \quad y = \omega; \quad u = \begin{bmatrix} T_L \\ V_M \end{bmatrix}$$

(13.17)

For the brake function where the motor function is off, the model can be derived. According to the properties of MR fluid and its relationship between the flux density and the yield shear stress, the brake torque can be represented as

$$T_B = K_H I_{mr} + K_\omega \omega \tag{13.18}$$

where K_H is the coefficient due to the electromagnetic field, and K_ω is the coefficient relating to the viscosity. It should be noted that these two coefficients are nonlinear.

The dynamic equation for brake function can be expressed as follows:

$$T_L - T_B = J_L \frac{d\omega}{dt} \tag{13.19}$$

where J_L is the equivalent moment of inertia of the load. The model of the brake function can then be derived in state–space form as

$$\begin{cases} \dot{x} = Ax + Bu \\ y = Cx + Du \end{cases}$$

where

$$A = \begin{bmatrix} -\dfrac{K_\omega}{J_L} & 0 \\ 0 & 0 \end{bmatrix}; \quad B = \begin{bmatrix} \dfrac{1}{J_L} & -\dfrac{K_H}{J_L} \\ 0 & 0 \end{bmatrix}; \quad C = \begin{bmatrix} 0 & -\dfrac{1}{K_\omega} \end{bmatrix}; \quad D = \begin{bmatrix} 0 & -K_H \end{bmatrix};$$

$$x = \begin{bmatrix} \omega \\ T_B \end{bmatrix}; \quad y = \omega; \quad u = \begin{bmatrix} T_L \\ I_{mr} \end{bmatrix} \tag{13.20}$$

For the clutch function, two cases should be considered. If the current applied on the inner coil is large enough, no slipping occurs between the actuator and load. In this state, the clutch will transfer the exact torque and angular velocity from the motor to the load. Therefore, the model in this case is the same as the motor function in Equation (13.17), provided that

$$T_C = T_M \leq K_H I_{mr} \tag{13.21}$$

On the other hand, if the current is not large enough and cannot transfer synchronous velocity, slipping occurs. The model of the clutch function is then the same as the brake function as in Equation (13.20) and the prerequisite is

$$T_C = K_H I_{mr} + K_\omega \omega < T_M \tag{13.22}$$

Control of the multifunctional actuator is easy to implement. When positive power is required, the motor function is on; when negative power is required, the brake function is on; the clutch function works as a switch between these two functions. By adjusting the current on the inner coil, the output torque is controllable.

13.5 Prototype Testing

A prototype as shown in Figure 13.12 was fabricated according to the above design and analysis. Experiments were conducted to investigate each function of the actuator and torque tracking in the brake function. The main specifications of the prototype are given in Table 13.2. The experimental setup is shown in Figure 13.13. A dynamic torque sensor (Model RST-C4A-30-1-A, RSTSensor Inc., Shenzen, China) was utilized to measure the output torque produced by the prototype. By changing the payload for motor function, the output torque versus applied stator current and the output torque versus output speed were investigated. If the output torque of the payload is kept constant, the rotor is driven by the motor at a constant speed. Therefore, by changing the current on the inner coil, the output torque of the brake function was measured. In this case, if the current in the inner coil was input as a

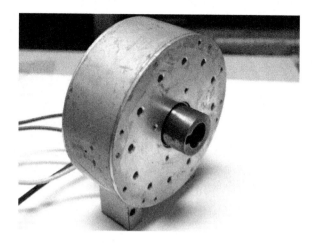

FIGURE 13.12
Prototype of the multifunctional actuator.

step signal, the response of the clutch function was then tested. In the experiments, the signals were processed by the dSPACE system (DS 1104, dSPACE Inc., Paderborn, Germany), which also commands control voltage signal to drive the actuator.

For motor function, the output torque versus applied stator current and the output torque versus output speed are the most important characteristics. Figure 13.14 shows the measured torque at different currents and speeds. The torque/current as well as torque/speed curves are nearly straight lines. Figure 13.15 shows the output power and power efficiency of the motor part. The efficiency was about 74.3%.

TABLE 13.2

Prototype Specifications of the Multifunctional Actuator

Parameters	Values
Weight	1.7 kg
Length	40 mm
Diameter	100 mm
Amount of MR fluids used	$0.24 \times 10^{-6} \, m^3$
Plate pairs in the clutch/brake	5 Pairs
Number of turns of the inner coil	350 Turns
Voltage applied on the outer coil	24 V
Voltage applied on the inner coil	24 V
Maximum current applied on the inner coil	2.4 A
Magnetic materials used	Pure iron
Nonmagnetic materials used	Al, stainless steel

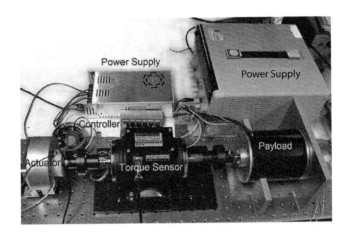

FIGURE 13.13
Experimental setup for testing the multifunctional actuator.

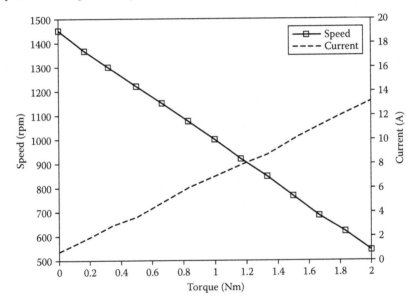

FIGURE 13.14
Torque vs. current and speed in motor function.

For the brake function, the torque generated from the clutch/brake with an interior inner coil is shown in Figure 13.16. The rotor was rotated at a speed of 600 rpm and step current was applied to the inner coil gradually. With the current augmented from 0 to 2.5 A, the measured torque increased until it reached a maximum value of 0.48 Nm. Although the torque was not sufficient to be applied to the human body directly, it is promising for use in assistive knee braces with a transmission mechanism. As shown in

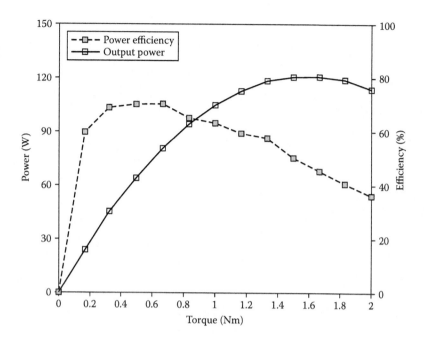

FIGURE 13.15
Output power and power efficiency in motor function.

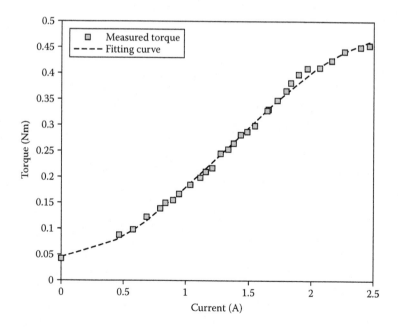

FIGURE 13.16
Measured torque vs. applied current in the brake function.

Figure 13.16, in the range of 0.5 to 2.5 A, the output torque was approximately linear with respect to the applied current. Therefore, the model of the brake function can be expressed as a first-order single-input, single-output linear plant.

The response of the clutch function was investigated. Figure 13.17 shows the response of the clutch/brake under a pulse signal. The response time was about 0.1 second, compared with the reaction time of an average person (0.15–0.4 seconds), so it is capable of stopping the torque transfer from the motor to the assistive knee brace in case of emergency.

Motor braking is an issue for motor control. The commonly used methods for motor braking consume large amounts of power and can damage the device with prolonged usage. For normal walking, the knee power is mainly passive and usually occurs during the bending of the knee joint. As discussed above, with MR fluids, output torque in the brake function of the actuator is approximately proportional to the current applied to the inner coil. By adjusting the current, the braking torque control is easy to implement. Experiments on torque tracking of the brake function were conducted, and the results are shown in Figure 13.18. It can be seen that the actuator can track the reference well in the brake function.

13.6 Conclusion

In this research, an MR fluids-based multifunctional actuator for assistive knee braces was designed. To decrease the dimension of the actuation device while enhancing its performance, a motor and MR fluids were integrated into a single device. By applying current on different coils on each part, the actuator has multiple functions as a motor, clutch, and brake. Design details of the motor and clutch/brake were considered. The motor was designed based on an interior rotor BLPM DC motor, and the clutch/brake was in the form of input–output plates. Possible combinations of these two parts were discussed. Because the actuator was composed of permanent magnets and MR fluids, the magnetic interaction force, influence of the permanent magnet on MR fluids, and magnetic flux distribution were analyzed using FEM. Modeling of the actuator for different functions was developed. A prototype was fabricated and tested, and characteristics of each function were investigated. Torque tracking in the brake function was investigated. Although the measured torque was not high, by adding transmission mechanisms, the torque can be increased while the speed is reduced. Therefore, the new multifunctional actuator is promising for assistive knee braces.

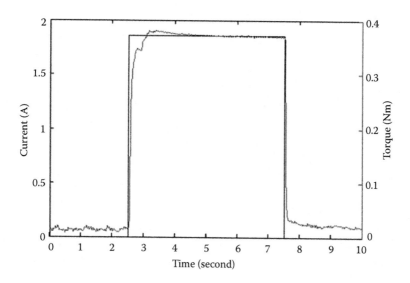

FIGURE 13.17
Pulse response in clutch function.

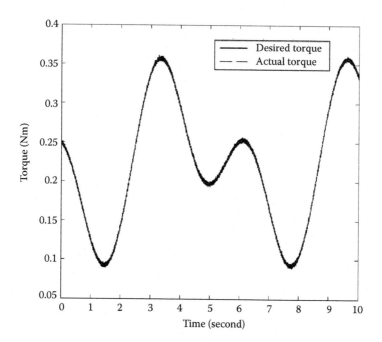

FIGURE 13.18
Torque tracking in the brake function of the actuator.

Acknowledgments

The work described in this chapter was supported by grants from the Innovation and Technology Commission (Project No. ITS/308/09) and Research Grants Council (Project No. CUHK 414810) of the Hong Kong Special Administrative Region, China.

References

Ahmadkhanlou, F., Zite, J., and Washington, G. 2007. A magnetorheological fluid-based controllable active knee brace. *Proceedings of SPIE on Industrial and Commercial Applications of Smart Structures Technologies*, 6527: 65270O-1–65270O-10.

Chen, F., Yu, Y., Ge, Y., Sun J., and Deng, X. 2007. WPAL for enhancing human strength and endurance during walking. Paper read at the International Conference on Information Acquisition, Seogwipo-zi, Korea.

Chen, J.Z. and Liao, W.H. 2010. Design, testing and control of a magnetorheological actuator for assistive knee braces. *Smart Materials and Structures*, 19: 035029, doi: 10.1088/0964-1726/19/3/035029.

Damiano, D.L., Martellotta, T.L., Sullivan, D.J., Granata, K.P., and Abel, M.F. 2000. Muscle force production and functional performance in spastic cerebral palsy: Relationship of cocontraction. *Archives of Physical Medicine and Rehabilitation*, 81(7): 895–900.

Guo, H.T. and Liao, W.H. 2009. Integrated design and analysis of smart actuators for hybrid assistive knee braces. *Proceedings of SPIE Conference on Smart Structures and Materials: Active and Passive Smart Structures and Integrated Systems*, 7288: 72881U1-11.

Hendershot, J. and Miller, T. 1994. *Design of Brushless Permanent-Magnet Motors*. Lebanon, OH: Magna Physics Publishing.

Honda Worldwide, April 2008. Available at http://world.honda.com/news/2008/c080422Experimental-Walking-Assist-Device/.

Kawamoto, H. and Sankai, Y. 2002. Comfortable power assist control method for walking aid by HAL-3. *IEEE International Conference on Systems, Man and Cybernetics*, 4: 6.

Kazerooni, H. and Steger, R. 2006. The Berkeley lower extremity exoskeleton. *Transactions of the ASME, Journal of Dynamic Systems, Measurements, and Control*, 128: 14–25.

Kordonsky, V., Shulman, Z., Gorodkin, S., Demchuk, S., Prokhorav, I., Zaltsgendler, E., and Khusid, B. 1990. Physical properties of magnetizable structure-reversible media. *Journal of Magnetism and Magnetic Materials*, 85: 1–3.

Lord Corporation. 2008. Available at http://www.lordfulfillment.com/.

Nakamura, T., Saito, K., and Kosuge, K. 2005. Control of wearable walking support system based on human-model and GRF. Paper read at the International Conference on Robotics and Automation, Barcelona, Spain, April 18, 2005.

Nikitczuk, J., Weinberg, B., and Mavroidis, C. 2005. Rehabilitative knee orthosis driven by electro-rheological fluid based actuators. Paper read at the IEEE International Conference on Robotics and Automation,Barcelona, Spain, April 18, 2005.

Phillips, R.W. 1969. Engineering applications of fluids with a variable yield stress. Ph.D. dissertation, University of California, Berkeley.

Pratt, J.E., Krupp, B.T., Morse, C.J., and Collins, S.H. 2004. The RoboKnee: An exoskeleton for enhancing strength and endurance during walking. Paper read at the IEEE International Conference on Robotics & Automation, New Orleans, LA, April 26–May 1, 2009.

Teixeira-Salmela, L.F., Olney, S.J., Nadeau, S., and Brouwer, B. 1999. Muscle strengthening and physical conditioning to reduce impairment and disability in chronic stroke survivors. *Archives of Physical Medicine and Rehabilitation*, 80: 1211–1218.

Wikenfeld, A. and Herr, H. 2003. User-adaptive control of a magnetorheological prosthetic knee. *Industrial Robot: An International Journal*, 30(1): 42–55.

Zoss, A. and Kazerooni, H. 2006. Design of an electrically actuated lower extremity exoskeleton. *Advanced Robotics*, 20(9): 967–988.

14

Mathematical Modeling of Brain Circuitry during Cerebellar Movement Control*

Henrik Jörntell, Per-Ola Forsberg, Fredrik Bengtsson, and Rolf Johansson

Lund University
Lund, Sweden

CONTENTS

14.1 Introduction 264
14.2 Problem Formulation 265
14.3 Materials and Methods 266
14.4 Results 266
14.4 Discussion 273
14.5 Conclusions 274
References 275

Abstract

Reconstruction of movement control properties of the brain could result in many potential advantages for application in robotics. However, a hampering factor so far has been the lack of knowledge of the structure and function of brain circuitry in vivo during movement control. Much more detailed information has recently become available for the area of the cerebellum that controls arm–hand movements. In addition to previously obtained extensive background knowledge of the overall connectivity of the controlling neuronal network, recent studies have provided detailed characterizations of local microcircuitry connectivity and physiology in vivo. In the present study, we study one component of this neuronal network, the cuneate nucleus, and characterize its mathematical properties using system identification theory. The cuneate nucleus is involved in the processing of the sensory feedback evoked by movements. As a substrate for our work, we use a characterization of

* © 2009 IEEE. Reprinted, with permission, from Proceedings of the 2009 IEEE International Conference on Robotics and Biomimetics (ROBIO2009), December 19–23, 2009, Guilin, China, pp. 98–103.

incoming and outgoing signals of individual neurons during sensory activation as well as a recently obtained microcircuitry characterization for this structure. We find that system identification is a useful way to find suitable mathematical models that capture the properties and transformation capabilities of the neuronal microcircuitry that constitutes the cuneate nucleus. Future work will show whether specific aspects of the mathematical properties can be ascribed to a specific microcircuitry and/or neuronal property.

14.1 Introduction

In order to understand and describe how the brain organizes limb movement control, we aim to design a mathematical model of this control. The study is based on a comprehensive neurophysiological characterization of the cerebellar system for voluntary arm–hand control as described in Apps and Garwicz (2005). This system may be viewed as a vast network of interconnected neurons that involves many parts of the brain, which all are interconnected through a specific area of the cerebellum (Bengtsson and Jörntell 2009; Jörntell and Ekerot 1999). A foundation for the model system is a previous, detailed characterization of all constituent neuron types and a systematic description of connectivity patterns both within the cerebellum and in those brain regions outside the cerebellum, which are part of the network devoted to this specific control as shown in previous publications from our group (Bengtsson and Jörntell 2009; Ekerot and Jörntell 2001, 2003; Jörntell and Ekerot 2002, 2006; Jörntell and Hansel 2006).

As for detailed electrophysiological neuron modeling, the Goldman–Hodgkin–Katz voltage equation (or the Goldman equation) is the standard model used in cell membrane physiology to determine the equilibrium potential across a cell membrane, taking into account all of the relevant ion species active through that membrane (Junge 1981).

Brain function may be viewed as a result of the transformation functions of individual neurons and their precise interconnections. However, the network of neurons that constitute the brain is very well organized into discrete subcomponents. Each subcomponent is connected to a limited set of other subcomponents in specific, well-conserved connectivity patterns. Viewed in this way, it is possible to make a control system-inspired interpretation of the function of the brain in movement control (Fujita 1982; Ito 1972; Kawato and Gomi 1992; Miall and Wolpert 1996; Schweighofer, Arbib, and Kawato 1998; Schweighofer et al. 1998; Wolpert, Miall, and Kawato 1998) and we can interpret the neuronal system for arm–hand movement control as being organized into a number of distinct functional units, in a similar fashion as a control system. Each functional unit, or subcomponent of brain circuitry, hence has a specific function, which can be expressed in mathematical terms. In the case of the brain, this function is carried out by a limited set of neuron types, which typically can have relatively simple internal circuitry connectivity.

Conversely, a mathematical problem formulation of optimal control problem and related adaptive control with tentative solutions was published in Johansson (1990a, 1990b).

In the present study, we aim to provide a mathematical description of the function of one of these functional subunits, namely, the cuneate nucleus, which carries out the first-order processing of movement-generated sensory feedback. We illustrate the firing patterns of the primary afferents, main cuneate neurons, and local inhibitory interneurons and how system identification methods can be used to obtain a mathematical expression of the function carried out by the cuneate nucleus. In ongoing work, we also simulate in detail how the underlying neuronal information processing is carried out, with the aim of providing neuroscientific correlates for specific features in these mathematical expressions.

14.2 Problem Formulation

Because our approach rests on the understanding of the biological system, that is, the brain, much work needed to be devoted the collection of the biological data. The data collection should be from primary afferents; that is, nerve fibers that mediate sensory input from peripheral receptors to the central nervous system, from the main neurons of the cuneate, which project the processed sensory information to the cerebellum (Bengtsson and Jörntell 2009). Ideally, we should record from the primary afferent and its target cuneate neuron simultaneously, but this is technically very difficult. An approximation is to record from primary afferents and cuneate neurons driven by the same inputs. To compare the primary afferent data with the data from the cuneate neurons, comparisons should only be made between primary afferents and neurons that are activated by the same modality of sensory information and from sensory input activated from the same topological area (on the skin or in the joints/muscles). If we can fulfill these criteria, we can take advantage of previous findings suggesting that single primary afferents can have a dominant influence on the cuneate neuron (Ferrington, Rowe, and Tarvin 1987). The transformation taking place between the primary afferent input and the cuneate neuron output for a given stimulus can then be characterized through system identification.

In order to verify that the mathematical model obtained accurately represents the transformation between the primary afferent and the cuneate neuron in the more general case, data from both the primary afferent and cuneate neuron should also be obtained from a very different type of stimulus. If the mathematical model is correct, it should also be able to reproduce the input–output transformation in this case.

14.3 Materials and Methods

The experiments were carried out with single-unit metal microelectrodes and patch clamp recordings in the acute animal preparation of the decerebrated cat as described in Bengtsson and Jörntell (2009) and Jörntell and Ekerot (2003). Primary afferent axons were recorded on their pathway into the cuneate nucleus and cuneate neurons were recorded inside the cuneate nucleus. Stimuli were delivered in two different ways. The first, which was used to produce the model through the system identification, was a standardized manual skin stimulation. A miniature strain-gauge device was mounted on the tip of the investigator in order to control that the same amount of force and the same stimulation time were used. A second mode of stimulus was electrical skin stimulation applied through a pair of needle electrodes inserted into the skin with a spacing of 3 mm. Stimulation intensity was 1.0 mA with a duration 0.1 ms.

As for empirical model estimation, standard methods and validation methods of system identification were used (Johansson and Magnusson 1991).

Then, the recorded data were processed using an action potential pattern recognition software, in order to reduce noise. For every action potential, only the time after stimulation was determined, transforming data to spike-time data. This in turn could be added over several stimulations, yielding histogram data. This was then exported to MATLAB (The Mathworks, Inc., Natick, MA, USA). For the mathematical modeling of the neuron transmission, the MATLAB System Identification Toolbox was used (Ljung 2002). Various different model structures were tested—e.g., prediction error estimate (PEM), ARX, ARMAX, OE, BJ, N4SID (Ljung 2002)—to determine the model that provided the most accurate representation. The starting point was to find the model that most accurately represented the transformation for a standardized manual skin stimulation. Subsequently, we simulated the primary afferent input evoked by electrical skin stimulation and compared the simulated cuneate neuron response with actual responses recorded from the cuneate neuron with the same electrical skin stimulation.

14.4 Results

Figure 14.1 illustrates the spike responses of a primary afferent and a cuneate neuron to manual skin stimulation. The data are displayed as peristimulus histograms; that is, the same stimulation was repeated many times and the spike counts for each bin represent the sum of spike responses for thirty to fifty consecutive, nearly identical stimuli. All stimuli were aligned so that they started at 0 ms and ended at 50 ms. The primary afferent, which conveys

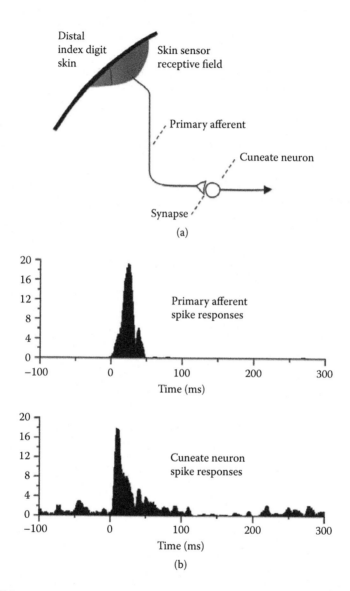

(a)

(b)

FIGURE 14.1

(a) Cartoon illustrating the central parts of the experimental setup. Cuneate neurons receive input from primary afferents, which in turn are excited from peripheral receptors (in this case the skin of the distal index finger or digit) and make excitatory synapses on the cuneate neuron. (b) Using the same standardized manual skin stimulation, data for the spike responses evoked in primary afferents and cuneate neurons were stored as peristimulus histograms (bin width 1 ms, stimulation started at time 0). The duration of the stimuli in this case was indicated to be 50 ms by the strain gauge device.

the input to the cuneate neuron via a synapse (Figure 14.1a), displays spike only on stimulation. Therefore, the time before the stimulation is devoid of spikes, even though the spike response to the stimulation is quite intense (Figure 14.1b, top). In contrast, the cuneate neuron has a spontaneous activity, and hence the spike activity before the stimulation, and in addition it seems to have a more intense spike response to stimulation (note the steep increase in spike activity immediately after the onset of the stimulation; Figure 14.1b, bottom).

In the next step, we simulated that the primary afferent input was driven by electrical skin stimulation. This type of stimulation evokes a precisely timed primary afferent spike, about 4.5 ms after the stimulation, with a near 100% fidelity and a coefficient of variation of 0% (at 0.1 ms resolution; data not shown). Figure 14.2 illustrates the actual cuneate neuron response when this primary afferent spike input was evoked experimentally.

Figure 14.2 illustrates the actual cuneate neuron response when this input was evoked experimentally (upper diagram) and the experimental response (lower diagram) evoked by a single pulse input comparable to the spike response of the real primary afferents (Figure 14.1b).

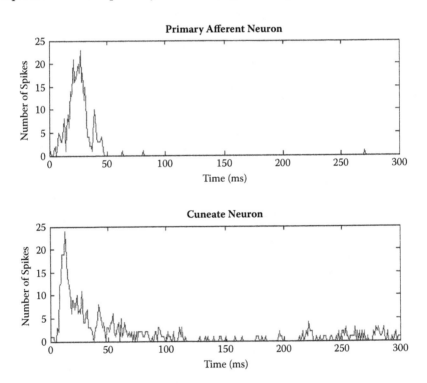

FIGURE 14.2
Primary afferent spike responses (top) and cuneate neuron spike responses (bottom) to electrical skin stimulation.

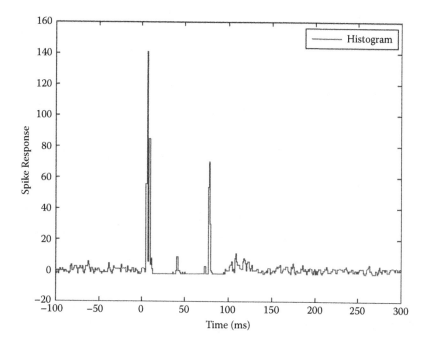

FIGURE 14.3
Spike response recorded from a cuneate neuron subject to electrical skin stimulation.

Figure 14.3 exhibits the spike response recorded from a cuneate neuron subject to electrical skin stimulation.

The traces illustrated in Figure 14.4 show the simulated response of the mathematical model with the best fit. Interestingly, this model captured the fast variations in the initial part of the response quite well but failed to capture the subsequent inhibitory response that followed the initial excitation. It also failed to capture the release from the inhibitory response (at 200 ms+). These two late phases of the response are likely generated by the local inhibitory interneurons of the cuneate nucleus.

With the necessary data at hand, we next attempted to use system identification to find an appropriate mathematical model representing the transformation of the information conveyed by the primary afferent to the cuneate neuron. We found that a PEM, discrete-time state–space model of fifth order gave the best fit, in the form of a state–space model:

$$x_{k+1} = Ax_k + Bu_k + Kw_k$$

$$y_k = Cx_k + w_k$$

The fit for the PEM, ARX, ARMAX, OE, and BJ models were 66, 61, 66, 64, and 64%, respectively.

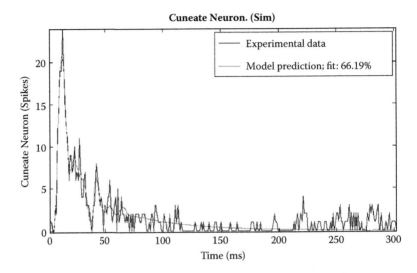

FIGURE 14.4
Recorded (black trace) and simulated response (gray trace) of a cuneate neuron to primary afferent response shown in Figure 14.1b.

The estimated state–space model is as follows:

$$x_{k+1} = Ax_k + Bu_k + Kw_k$$

$$y_k = Cx_k + w_k$$

with the system matrices

$$
A = \begin{bmatrix}
1.0281 & 0.1103 & -0.0329 & -0.0179 & -0.0476 \\
0.0078 & 0.9167 & 0.1257 & -0.0376 & 0.5252 \\
-0.0744 & -0.0056 & 0.8474 & 0.3213 & -0.0070 \\
-0.0002 & -0.0528 & -0.4983 & 0.7843 & 0.0813 \\
-0.0207 & -0.1959 & -0.0113 & -0.3575 & 0.7903
\end{bmatrix}
$$

$$
B = \begin{bmatrix}
0.0027 \\
-0.0163 \\
-0.0004 \\
-0.0095 \\
0.0018
\end{bmatrix}, \quad
K = \begin{bmatrix}
0.0026 \\
0.0022 \\
0.0033 \\
0.0070 \\
-0.0039
\end{bmatrix} w
$$

$$C = \begin{bmatrix} 20.5466 & -9.6495 & 4.4225 & 1.8089 & 5.8488 \end{bmatrix}$$

Figure 14.5 shows the impulse response for the PEM in the form of a state–space model of the cuneate spike response. In this case, the fit between the experimental data and the prediction accuracy of the simulation appears to be very high, although the temporal relationships seem to need some further refinements of the model. In the recorded data (see Figure 14.3) the spontaneous firing activity of the cuneate neuron provides a background against which inhibitory effects in the neuron can also be recorded (as a temporary depression of the spontaneous firing activity). This occurs immediately after the initial excitatory response. In the model, inhibition is represented by negative output, something that is not possible in the brain for neurons that make excitatory synapses (which is the case for the cuneate neurons that make excitatory synapses with neurons of the cerebellum and thalamus). However, spontaneous background activity also participates in determining the spike output of the downstream neurons (i.e., in the cerebellum and thalamus), so the reduction of this background activity can actually be viewed as being equivalent to negative

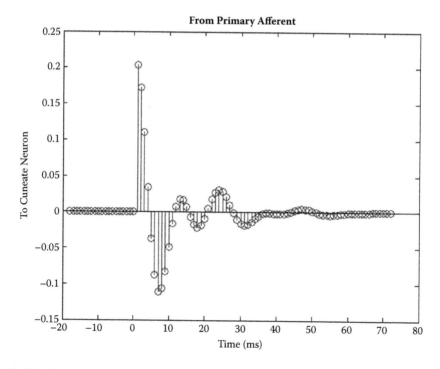

FIGURE 14.5
Impulse response for the PEM in the form of a state–space model of the cuneate spike response.

output. Therefore, we can conclude that the mathematical model reflects the response properties of the primary afferent-to-cuneate neuron junction well. Because it is able to do so for two widely different inputs (manual skin stimulation that evokes a primary afferent spike response lasting 50 ms and electrical skin stimulation that evokes a spike response lasting for 0.1 ms), it promises to be able to account for the response properties over a wide range of inputs and perhaps covering the majority of the physiological range of inputs.

As an illustration of model variability, Figure 14.6 shows the impulse response corresponding to electrical skin stimulation for the ARX model. It is evident that these models do not capture the cuneate neuron firing mechanics in response to electrical stimulation as the PEM model did. These empirical mathematical models are of the form

- ARX:
$$A(z)y_k = B(z)u_k + w_k$$

- OE:
$$y_k = \frac{B(z)}{F(z)} u_k + w_k$$

Figure 14.7 shows the Bode diagram of the PEM model. Interestingly, the diagram shows deriving properties for a large part of the spectrum with

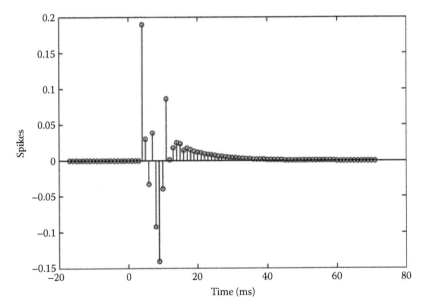

FIGURE 14.6
Impulse response for the ARX model.

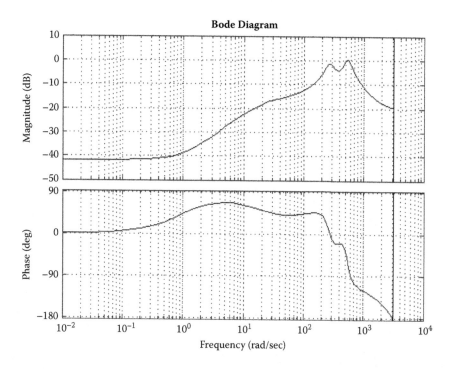

FIGURE 14.7

Bode diagram of the PEM model of the cuneate spike response. It is interesting to note that the model exhibits differentiating properties and phase lead for a part of the spectrum, indicating that these properties could be important features of the cuneate neuron.

phase lead. These are favorable properties from a control systems point of view. This indicates that these properties could be important features of the cuneate neuron in its role of transforming sensory information from primary afferent neurons to the cerebellum, which in turn can be viewed as a controller of body movements.

Finally, a Ho-Kalman impulse response model reproducing cuneate histogram spike-response data was made with high modeling accuracy (Figure 14.8). Note that a long-term response was reproduced by the model.

14.4 Discussion

Based on the findings of Figures 14.5, 14.7, and 14.9, the empirical cuneate model exhibits differentiating characteristics, suggesting a phase lead action of the cuneate response. When a longer impulse response is considered (see Figure 14.9), the differentiating aspects are less pronounced.

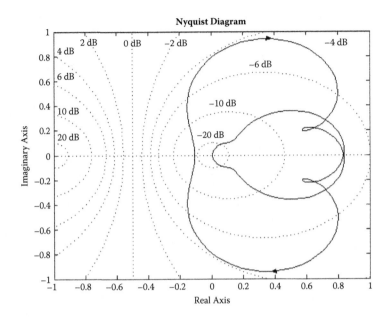

FIGURE 14.8

Nyquist diagram of the PEM model of the cuneate spike response including closed-loop gain-level surfaces for the cuneate spike response. It is interesting to note that the model shows differentiating properties and phase lead for a part of the spectrum, indicating that these properties could be important features of the cuneate neuron.

14.5 Conclusions

Our preliminary findings suggest that system identification can be used to identify the mathematical properties of a local neural structure with an uncomplicated network structure. The failure to reproduce the later phases of the response to manual skin stimulation (see Figure 14.2) can be explained by the fact that this response occurred well after the cessation of the primary afferent spike train. In the brain, this type of response is likely created by the local inhibitory interneurons, which is an input that was not known to the model. Future modeling experiments will show whether the addition of this factor can make the model reproduce this aspect of the response.

Based on these findings and the previous experimental results of Ekerot and Jörntell (2001, 2003), Bengtsson and Jörntell (2009), Jörntell and Ekerot (1999, 2002, 2003, 2006), and Jörntell and Hansel (2006), further modeling of neural structures—inside and outside the cerebellum, in order to understand control system aspects—could potentially give new insights into cerebellar movement control. This aspect—that is, how the cerebellum achieves movement control—could be of great interest not only in the field of neuroscience but in robotics and other control applications as well.

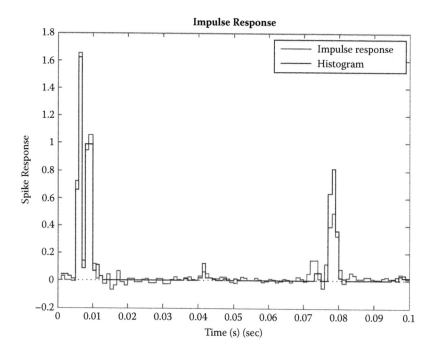

FIGURE 14.9

Ho-Kalman impulse response model reproducing cuneate histogram spike-response data.

References

Apps, R. and Garwicz, M. 2005. Anatomical and physiological foundations of cerebellar information processing. *Nature Reviews Neuroscience*, 6: 297–311.

Bengtsson, F. and Jörntell, H. 2009. Sensory transmission in cerebellar granule cells relies on similarly coded mossy fiber inputs. *Proceedings of the National Academy of Sciences USA*, 106: 2389–2394.

Ekerot, C.F. and Jörntell, H. 2001. Parallel fibre receptive fields of Purkinje cells and interneurons are climbing fibre-specific. *European Journal of Neuroscience*, 13: 1303–1310.

Ekerot, C.F. and Jörntell, H. 2003. Parallel fiber receptive fields: A key to understanding cerebellar operation and learning. *Cerebellum*, 2: 101–109.

Ferrington, D.G., Rowe, M.J., and Tarvin, R.P. 1987. Actions of single sensory fibres on cat dorsal column nuclei neurones: vibratory signalling in a one-to-one linkage. *Journal of Physiology*, 386: 293–309.

Fujita, M. 1982. Adaptive filter model of the cerebellum. *Biological Cybernetics*, 45: 195–206.

Ito, M. 1972. Neural design of the cerebellar motor control system. *Brain Research*, 40: 81–84.

Ito, M. 2008. Control of mental activities by internal models in the cerebellum. *Nature Reviews Neuroscience*, 9: 304–313.

Johansson, R. 1990a. Adaptive control of robot manipulator motion. *IEEE Transactions on Robotics and Automation*, 6(4): 483–490.

Johansson, R. 1990b. Quadratic optimization of motion coordination and control. *IEEE Transactions on Automatic Control*, 35(11): 1197–1208.

Johansson, R. 1993. *System Modeling and Identification*. Englewood Cliffs, NJ: Prentice Hall.

Johansson, R. and Magnusson, M. 1991. Optimal coordination and control of posture and locomotion. *Mathematical Biosciences*, 103: 203–244.

Jörntell, H. and Ekerot, C.F. 1999. Topographical organization of projections to cat motor cortex from nucleus interpositus anterior and forelimb skin. *Journal of Physiology (London)*, 514(Pt. 2): 551–566.

Jörntell, H. and Ekerot, C.F. 2002. Reciprocal bidirectional plasticity of parallel fiber receptive fields in cerebellar Purkinje cells and their afferent interneurons. *Neuron*, 34: 797–806.

Jörntell, H. and Ekerot, C.F. 2003. Receptive field plasticity profoundly alters the cutaneous parallel fiber synaptic input to cerebellar interneurons in vivo. *Journal of Neuroscience*, 23: 9620–9631.

Jörntell, H. and Ekerot, C.F. 2006. Properties of somatosensory synaptic integration in cerebellar granule cells in vivo. *Journal of Neuroscience*, 26: 11786–11797.

Jörntell, H. and Hansel, C. 2006. Synaptic memories upside down: Bidirectional plasticity at cerebellar parallel fiber-Purkinje cell synapses. *Neuron*, 52: 227–238.

Junge, D. 1981. *Nerve and Muscle Excitation* (2nd ed.). Sunderland, MA: Sinauer Associates.

Kawato, M. and Gomi, H. 1992. A computational model of four regions of the cerebellum based on feedback-error learning. *Biological Cybernetics*, 68: 95–103.

Ljung, L. 2002. *System Identification Toolbox for Matlab*. Natick, MA: MathWorks.

Miall, R.C. and Wolpert, D.M. 1996. Forward models for physiological motor control. *Neural Networks*, 9: 1265–1279.

Schweighofer, N., Arbib, M.A., and Kawato, M. 1998. Role of the cerebellum in reaching movements in humans. I. Distributed inverse dynamics control. *European Journal of Neuroscience*, 10: 86–94.

Schweighofer, N., Spoelstra, J., Arbib, M.A., and Kawato, M. 1998. Role of the cerebellum in reaching movements in humans. II. A neural model of the intermediate cerebellum. *European Journal of Neuroscience*, 10: 95–105.

Wolpert, D.M., Miall, R.C., and Kawato, M. 1998. Internal models in the cerebellum. *Trends in Cognitive Science*, 2: 338–347.

15

Development of Hand Rehabilitation System Using Wire-Driven Link Mechanism for Paralysis Patients

Hiroshi Yamaura
Panasonic Corporation
Osaka, Japan

Kojiro Matsushita
Osaka University Medical School
Osaka, Japan

Ryu Kato and Hiroshi Yokoi
The University of Electro-Communications
Tokyo, Japan

CONTENTS

15.1 Introduction 278
15.2 Proposed Design 280
    15.2.1 Four-Link Mechanism with the Wire-Driven Mechanism 280
    15.2.2 Coupled Mechanism for the Distal Interphalangeal and
    Proximal Interphalangeal Joints 285
15.3 Actual Hand Rehabilitation Machine 285
15.4 Working of the Hand Rehabilitation Machine 288
15.5 Working of the Hand Rehabilitation System 289
15.6 Conclusions and Future Works 291
References 292

Abstract

In this chapter, we present a hand rehabilitation system for patients suffering from paralysis or contracture. This system consists of two components: a hand rehabilitation machine, which moves human finger joints by using motors, and a data glove, which enables control of the movement of the finger joints attached to the rehabilitation machine. The machine is based on the arm structure type of hand rehabilitation machine; a motor indirectly moves a finger joint via a closed four-link mechanism. We used a wire-driven mechanism and a coupled mechanism for the distal interphalangeal (DIP) and proximal interphalangeal (PIP) joints. These mechanisms render the machine lightweight, resulting in a wider range of motion than that obtainable in conventional systems. The design specifications for the mechanisms and the experimental results are described in this chapter.

15.1 Introduction

As the development of various technologies in medical applications becomes more rapid, machine-assisted physical rehabilitation, which requires long-term recurrent movements, is in increasing demand. For example, hand rehabilitation is an important process because hand movement is one of the most basic actions performed in daily life. Generally, hand paralysis or contracture is treated with the assistance of a physical therapist. The therapist holds and repeatedly moves the fingers affected by paralysis or contracture through the maximum range of their joint angles (Figure 15.1). A few months are usually required to improve the range through which the fingers can move. As a result, hand rehabilitation is expensive and time consuming. Furthermore, the unavailability of physical therapists underscores the requirement for engineering solutions for physical rehabilitation. A hand rehabilitation machine that can act as a substitute for physical therapists would be beneficial (Burger et al. 2000).

Conventional hand rehabilitation machines are categorized into two types: endoskeleton and exoskeleton. The main difference between these two types

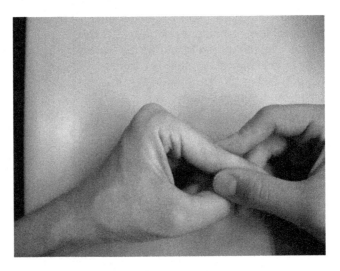

FIGURE 15.1
Rehabilitation of the injured finger.

of machines is the manner in which the machine is attached to the human body. With the endoskeleton type, actuators are attached directly to the skeleton and the joints are actuated by the actuators directly. With the exoskeleton type, a link mechanism is attached to the body and the joints are actuated by the actuators, which are operated by a link mechanism. The endoskeleton-type machines generally use pneumatic actuators as substitutes for human muscles. A pneumatic actuator consists of rubber, a tube, and an air compressor. Because the drive unit (i.e., the rubber) is assembled separately, the pneumatic actuator has the advantages of high driving capability and a lightweight drive source (i.e., the air compressor; Noritsugu 2008). However, the actuator shape limits the number of places where the actuator can be attached; that is, this type of machine is not suitable for hand rehabilitation because it is difficult to attach a pneumatic actuator within the limited space available on a human finger. Exoskeleton-type machines are generally heavier than endoskeleton-type machines. However, the link mechanism enables the placement of the actuators anywhere on the human body. Thus, exoskeleton-type machines are potentially suitable for use for any part of the human body; therefore, we used an exoskeleton-type machine for our hand rehabilitation system.

Exoskeleton-type machines are mechanically categorized on the basis of their structure, including joint structure, arch structure, and arm structure types of machines (Figure 15.2). The joint structure type is characterized by actuators set along the fingers. It has high controllability because the actuators move the paralyzed finger joint. However, the joint structure is placed along the sides of the finger and is available for only the first, second, and fifth fingers; that is, this machine cannot be placed between fingers. Hasegawa et al. (2008) developed a power assist glove based on joint structure. The glove uses motors and wire-driven mechanisms as drive sources; it is lightweight and has high drive (the grasping force of the glove is 15[N]). The third and fourth fingers, which cannot be attached to the machine, are moved by coupling them with the fifth finger. The arch structure type is characterized by an arc slider placed on the finger joint; the finger is moved by actuating the slider. Because the slider is placed on the finger, the machine can be used on all fingers (i.e.,

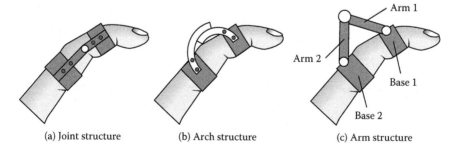

(a) Joint structure   (b) Arch structure   (c) Arm structure

FIGURE 15.2
Mechanisms of exoskeleton-type machines.

the arch structure resolves the problem faced when using the joint structure type of machine). Fu, Wang, and Wang (2008) developed a hand rehabilitation machine with an arch structure, and they were able to successfully control four joints in a single finger. The above-mentioned examples show that machines can possibly substitute for physical therapists because they can suitably control finger movement. A disadvantage of both the joint and arch structure type of machines is the difficulty involved in attaching them to the fingers; that is, the rotational centers of the joints of these structures should match that of the corresponding finger joint. Moreover, each finger has a different length; hence, the structure of the machine must be suitably modified for each user and different finger lenths. One of the solutions to this problem is the arm structure type of machine, which was proposed by Fu, Zhang, and Wang (2004); Kawasaki et al. (2007) developed an arm structure consisting of a closed four-link mechanism: four links (i.e., two metal links and two human finger links) and four joints (one actuated joint, two free joints, and one human finger joint). The finger joint is not directly controlled by the actuated joint. The geometry of the links indirectly controls the finger. In the closed four-link mechanism, the distance between Base 1 and Base 2 (Figure 15.2c) is adjustable because of the free joints. Thus, this structure can be adjusted to suit any user without any design modification, which enhances its practical usability.

However, the closed four-link mechanism has three structural problems: (1) The finger joint has two possible configurations for an angle of the actuated joint. Thus, it becomes necessary to avoid some angles of the actuated joint; that is, this mechanism limits the range of joint motion. (2) The machine is heavy because the motor is placed inside the mechanism. Thus, this structure is not suitable for long-term use. (3) The mechanism overloads the finger joint when the finger joint bends more than 90 degrees. This is because the free joints cannot generate rotational torque; instead, they apply shear forces to the finger joint. This, too, limits the range of the joint angle.

In this study, we developed a new hand rehabilitation machine that is based on arm structure. We aimed to reduce the weight of the machine and increase the range of joint motion by using a wire-driven mechanism. Furthermore, we propose a hand rehabilitation system in which fingers affected by paralysis can be moved using the proposed hand rehabilitation machine, and the finger joints can be controlled using a data glove worn on the healthy hand.

15.2 Proposed Design

15.2.1 Four-Link Mechanism with the Wire-Driven Mechanism

The arm structure type of hand rehabilitation machine uses a closed four-link mechanism, and this machine can be attached to fingers of any length. To the best of our knowledge, this is the most convenient hand rehabilitation machine available at present. Therefore, we focused on the arm structure type of machine and endeavored to improve its performance; specifically, we aimed to increase the range of joint motion and improve the control of finger movement. To achieve this, we propose a design that combines the closed four-link mechanism with a wire-driven mechanism.

Our basic design is based on the arm structure type of machine (Figure 15.2c), which has three joints—one motor joint and two free joints—in the closed four-link mechanism. We substituted the motor joint with a free joint and attached three pulleys to the three free joints. The pulleys are connected by two wires (Figure 15.3a); the gray line represents a flexion wire, and the black line represents an extension wire. One end of each wire is attached to Base 1, and the other end is attached to a motor. The rehabilitation machine bends the finger when the flexion wire is pulled (Figure 15.3b) and extends the finger when the extension wire is pulled (Figure 15.3c). A conceptual diagram of the rehabilitation machine is shown in Figure 15.4. The wire-driven mechanism allows spatial separation of the drive from the actuator. In this mechanism, the motor is not placed on the fingers, thereby reducing the weight of the machine on the finger. Furthermore, because the motor does not occupy space on the finger, we can add three arm

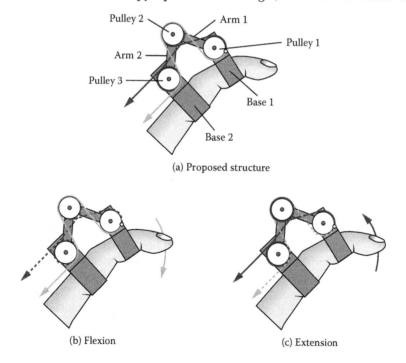

(a) Proposed structure

(b) Flexion

(c) Extension

FIGURE 15.3
Proposed design.

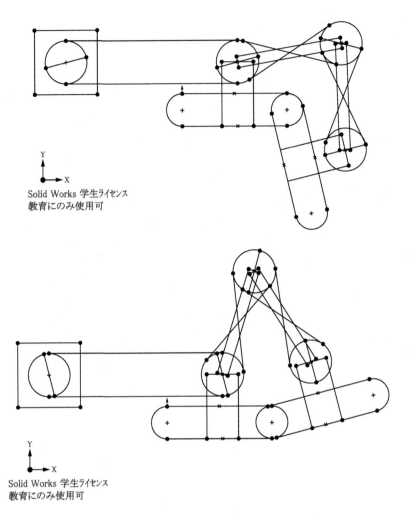

FIGURE 15.4
Flexion and extension actuated by a single motor.

structures on a finger, thus affording multiple degrees of freedom (DOFs). Therefore, it is possible to use a motor with a higher drive, which is heavier. Our proposed design is advantageous because this system would have a lighter weight, higher drive, and thus greater DOFs than do conventional machines. This mechanism can adjust to various hand sizes (Figure 15.5).

The combination of the wire-driven mechanism and closed four-link mechanism overcomes the limitations of the arm structure. In the original arm structure design, the motor could not rotate when the three joints were in a straight line. However, in the proposed design, all three joints can be coupled and actuated with one motor. Therefore, even when the joints are in a straight line, the motor continues to rotate easily; that is, the proposed design

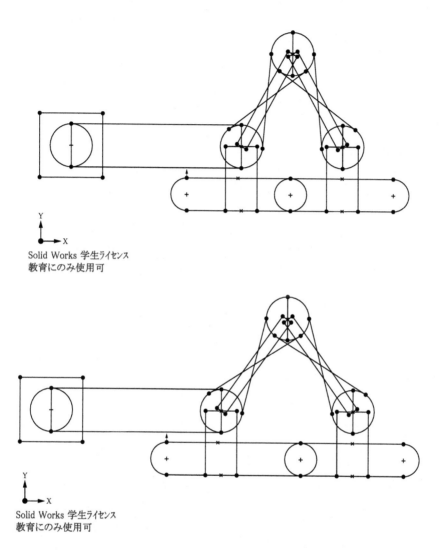

FIGURE 15.5
Adjustment of structure to various hand sizes.

enables a wider range of joint motion than does the original arm structure. In summary, the proposed hand rehabilitation machine is designed to be practically applicable. Its light weight will enable patients to use it for a long period. It offers multiple DOFs and high drive, which enhance the control of the fingers; this machine can therefore be used for various rehabilitation plans. To analyze the range of joint angles achievable using our proposed design, we constructed a mathematical model of the proposed machine (Figure 15.6). It consists of three pulleys, two links, and two wires. A wire runs from Base 1 to Pulley 3. Point A on Base 1 indicates the starting point of

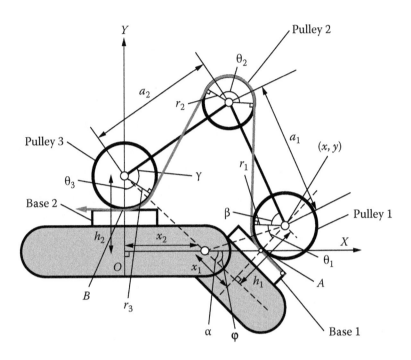

FIGURE 15.6
Schematic diagram of wire-driven mechanism.

the wire, and point A on Pulley 3 indicates its end point. The length l_{AB} of the wire between the two pulleys is given by Equation (15.1).

$$l_{AB} = r_1\theta_1 + r_2\theta_2 + r_3\theta_3 + \sqrt{a_1^2 - (r_1 + r_2)^2} + \sqrt{a_2^2 - (r_2 + r_3)^2} \qquad (15.1)$$

The point (x,y) is expressed as shown in Equations (15.2) and (15.3):

$$x = x_2 + L\cos(\alpha - \varphi)$$
$$= a_2\sin(\theta_3 + \gamma) - a_2\sin(\theta_2 - \theta_3 - \beta) \qquad (15.2)$$

$$y = L\sin(\alpha - \varphi)$$
$$= h_2 - a_2\cos(\theta_3 + \gamma) + a_1\cos(\theta_2 - \theta_3 + \beta) \qquad (15.3)$$

L, α, β, and γ are expressed as follows:

$$L = \sqrt{{x_1}^2 + {h_1}^2}$$

$$\alpha = \arctan \frac{h_1}{x_1}$$

$$\beta = \arccos \frac{r_1 + r_2}{a_1}$$

$$\gamma = \arccos \frac{r_2 + r_3}{a_2}$$

The geometrical relation yields the following equation:

$$\varphi = \pi - \theta_1 + \theta_2 - \theta_3 \qquad (15.4)$$

The relation between l_{AB} and φ is obtained by removing θ_1, θ_2, and θ_3 in Equations (15.1) to (15.4); that is, the result indicates that the traction distance of the wire controls the human finger joint.

15.2.2 Coupled Mechanism for the Distal Interphalangeal and Proximal Interphalangeal Joints

Physiological studies have revealed that the distal interphalangeal (DIP) and proximal interphalangeal (PIP) joints in a human finger are actuated with the same muscles, and the movements are coupled. We used a similar coupled mechanism in our hand rehabilitation machine in order to enhance its mobility; that is, reducing the number of motors results in a lighter and smaller machine that is long lasting. The conceptual design of the coupled mechanism is shown in Figure 15.7: (1) the wire-driven four-link mechanism is set on the DIP and PIP joints; (2) the wire that bends the DIP joint is connected to the wire that bends the PIP joint; and (3) the wire that extends the DIP joint is connected to the wire that extends the PIP joint. Thus, both the DIP and PIP joints are both subjected to the same directional force through the connected wires, and the movements are coupled.

15.3 Actual Hand Rehabilitation Machine

A computer-aided design (CAD) image and a photograph of the proposed rehabilitation machine are shown in Figures 15.8 and 15.9, respectively. The machine is designed such that there are three arm structures for the metacarpophalangeal

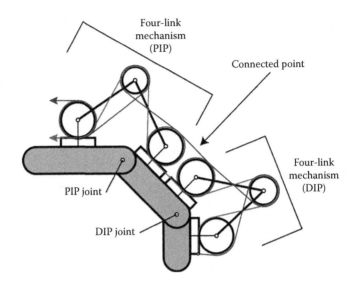

FIGURE 15.7
Coupled mechanism for the DIP and PIP joints.

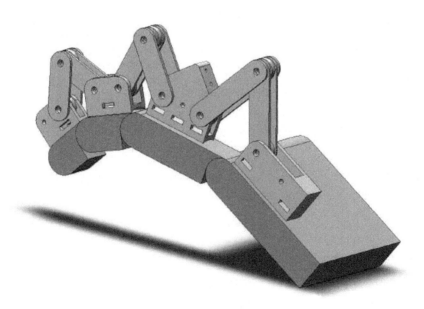

FIGURE 15.8
CAD image of the exoskeleton of the proposed machine for one finger.

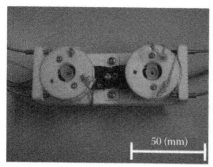

Motor unit

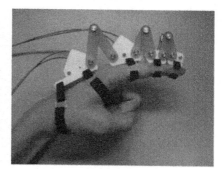

Exoskeleton

FIGURE 15.9
Prototype of the exoskeleton for one finger.

(MP), PIP, and DIP joints. The arm structure for the MP joint is actuated with a radio control (RC) servo; the arm structures for the PIP and DIP joints are coupled using two wires so that these joints are actuated with another RC servo (i.e., interference mechanism). Thus, this machine uses two RC servos to move three finger joints. The arm structure is made of two materials: the base is made of fine nylon, and the arm is made of glass epoxy. The weight of the arm structure is 51 g. We used Velcro tape to attach the arm structure to the fingers, because it is easy to attach and remove. We used the wire-driven mechanism to make the structure light. This mechanism allows the user to place the actuators on arbitrary locations. We plan to place the motor unit on the user's shoulder or the lower back of the user so that long-term usage is possible. The arm structure is actuated with the RC servo through two wires. The wires are made of polyethylene, and they are connected to the motor through a metal spring tube. A motor unit is shown in Figure 15.9. It consists of two RC servos, two pulleys, and one RC servo case with a tube attachment made of fine nylon. Its weight is 83 g. The motor is an RC servo (GWS Micro 2BBMG [Grand Wing System U.S.A. Inc., City of Industry CA, USA]; torque, 5.4 kg · cm; weight, 28 g; dimensions, 28 × 30 × 14 mm^3). The specifications of the hand rehabilitation machine are listed in Table 15.1.

TABLE 15.1

Specifications of Hand
Rehabilitation System

Weight	Exoskeleton: 51 g
	Motor unit: 83 g
Arm length	DIP: 20.0 mm
	PIP: 25.0 mm
	MP: 35 mm
Width	17.5 mm

15.4 Working of the Hand Rehabilitation Machine

The attachment of the hand rehabilitation machine to a hand is shown in Figure 15.9. The machine is suitably attached to the second finger (finger length, 69 mm; Figure 15.10a-1) and to the fifth finger (finger length, 58 mm; Figure 15.10b-1); after attachment, the machine can move these fingers. The time required to adjust the arm structure according to the finger length is within 1 min.

The machine could successfully bend the finger joints (Figures 15.10a-2 and 15.10b-2); the ranges of motion are listed in Table 15.2. In both cases, the machine could smoothly bend the DIP joints at sufficient angles. This indicates that the coupled mechanism for DIP and PIP joints works properly. Moreover, because the pulleys on the arm structure simultaneously rotate with the wire-driven mechanism, the user feels less loading on the finger. Furthermore, the combination of the closed four-link mechanism and the wire-driven mechanism results in a one-to-one positional relationship between the motor joint and the human finger joint, which offers better control than that provided by the original arm structure.

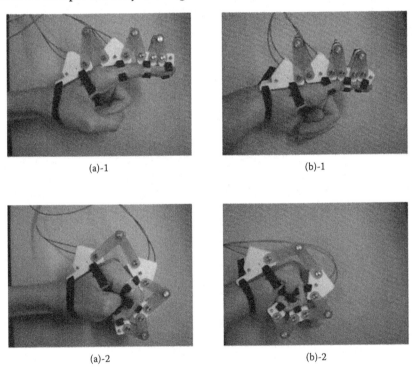

(a)-1   (b)-1

(a)-2   (b)-2

FIGURE 15.10
Operation of the (a) index finger and (b) little finger.

TABLE 15.2

Supported Range of Motion for the Little/Index Finger Joints

	Little Finger		Index Finger	
	Extension	Flexion	Extension	Flexion
MP (°)	0	85	0	85
PIP (°)	0	90	0	90
DIP (°)	0	65	0	65

© 2009 IEEE.

15.5 Working of the Hand Rehabilitation System

Generally, hand paralysis affects only one hand. Therefore, some hand rehabilitation systems involve the use of the unaffected healthy hand. This is known as *self-motion control*.

For example, Kawasaki et al. (2007) developed a hand rehabilitation system that acquires information about the joint angles of the healthy hand and controls the paralyzed hand with a machine by using this information.

In this study, we applied the same concept to our hand rehabilitation system (Figure 15.11). The hand rehabilitation system is used in the following sequence: (1) The user wears the data glove on the healthy hand (Figure 15.12). (2) The rehabilitation machine is attached to the target finger of the affected hand. (3) The machine is calibrated for maximum flexion and extension of the finger (Figure 15.12). (4) The target finger joints are controlled by the finger joints on the data glove (i.e., mirror motion). Thus, hand rehabilitation is performed without the help of a physical therapist. In addition, this system has a motion playback function that can be used without the help of a therapist.

The data glove system measures the angles of the DIP and PIP joints on the index finger of the left hand. This information is fed as control input to the hand rehabilitation machine, and this input controls the angles of the DIP and PIP joints on the index finger of the right hand. The workings of the data glove system are shown in Figure 15.13: the DIP and PIP joints on the index finger of the right hand are controlled using the index finger on the left hand. Thus, the hand rehabilitation machine, which is controlled by the data glove, enables the user to achieve complex finger movements (Figure 15.14). This system greatly contributes to hand rehabilitation and can be used without the aid of a therapist. In addition, because this system has a motion playback function, the user can record finger movements for a maximum of 10 seconds and play back the finger movements cyclically. Thus, long-term passive rehabilitation can be provided.

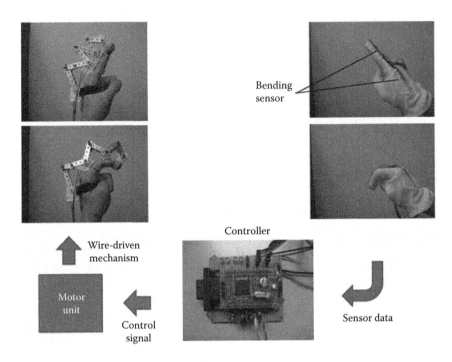

FIGURE 15.11
Control system of the hand rehabilitation system for hemiplegic patients.

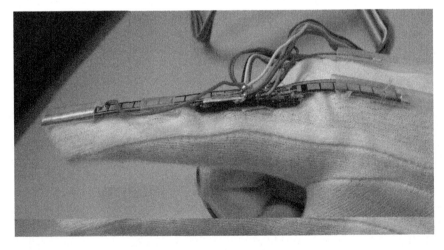

FIGURE 15.12
Data glove used for measurement of DIP and PIP joint angles.

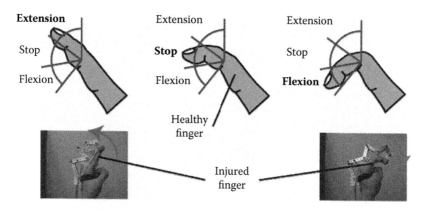

FIGURE 15.13
Determination of the range of motion.

15.6 Conclusions and Future Works

We have developed a hand rehabilitation system for patients affected by paralysis or contracture. It consists of 2 two components: a hand rehabilitation machine, which moves human finger joints using motors, and a data glove, which provides control of the finger joints attached to the rehabilitation machine. The machine is based on the arm structure type of rehabilitation machine; a motor indirectly moves a finger joint via a closed four-link mechanism. We have employed a wire-driven mechanism and have developed a compact design that can control all three joints (i.e., PIP, DIP, and MP joints) of a finger; the design renders the machine lightweight and offers a wider range of joint motion than conventional systems. Further, we have demonstrated the hand rehabilitation process in which the finger joints of the left hand attached to the machine are controlled by the finger joints of the right hand wearing the data glove.

We intended to resolve the following issues in future studies in order to improve the practical application of our proposed system: (1) The range of motion of the machine needs to be improved because a certified hand rehabilitation machine is required to move human fingers through the following angles: 85 degrees at the MP joint, 110 degrees at the PIP joint, and 65 degrees at the DIP joint (Fu, Zhang, and Wang 2004). (2) A rehabilitation machine that can be used with all five fingers needs to be developed and its performance evaluated by testing it on actual patients. (3) A method that enables hemiplegic and paraplegic patients to control the system without the aid of therapists needs to be developed because these patients cannot achieve self-motion control.

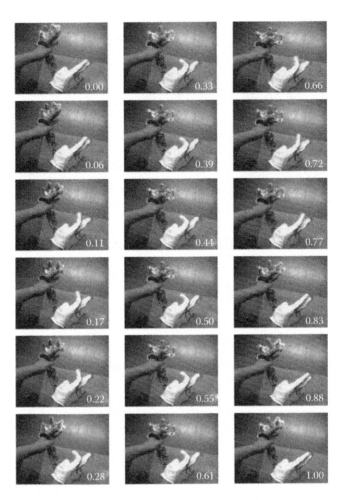

FIGURE 15.14
Demonstration of the data glove system.

References

Burger, C.G., Lum, P.S., Shor, P.C., and Machiel Van der Loos, H.F. 2000. Development of robots for rehabilitation therapy: The Palo Alto VA/Stanford experience. *Journal of Rehabilitation Research and Development*, 37(6): 663–673.

Fu, Y., Wang, P., and Wang, S. 2008. Development of a multi-DOF exoskeleton based machine for injured fingers. Paper presented at the IEEE/RSJ International Conference on Intelligent Robots and Systems, Nice, France, September 22–26, 2008, 1946–1951.

Fu, Y., Zhang, F., and Wang, S. 2004. Structure types design and genetic algorithm dimension synthesis of a CPM machine for injured fingers. Paper read at the International Conference on Robotics and Biomimetics, Shenyang, China, August 22–26, 640–644.

Hasegawa, Y., Mikami, Y., Watanabe, K., and Sankai, Y. 2008. Five-fingered assistive hand with mechanical compliance of human. Paper presented at the IEEE International Conference on Robotics and Automation, Pasadena, CA, May 19–23, 2008, 718–729.

Kawasaki, H., Ito, S., Ishigure, Y., Nishimoto, Y., Aoki, T., Mouri, T., Sakaeda, H., and Abe, M. 2007. Development of a hand motion assist robot for rehabilitation therapy by self-motion control. Paper presented at the IEEE 10th International Conference on Rehabilitation Robotics, 12–15 June, Noordwijk, The Netherlands, June 12–15, 2007, 234–240.

Noritsugu, T., Yamamoto, H., Sasaki, D., and Takaiwa, M. 2008. Wearable power assist device for hand grasping using pneumatic artificial rubber muscle. Paper presented at the SICE Annual Conference, Sapporo, Japan, August 4–6, 2004, 420–425.

16

A Test Environment for Studying the Human-Likeness of Robotic Eye Movements*

Stefan Kohlbecher, Klaus Bartl, and Erich Schneider
University of Munich Hospital
Munich, Germany

Jürgen Blume, Alexander Bannat, Stefan Sosnowski,
Kolja Kühnlenz, and Gerhard Rigoll
Technische Universität München
Munich, Germany

Frank Wallhoff
Jade University of Applied Sciences
Oldenburg, Germany

CONTENTS

16.1 Introduction 296
    16.1.1 State of the Art 298
    16.1.2 Motivation 299
    16.1.3 Objectives 299
16.2 Methods 300
    16.2.1 Robots 300
        16.2.1.1 ELIAS 300
        16.2.1.2 EDDIE 301
    16.2.2 Camera Motion Device 302
    16.2.3 Eye and Head Tracker 304
    16.2.4 Teleoperation Channel 305
16.3 Discussion and Results 306
    16.3.1 Handling of Eye Vergence 306
    16.3.2 Camera Motion Device 306
    16.3.3 Eye and Head Tracker 308
16.4 Conclusion and Future Work 309
Acknowledgments 310
References 310

* Portions reprinted, with permission, from "Experimental Platform for Wizard-of-Oz Evaluations of Biomimetic Active Vision in Robots," 2009 IEEE International Conference on Robotics and Biomimetics (ROBIO), © 2009 IEEE.

Abstract

A novel paradigm for the evaluation of human–robot interaction is pro-posed, with special focus on the importance of natural eye and head movements in nonverbal human–machine communication scenarios. We present an experimental platform that will enable Wizard-of-Oz experi-ments in which a human experimenter (*wizard*) teleoperates a robotic head and eyes with his own head and eyes. Because the robot is ani-mated based on the nonverbal behaviors of the human experimenter, the whole range of human eye movements can be presented without having to implement a complete gaze behavior model first. The experimenter watches and reacts to the video stream of the participant, who directly interacts with the robot. Results are presented that focus on those tech-nical aspects of the experimental platform that enable real-time and human-like interaction capabilities. In particular, the tracking of ocular motor dynamics, its replication in a robotic active vision system, and the involved teleoperation delays are evaluated. This setup will help to answer the question of which aspects of human gaze and head move-ment behavior have to be implemented to achieve humanness in active vision systems of robots.

16.1 Introduction

How important is it to resemble human performance in artificial eyes and which aspects of ocular and neck motor functionality are key to people's attribution of humanness to robot heads? In a first step toward answering this question, we have implemented an experimental platform that facili-tates evaluations of human-like robotic eye and head movements in human–machine interactions. It is centered around a pair of artificial eyes exceeding human performance in terms of acceleration and angular velocity. Due to their modular nature and small form factor, they were already integrated into two different robots.

We also provide two distinct ways to control the robotic eye and head movements. There is a simple MATLAB (The MathWorks, Natick, MA, USA) interface that allows easy implementation of experiments in controlled envi-ronments. But we also wanted to be able to examine eye and head movements in the context of natural conversation scenarios. Facing the challenging task of implementing a complicated conversation flow model that involves speech recognition, synthesis, and semantic processing, we decided to take a short-cut and put a real human "inside" the robot who would not only speak and listen through the robot but also be able to naturally control the robot's eyes and head with his own eyes and head.

This novel Wizard-of-Oz scenario, in which the experimenter (wizard) teleoperates the head and eye movements of a robot (see Figure 16.1), ensures

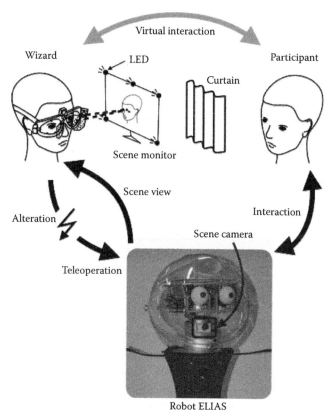

FIGURE 16.1
Experimental platform for Wizard-of-Oz evaluations of gaze-based human–robot interaction. The hidden experimenter (wizard, left) teleoperates a robot (bottom) with his head and eyes. Equipped with a head-mounted eye tracker and a LED-based head tracker, the wizard sits in front of a calibrated computer screen that displays the video stream of the robot scene camera. Thereby, the wizard—and hence the robot—can observe and react to the actions of the human participant (right). With this setup, a natural gaze-based and nonverbal interaction can be established between the robot and a human participant. In future experiments the teleoperation channel will be systematically altered (denoted by a flash) in order to examine the effects of artificial changes in ocular motor functionality on, for example, participant–robot interaction performance. © 2009 IEEE.

that the robot is equipped with natural, human-like eye movements from the beginning, without the need to implement a gaze model first.

Direct communication between humans normally occurs through speech. But there are other, nonverbal channels, too, such as body language, gestures, facial expressions, and eye contact. Eye movements are a vital component of communication (Argyle, Cook, and Argyle 1976; Emery 2000; Langton, Watt, and Bruce 2000). An overview of the different roles of gaze in human communication can be found in Argyle et al. (1973).

The basis for verbal communication has previously been implemented in robotic systems. Speech recognition and synthesis are an accepted means of human–machine interaction, used, for example, in call centers. For eye contact, however, there does not exist such a sophisticated infrastructure, yet.

In our work, we focus on the nonverbal part, in particular on eye and head movements. Because a number of robotic vision systems already exist and can be found in the literature, we will give a short overview of the state of the art in this field.

16.1.1 State of the Art

The most obvious purpose a vision system fulfills is that of a sensor system for visual perception. For this purpose, simple systems with fixed stereo cameras can be used. Humanoid robots in this category include HRP-2 (Kaneko et al. 2004), Johnnie (Cupec, Schmidt, and Lorch 2005), and Justin (Ott et al. n.d.). Robots can also use their eyes as a display for natural human–robot interaction. Eye movements are understood by any human and their meaning does not have to be learned. The eyes must be moveable but do not have to provide actual vision for the robot. Androids like ROMAN (Berns and Hirth 2006), Geminoid HI-1 (Ishiguro and Nishio 2007), and Repliee R1/Q2 (Matsui et al. 2005; Minato et al. 2004) are included in this category. Ideally, the vision system of the robot is used for both purposes. This is demanding, because the eyes have to be fast and precise to minimize motion blur and their motions have to be independent of each other to support vergence movements, even when the head rotates around the line of sight (torsional movement). For human-like foveated vision, often peripheral cameras are used, which are either moved with the foveated cameras or are fixed. Cog (Brooks et al. 1999) and Kismet (Breazeal 2003; Breazeal et al. 2000, 2001) from the Massachusetts Institute of Technology (MIT) both support a moveable head with eyes that are able to rotate around two independent vertical axes but with only one coupled horizontal axis, which limits vergence movements (as long as the head is not rolled). Whereas Cog has two cameras per eye for both foveal and peripheral vision, Kismet has only moveable foveal vision, with two head-fixed peripheral cameras. The SARCOS robots DB and CB at Advanced Telecommunications Research Institute International (ATR) have biomimetic oculomotor control (Shibata and Schaal 2001; Shibata et al. 2001; Ude, Gaskett, and Cheng 2006). Domo (Edsinger-Gonzales and Weber 2004) uses only wide-angle cameras, whereas ARMAR has foveal/peripheral vision. Other robots with active vision are iCub (Beira et al. 2006) and WE-4RII (Miwa et al. 2004). Stand-alone systems have been developed as well (Samson et al. 2006). There have also been efforts to move from the foveal/peripheral camera pair to a more anthropomorphic eye (Samson et al. 2006). Apart from DB/CB none of the robots implement two fully independent eyes, but they share at least one common rotation axis. With the exception of stand-alone vision systems (Samson et al. 2006), no other system so far has considered ocular torsion.

16.1.2 Motivation

In human–robot interaction, gaze-based communication with human performance on the robot side has a great advantage: humans do not have to learn how to use an artificial interface such as a mouse or a keyboard, but they can communicate immediately and naturally just like with other humans. This is especially important for service robots who directly interact with people, some of whom might be older or disabled.

To our knowledge, human likeness of robotic gaze behavior has not yet been examined with a gaze-based telepresence setup. In contrast to the few studies that have applied only simple and stereotyped eye movements, in either virtual reality environments (Garau et al. 2001; Lee, Badler, and Badler 2002) or with real robots (MacDorman et al. 2005; Sakamoto et al. 2007), our approach bears the potential to open up a new field by providing the whole range of coordinated eye and head movements. Although in this work we only present technical aspects of our experimental platform, our long-term aim is not a telepresence system per se but rather to use it as a tool to identify which aspects of gaze a social robot should implement. The reduction of critical aspects and the omission of unimportant functionalities will eventually simplify the final goal of an autonomous active vision system.

Instead of building a model for robotic interaction from scratch, as has been done, for example, in Breazeal (2003), Lee, Badler, and Badler (2002), and Sidner et al. (2004), we use a top-down approach, in which we have a complete cognitive model of a robotic communication partner (controlled by a human). Then, we can restrict or alter its abilities bit by bit (see flash in Figure 16.1) to elucidate the key factors of gaze and head movement behavior in human–robot interactions.

16.1.3 Objectives

We provide two different modes for controlling the eye and head movements. For scripted experiments, three-dimensional coordinates can directly be fed to the robot. Also, laser pointers can be attached to the robotic eyes, thus visualizing the lines of sight in both the real world and the scene camera. By manually moving the eyes with the mouse, target points can be selected and later played back by a script.

In the experimental Wizard-of-Oz setup outlined in Figure 16.1, the ability to replicate the whole range of ocular motor functionality and to manipulate different aspects is mandatory for enabling examinations of gaze-based human–robot interactions. The platform needs to provide human-like interaction capabilities and, in particular, the dynamics of the motion devices at least need to achieve human performance in terms of velocity, acceleration, and bandwidth. Most importantly, the critical delays introduced by the eye tracker and the motion devices as well as the teleoperation and video channels need to be short enough for operating the platform in real time. To quantify these requirements, human eye movements are characterized by rotational speeds of up to 700 degrees and accelerations of 25,000 deg/s² (Leigh and Zee 1999), with saccades, the fastest of all eye movements, occurring up to five times per second (Schneider et al. 2003). The cutoff frequency is in the range of 1 Hz (Glasauer 2007) and the delay (latency) of the fastest (vestibulo ocular) reflex is on the order of 10 ms (Leigh and Zee 1999). In addition, the total delay in the virtual interaction loop of Figure 16.1 must not exceed typical human reaction times of about 150 ms. Results are presented that focus on those technical aspects that help to fulfill these requirements, thereby providing human-like interaction capabilities.

16.2 Methods

The experimental Wizard-of-Oz platform (see Figure 16.1) mainly consists of an eye and head tracker, a robot head, a pair of camera motion devices (robot eyes), and a teleoperation link that connects the motion tracker with the motion devices. In addition, there is a video channel that feeds back a view of the participant in the experimental scene. In view of the required dynamics and real-time capabilities, the motion trackers and the robot eyes as well as the bidirectional data transmission channels were identified as the critical parts of this chain. We will therefore present implementation details of our eye and head tracker and of our novel camera motion devices in subsequent sections.

16.2.1 Robots

We have integrated the artificial eyes into two different robotic platforms, each with their specific fields of use.

16.2.1.1 ELIAS

ELIAS (see Figure 16.1) is based on a commercially available robotic platform SCITOS G5 (MetraLabs GmbH, Ilmenau, Germany) and serves as a research platform for human–robot interaction. It consists of a mobile base with a differential drive accompanied by a laser scanner and sonar sensors used for navigation. The robotic platform is certified for use in public environments. The built-in industrial PC hosts the robotic-related services, like moving the platform. Furthermore, this base is extended with a human–machine interface (HMI) featuring a robotic head, a touch screen, cameras, speakers, and microphones. The touch screen is used for direct haptic user input; the cameras can provide visual saliency information, and the microphones are used for speech recognition and audio-based saliency information. The modules for the interaction between the human and the robot are run on an additional PC, which is powered by the on-board batteries (providing enough power for the robot to operate for approximately 8 hours). For the communication between and within these computing nodes, two middlewares are applied and the services can be orchestrated using a knowledge-based controller as in Wallhoff et al. (2010). However, the services can be additionally advertised using the Bonjour protocol and thereby allow other modules, such as the Wizard-of-Oz module, to request information (e.g., current head position) or send control commands.

The robotic head itself has two degrees of freedom (DOF; pan/tilt) and was originally equipped with 2-DOF pivotable eyes, which, however, did not meet our requirements and were therefore replaced. We chose this particular robot head because, in contrast to a more human-like android platform, it possesses stylized facial features. This allowed leaving aside uncanny valley effects that are likely to appear as soon as the robot looks almost human (Mori 1970). Furthermore, this choice reduced human likeness even more to eye and head movement behavior, as opposed to comparing the overall appearance.

16.2.1.2 EDDIE

EDDIE (see Figure 16.2) is a robot head that was developed at the Institute of Automatic Control Engineering to investigate the effect of nonverbal communication on human–robot interaction, with the focus on emotional expressions (Sosnowski, Kühnlenz, and Buss 2006). A distinctive feature of this robot head is that it includes not only human-like facial features but also animal-like features (Kühnlenz, Sosnowski, and Buss 2010). The ears can be tilted as well as folded/unfolded and a crown with four feathers is included. Accounting for the uncanny valley effect, the design of the head resembles a reasonable degree of familiarity to a human face while remaining clearly machine-like. EDDIE has a total of 28 degrees of freedom, with 23 degrees of freedom in the face and 5 degrees of freedom in the neck. The 5 degrees of freedom in the neck provide the necessary redundancy to approximate the flexibility and redundancy of the human neck when looking at given coordinates. It utilizes an experimentally derived humanoid motion model, which solves the redundancy and models the joint trajectories and dependencies. For the Wizard-of-Oz scenario, the head tracker data can be directly mapped to the joints of the neck, circumventing the motion model.

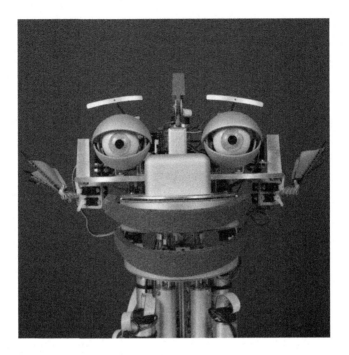

FIGURE 16.2
Robot EDDIE.

Both robots have their unique advantages: ELIAS is a mobile robot that can be operated securely even in large crowds. We added the option to control this robot wirelessly for scenarios in which a certain latency is tolerable.

EDDIE is currently better suited for static experiments but has more human features and his neck is able to reproduce human head movements correctly.

16.2.2 Camera Motion Device

The most critical parts of the proposed Wizard-of-Oz platform are the camera motion devices that are used as robotic eyes. On the basis of earlier work (Schneider et al. 2005, 2009; Villgrattner and Ulbrich 2008a, 2008b; Wagner, Günthner, and Ulbrich 2006), we have developed a new 2-DOF camera motion device that was considerably reduced in size and weight (see Figure 16.3). At the center of its design there is a parallel kinematics setup with two piezo actuators (Physik Instrumente, Karlsruhe, Germany) that rotate the camera platform around a cardanic gimbal joint (Mädler, Stuttgart, Germany) by means of two push rods with spherical joints (Conrad, Hirschau, Germany). The push rods are attached to linear slide units (THK, Tokyo, Japan), each of which is driven by its own piezo actuator. The position of each slide unit is measured by a combination of a magnetic position sensor (Sensitec, Lahnau, Germany) and a linear

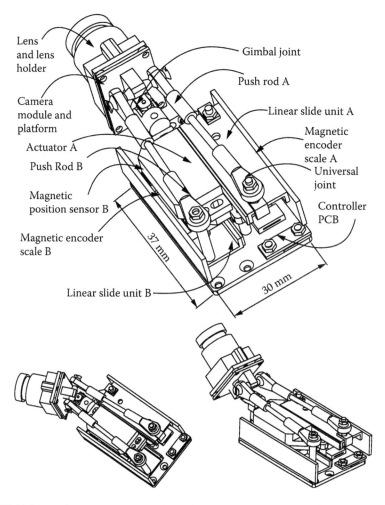

FIGURE 16.3
Camera motion device (robot eye) with the most important parts and dimensions annotated (top). The camera is shown in different orientations: straight ahead (top), up (bottom left), and to the right (bottom right). © 2009 IEEE.

magnetic encoder scale with a resolution of 1 μm (Sensitec) that is glued to the slide unit. The microprocessor (PIC, Microchip, Chandler, AZ) on the printed circuit board (PCB) implements two separate proportional-integral-derivative controllers, one for each actuator–sensor unit. The controller outputs are fed into analog driver stages (Physik Instrumente), which deliver the appropriate signals to drive the piezo actuators. The transformation of desired angular orientations to linear slide unit positions is performed by means of an inverse kinematic, which has been presented before (Villgrattner and Ulbrich 2008b).

In the Results section we will report on the dynamical properties of the new camera motion device with special focus on the delay that is achieved between the movement of the wizard's eye and its replication in the artificial robot eye.

16.2.3 Eye and Head Tracker

The wizard sits in front of a video monitor that displays the image of the scene view camera that is attached to the robot's neck (see Figure 16.1). A head-mounted eye and head tracker with sampling rates of up to 500 Hz was implemented and used to calculate the intersection of the wizard's gaze with the video monitor plane (see Figures 16.1 and 16.4). Details of the eye-tracking part have been presented before (Boening et al. 2006; Schneider et al. 2009). For head-tracking purposes, the eye tracker was extended by

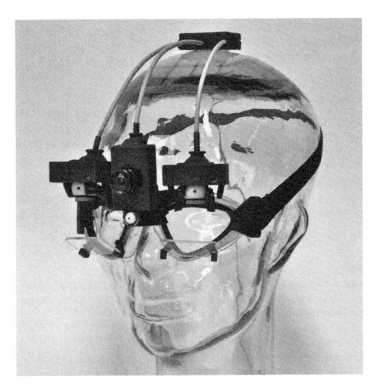

FIGURE 16.4
Eye and head tracker. Eye positions are measured by laterally attached FireWire (IEEE 1394) cameras. The eyes are illuminated with infrared light (850 nm) that is reflected by the translucent hot mirrors in front of the eyes. Another wide-angle camera above the forehead is used to determine head pose with respect to bright infrared LEDs on the video monitor (see Figure 16.1). A calibration laser with a diffraction grating is mounted beneath this camera. All cameras are synchronized to the same frame rate, which can be up to 500 Hz.

a forward-facing, wide-angled scene camera operating in the near-infrared spectrum. The wizard's screen has five infrared light-emitting diodes (LEDs) arranged in a predefined geometrical setup. These LEDs are detected by the eye tracker's calibrated scene camera, so it is possible to calculate the goggles' position and with it the head pose.

After a simple calibration procedure, which requires the subject to fixate on five different calibration targets projected by a head-fixed laser, the eye tracker yields eye directions in degrees. The fixation points are generated by a diffraction grating at equidistant angles, regardless of the distance to the projection. Because at small distances a parallax error would be generated by the offset between eye and calibration laser, the laser dots are projected to a distant wall. At a typical distance of 5 meters, the error decreases to 0.4 degrees. In view of the refixation accuracy of the human eye of about 1 degrees (Eggert 2007), this is a tolerable value.

In an additional step, the wizard's origin of gaze, that is, the center of the eyeballs, with respect to the head coordinate system, has to be calculated. This is done by letting the wizard fixate on two known points on the screen without moving his head. The results are two gaze vectors per eye from which the eyeball center can be calculated in head coordinates. After complete calibration, the point of gaze in the screen plane can be determined together with the head pose.

During normal operation, the wizard is shown two markers on his screen as a feedback. The calculated eye position is displayed together with the intersection of the head direction vector and the screen plane. This is used to validate the calibration during the experiment. Furthermore, the wizard has better control over the robot, because he sees where the robot's head points to.

Depending on the robot's capabilities two, respectively five, head angles plus two eye angles for each eye are sent.

In the Results section we will report on the accuracy, resolution, and real-time capable delays that we achieved with this eye tracker.

16.2.4 Teleoperation Channel

The robot head (see Figure 16.1) is equipped with a forward-facing, wide-angle camera mounted on the neck. The camera is tilted slightly upwards to point to the face level of humans in front of the robot. The image of the scene camera is displayed on the wizard's video monitor.

To keep the latency low, we decided to use two different transmission channels: a USB connection for the eye and head position signals and standard analog video equipment for the scene view, consisting of an analog video camera and a CRT video monitor, both operating at a 50 Hz PAL frame rate.

This setup is well suited for static experiments, but if the robot is mobile, a wireless link is needed. Therefore, we added the option to transmit the scene view video as well as the motor commands over a WiFi connection at the cost of a higher overall latency.

In the Results section we will report on the measured latencies for each method. A short total delay, preferably at only a fraction of the time of human reactions, is of particular importance for future experiments, because we intend to manipulate the teleoperation channel by introducing, for example, additional systematic delays (see flash in Figure 16.1) and test their effects on interaction performance. Therefore, the baseline delay needs to be as close to zero as possible.

16.3 Discussion and Results

We have developed a novel experimental platform for Wizard-of-Oz evaluations of biomimetic properties of active vision systems for robots. The main question was how well this platform is suited for the envisioned types of experiments. Evidently, human eye movements have to be replicated with sufficient fidelity, and the combination of an eye tracker with camera motion devices has to fulfill rigid real-time requirements. In this section we quantify how well the overall design meets these requirements.

16.3.1 Handling of Eye Vergence

One fundamental challenge was the question of how to handle vergence eye movements, which occur when points at different depths are fixated on. Given the geometry of the robot, in particular the eye positions and the kinematics of the head, it is possible to direct both lines of sight at one specific point in three-dimensional space. This poses a problem in the Wizard-of-Oz scenario, where the wizard is only able to look at a flat surface (i.e., his screen). If the distance to the fixated object is sufficiently large (>6 m), the eyes are nearly parallel, but the nearer the fixation is, the more eye vergence becomes noticeable. For now, we have resolved this problem by preselecting the distance at which the wizard fixates. This is an adequate solution for dialog scenarios, where the robot interacts with one or a few persons at roughly the same distance. If the scene is static and more control is needed, regions of interest on the wizard's monitor could be mapped to distinct distances. To reproduce eye vergence in its entirety, though, a binocular eye tracker combined with a stereoscopic monitor or head-mounted display would be needed.

16.3.2 Camera Motion Device

The piezo actuators chosen for the new camera motion device proved particularly beneficial in the overall design. They are backlash free and each piezo

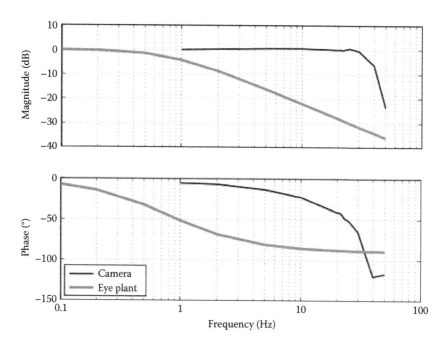

FIGURE 16.5
Bode plot of the frequency response of the camera motion device (black). For comparison, the frequency response of a human eye plant is also plotted (gray). © 2009 IEEE.

actuator can generate a force of up to 2 N, which is sufficient for rotating the cameras with the required dynamics. We have measured the frequency response in a range of 1 to 30 Hz at a deflection amplitude of 2 degrees. The results are plotted in Figure 16.5. The bandwidth is characterized by a corner frequency of about 20 Hz, at which the phase shift reaches 45 degrees. It is therefore a magnitude above the human eye mechanics, with a corner frequency on the order of 1 Hz (Glasauer 2007).

In comparison with our previous designs, we were able to significantly reduce the dimensions of the camera motion device. This was mainly due to replacing the optical encoders in our previous design (Villgrattner and Ulbrich 2008b) with new magnetic sensors, which were not only more accurate but allowed for a more compact configuration of all parts (see Figure 16.3). We also decided to give up the previous symmetrical design in favor of an asymmetrical one, which helped to additionally reduce device dimensions to an area of 30 mm × 37 mm. This reduction in size also contributed to a reduction of weight to 72 g, and both contributed to improved dynamical properties in terms of achievable velocities and acceleration. The maximal angular velocity measured around the primary position was 3,400 deg/s for both the horizontal and vertical directions. Accelerations were on the order of 170,000 deg/s^2. These values are about five times above the values of the human ocular motor system.

In the mechanical configuration of Figure 16.3 the sensor resolution of 1 μm yields an angular resolution of 0.01 degrees in the primary position. The workspace is characterized by maximal deflections of 40 and 35 degrees in horizontal and vertical directions, respectively.

16.3.3 Eye and Head Tracker

Eye trackers are usually characterized by their accuracy as well as their spatial and temporal resolution. The accuracy of an eye tracker cannot exceed the accuracy with which the human eye is positioned on visual targets. Human refixations usually have a standard deviation on the order of 1 degrees (Eggert 2007). With our eye and head tracker we have measured differences of 0.6 ± 0.27 degrees between visual targets on the screen and the corresponding intersections of subjects' gaze vectors with the screen plane (Schneider et al. 2005). The spatial resolution, given as the standard deviation of eye position values during a fixation, is 0.02 degrees. The temporal resolution is determined by the high-speed FireWire cameras, which can be operated at frame rates of up to 600 Hz. Such a sampling rate allows measurement of saccades, the fastest human eye movements.

We used a USB-to-RS232 converter to connect the eye tracker with the camera motion device (see Figure 16.1). We then operated the eye tracker at frame rates of 100, 200, and 500 Hz and measured the delay between an artificial eye that was moved in front of an eye-tracker camera and the corresponding movement replicated by the robot eye. As expected, the total delay linearly depended on the time interval between two frames; that is, the inverse frame rate (see Figure 16.6). The delay at 500 Hz was 10 ms, which is on the order of the fastest ocular motor reflex latency in humans (Leigh and Zee 1999). We also measured the delays introduced by image

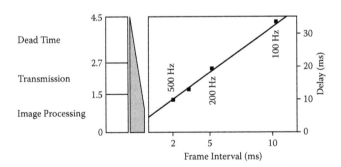

FIGURE 16.6
Delays between eye and corresponding camera movements at different eye tracker frame rates. The system delay depends linearly on the frame interval of the camera. At 500 and 100 Hz the delays are 10 and 32 ms, respectively. The intercept at 4.5 ms is the sum of the delays caused by image processing, signal transmission, and mechanical dead times. © 2009 IEEE.

processing, signal transmission, and dead times, which amounted to 1.5, 1.2, and 1.8 ms, respectively (see Figure 16.6).

In addition to the eye-tracker delay of 10 ms, the delay of the analog video transmission for the scene view (see Figure 16.1) needs to be considered. We measured this delay by using a flashing LED in front of ELIAS's scene camera and a photodiode on the wizard's video monitor. This delay amounted to 20 ms. The total delay in the virtual interaction loop was therefore 30 ms. This is just a fraction of the typical human reaction time of 150 ms.

For the wireless link, we measured a latency between 50 and 80 ms depending on synchronization of the camera and monitor, which led to an overall mean latency of 75 ms.

16.4 Conclusion and Future Work

In this work we proposed a novel paradigm for the evaluation of human–robot interaction, with special focus on the importance of natural eye and head movements in human–machine communication scenarios. We also presented a unique experimental platform that will enable Wizard-of-Oz experiments in which a human experimenter (wizard) teleoperates a robotic head and eyes with his own head and eyes. The platform mainly consists of an eye and head tracker and motion devices for the robot head and his eyes, as well as a feedback video transmission link for the view of the experimental scene. We demonstrated that the eye tracker can measure the whole dynamical range of eye movements and that these movements can be replicated by the novel robotic eyes with more than sufficient fidelity. The camera motion device developed combines small dimensions with dynamical properties that exceed the requirements posed by the human ocular motor system. In addition, by reducing all critical delays to a minimum, we met the rigid real-time requirements of an experimental platform that is designed to enable seamless human–machine interactions.

Preliminary evaluation with human subjects showed a high acceptance of the system. In future experiments we intend to answer the question of how important it is to resemble human performance in artificial eyes and which aspects of ocular and neck motor functionality are key to people's attribution of humanness to robotic active vision systems. Possible experiments might examine the effects on human–robot interaction performance while the teleoperation channel is manipulated, for example, with artificial delays.

We also plan to control even more aspects of the robot by the wizard, for example, the eyelids (which directly map to the wizard's eye lids) or mouth movements, which would require an additional camera that tracks the wizard's mouth area.

Acknowledgments

This work was supported in part within the DFG excellence initiative research cluster Cognition for Technical Systems–CoTeSys, by Deutsche Forschungsgemeinschaft (DFG: GL 342/1-3), by funds from the German Federal Ministry of Education and Research under the Grand code 01 EO 9091, and by the Institute for Advanced Study (IAS), Technische Universität München; see also http://www.tum-ias.de.

References

Argyle, M., Cook, M., and Argyle, M. 1976. *Gaze and Mutual Gaze*. Cambridge: Cambridge University Press.

Argyle, M., Ingham, R., Alkema, F., and McCallin, M. 1973. The different functions of gaze. *Semiotica*, 7: 10–32.

Beira, R., Lopes, M., Praça, M., Santos-Victor, J., Bernardino, A., Metta, G., Becchi, F., and Saltaren, R. 2006. Design of the Robot-Cub (iCub) head. Paper read at the IEEE International Conference on Robotics and Automation, May, Orlando, FL, May 15–19, 2006.

Berns, K., and Hirth, J. 2006. Control of facial expressions of the humanoid robot head ROMAN. Paper read at the IEEE/RSJ International Conference on Intelligent Robots and Systems, Beijing, China, October 9–15, 2006.

Boening, G., Bartl, K., Dera, T., Bardins, S., Schneider, E., and Brandt, T. 2006. Mobile eye tracking as a basis for real-time control of a gaze driven head-mounted video camera. In *Eye Tracking Research and Applications*. New York: ACM.

Breazeal, C. 2003. Toward sociable robots. *Robotics and Autonomous Systems*, 42(3–4): 167–175.

Breazeal, C., Edsinger, A., Fitzpatrick, P., and Scassellati, B. 2001. Active vision for sociable robots. *Systems, Man and Cybernetics, Part A*, 31(5): 443–453.

Breazeal, C., Edsinger, A., Fitzpatrick, P., Scassellati, B., and Varchavskaia, P. 2000. Social constraints on animate vision. *IEEE Intelligent Systems*, 15: 32–37.

Brooks, R., Breazeal, C., Marjanovic, M., Scassellati, B., and Williamson, M. 1999. The Cog Project: Building a humanoid robot. *Lecture Notes in Computer Science*, 52–87.

Cupec, R., Schmidt, G., and Lorch, O. 2005. Vision-guided walking in a structured indoor scenario. *Automatika-Zagreb*, 46(1/2): 49.

Edsinger-Gonzales, A., and Weber, J. 2004. Domo: a force sensing humanoid robot for manipulation research. Paper read at the 4th IEEE/RAS International Conference on Humanoid Robots, Santa Monica, CA, November 10–12, 2004.

Eggert, T. 2007. Eye movement recordings: Methods. *Developments in Ophthalmology*, 40: 15–34.

Emery, N. 2000. The eyes have it: The neuroethology, function and evolution of social gaze. *Neuroscience and Biobehavioral Reviews*, 24(6): 581–604.

Garau, M., Slater, M., Bee, S., and Sasse, M. 2001. The impact of eye gaze on communication using humanoid avatars. In *Proceedings of the SIGCHI Conference on Human Factors in Computing Systems*. New York: ACM.

Glasauer, S. 2007. Current models of the ocular motor system. *Developments in Ophthalmology*, 40: 158–174.

Ishiguro, H., and Nishio, S. 2007. Building artificial humans to understand humans. *Journal of Artificial Organs*, 10(3): 133–142.

Kaneko, K., Kanehiro, F., Kajita, S., Hirukawa, H., Kawasaki, T., Hirata, M., Akachi, K., and Isozumi, T. 2004. Humanoid robot HRP-2. Paper read at the IEEE International Conference on Robotics and Automation, New Orleans, LA, April 26–May 1, 2004.

Kühnlenz, K., Sosnowski, S., and Buss, M. 2010. Impact of animal-like features on emotion expression of robot head EDDIE. *Advanced Robotics*, 24(8–9): 1239–1255.

Langton, S., Watt, R., and Bruce, V. 2000. Do the eyes have it? Cues to the direction of social attention. *Trends in Cognitive Sciences*, 4(2): 50–59.

Lee, S., Badler, J., and Badler, N. 2002. Eyes alive. *ACM Transactions on Graphics*, 21(3): 637–644.

Leigh, R. J., and Zee, D. S. 1999. *The Neurology of Eye Movements*. New York: Oxford University Press.

MacDorman, K., Minato, T., Shimada, M., Itakura, S., Cowley, S., and Ishiguro, H. 2005. Assessing human likeness by eye contact in an android testbed. Paper read at the XXVII Annual Meeting of the Cognitive Science Society, Stresa, Italy, Juy 21–23, 2005.

Matsui, D., Minato, T., MacDorman, K., and Ishiguro, H. 2005. Generating natural motion in an android by mapping human motion. Paper read at the IEEE/RSJ International Conference on Intelligent Robots and Systems.

Minato, T., Shimada, M., Ishiguro, H., and Itakura, S. 2004. Development of an android robot for studying human–robot interaction. *Lecture Notes in Computer Science*, 424–434.

Miwa, H., Itoh, K., Matsumoto, M., Zecca, M., Takanobu, H., Roccella, S., Carrozza, M., Dario, P., and Takanishi, A. 2004. Effective Emotional Expressions with Emotion Expression Humanoid Robot WE-4RII. Paper read at International Conference on Intelligent Robots and Systems (IROS) Sendai, Japan, October 2, 2004.

Mori, M. 1970. The uncanny valley. *Energy*, 7(4): 33–35.

Ott, C., Eiberger, O., Friedl, W., Bauml, B., Hillenbrand, U., Borst, C., Albu-Schaffer, A., Brunner, B., Hirschmuller, H., Kielhofer, S. Konietschke, R., Suppa, M., Wimböck, T., Zacharias, F., and Hirginger, G. n.d. A humanoid two-arm system for dexterous manipulation. *Head and Neck* 2: 43.

Sakamoto, D., Kanda, T., Ono, T., Ishiguro, H., and Hagita, N. 2007. Android as a telecommunication medium with a human-like presence. In *Proceedings of the ACM/IEEE International Conference on Human–Robot Interaction*. New York: ACM.

Samson, E., Laurendeau, D., Parizeau, M., Comtois, S., Allan, J., and Gosselin, C. 2006. The agile stereo pair for active vision. *Machine Vision and Applications*, 17(1): 32–50.

Schneider, E., Bartl, K., Bardins, S., Dera, T., Boening, G., and Brandt, T. 2005. Eye movement driven head-mounted camera: It looks where the eyes look. Paper read at the IEEE International Conference on Systems, Man and Cybernetics.

Schneider, E., Glasauer, S., Brandt, T., and Dieterich, M. 2003. Nonlinear nystagmus processing causes torsional VOR nonlinearity. *Annals of the New York Academy of Sciences*, 1004: 500–505.

Schneider, E., Villgrattner, T., Vockeroth, J., Bartl, K., Kohlbecher, S., Bardins, S., Ulbrich, H., and Brandt, T. 2009. EyeSeeCam: An eye movement-driven head camera for the examination of natural visual exploration. *Annals of the New York Academy of Sciences*, 1164: 461–467.

Shibata, T., and Schaal, S. 2001. Biomimetic gaze stabilization based on feed-back-error-learning with nonparametric regression networks. *Neural Networks*, 14(2): 201–216.

Shibata, T., Vijayakumar, S., Conradt, J., and Schaal, S. 2001. Biomimetic oculomotor control. *Journal of Computer Vision*, 1(4): 333–356.

Sidner, C., Kidd, C., Lee, C., and Lesh, N. 2004. Where to look: A study of human-robot engagement. In *Proceedings of the 9th International Conference on Intelligent User Interfaces*. New York: ACM.

Sosnowski, S., Kühnlenz, K., and Buss, M. 2006. EDDIE—An emotion-display with dynamic intuitive expressions. Paper read at the 15th IEEE International Symposium on Robot and Human Interactive Communication..

Ude, A., Gaskett, C., and Cheng, G. 2006. Foveated vision systems with two cameras per eye. Paper read at the IEEE International Conference on Robotics and Automation.

Villgrattner, T., and Ulbrich, H. 2008a. Control of a piezo-actuated pan/tilt camera motion device. Paper read at the 11th International Conference on New Actuators, Bremen, Germany.

Villgrattner, T., and Ulbrich, H. 2008b. Piezo-driven two-degree-of-freedom camera orientation system. Paper presented at the IEEE International Conference on Industrial Technology.

Wagner, P., Günthner, W., and Ulbrich, H. 2006. Design and implementation of a parallel three-degree-of-freedom camera motion device. Paper read at the Joint Conference of the 37th International Symposium on Robotics ISR 2006 and the German Conference on Robotics.

Wallhoff, F., Blume, J., Bannat, A., Rösel, W., Lenz, C., and Knoll, A. 2010. A skill-based approach towards hybrid assembly. *Advanced Engineering Informatics*, 24(3): 329–339.

Index

3-DOF robotic neck
    hardware development, 108–111
    programming head movements for,
        111
    system overview, 107–108

A

Acceleration coupling torque, 60–61
Acoustic noises, generation of by head/
    neck movements, 106
Acoustic testing, robotic neck, 121–122
Active actuators, 241
Actuation, biologically inspired, 9
Actuators
    ionic conducting polymer film
        (ICPF), 86
    load capability of, 68–70
    multifunctional design, 241–243
    use of in assistive knee braces,
        240–241
    use of in hand rehabilitation
        machines, 279
    use of in hyperdynamic
        manipulators, 62
Added-mass hydro dynamic theory,
    93–94
AFM cantilevers
    fabrication of tips for nanoprobes,
        182–183
    stiffness measurements of single
        cells using, 179–182
Aging, effects of, 240
AIBO robotic dog, 4
AIST humanoid robot HRP-2, 2–3
Al-Jazari, 3
Albert HUBO serial neck, 106
Anguilliform propulsion, 87–89
Arch structure hand rehabilitation
    machine, 279–280
Arm structure hand rehabilitation
    machine, 279–280, 285–287
    proposed mechanism for, 280–285

Arm-hand movement control, neuronal
    system for, 264–265
ARMAR-III serial neck, 106, 298
Arterial blood flow, measurement of, 194
Artificial eyes
    human performance in, 296
    use of in robots, 300–302
Artificial muscles, 9
Asimo, 3
Assistive devices, 190
    control experiment results using
        hybrid sensor probe, 200–203
    control experiment using hybrid
        sensor probe, 198–199
Assistive knee braces, 240
    actuation devices in, 241
    prototype testing, 254–258
Automated single-cell loading and
    supply system, use of
    microfluidic technologies for,
    127–128
Automatic single-cell transfer model
    cell detection/tracking and control
        algorithm for, 134–138
    cell suction system, 130–131
    cell types and preparation, 129–130
    direction control in, 139–143
    manufacture of microfluidic chips
        for, 131–132
    materials and methods for, 128–129
    oocyte and fibroblast suction,
        138–139
    use of cell suction system in, 130–131
    valve control principle for, 132–133
    vision system for, 133–134
Autonomous robotic fish, 86. See also
    Robotic fish
Axial deformation, relationship with
    stretching force, 161

B

Bacterial chemotaxis algorithm, 97–101
Basic resistance, 46

BCF propulsion, 87–89
Behavior control, 5–9
Berkeley Lower Extremity Exoskeleton
        (BLEEX), 240
Bio-Cycle, 34–36
    design of compound resistance
        system for, 44–50
    design of the pedal crank and hand
        crank of, 40–41
    design of the saddle pole, 41–43
    detection of exercise motions, 47–50
    development and test, 51
    handle design, 43–44
Bio-robotics
    history of, 2–4
    modeling/analysis, 2
Bioelectrical signals, measuring, 191–192
Biologic systems, control of, 6
Biological cells, deformation response of
        in microinjection, 150
Biological fish, swimming behaviors of,
        87–89
Biologically inspired robotics
    definition of, 1–2
    designing mechanisms for, 5
    motion and behavior control, 5–9
Biomembrane, 148
    deformation behavior of, 150
Biomimetic robots, 3–4
Biomimetics, 1–2
Bioplant, 127
BIT humanoid robot BHR-2, 3
Blood information, measurement of in
        the brain using optical data,
        192–194
BLPM DC motors, design of, 243–244
Body and/or caudal fin propulsion. *See*
        BCF propulsion
Bottom surface treatment, use of in
        automatic single-cell transfer
        design, 130
Brain, measurement of blood
        information of, 192–194
Brain activities
    methods to measure, 191–194
    scanning, 190–191
Brain function, 264–265
Brain waves, biolectric signal
        measurement, 191–192

Brain-computer interface (BCI), 190
Brake function
    active actuators in assistive knee
        braces with, 241
    torque tracking in multifunctional
        actuator, 259
    torque *vs.* applied current in
        multifunctional actuator, 257
Breaking torque control, assistive knee
        braces with, 241
Buckling phenomenon of nanoprobes,
        173–174

C

Cable housings
    inverse kinematics and static
        analysis for, 114–116
    use of in low-noise robotic head
        system, 108
Camera motion device, use of in
        telepresence robotic control,
        302–304, 306–308
Cantilever tips, 180
    fabrication of for nanoprobes, 182–183
Capillary electrophoresis, 127–128
Capsule endoscopy, 206–208
Capsule endoscopy images. *See* CE
        images
Carangiform propulsion, 87–89
CE images
    computer-aided detection of, 208
    experimental results of computer-
        aided recognition, 213–215
    use of color for computer-aided
        recognition of, 210–212
    use of shape for computer-aided
        recognition, 212–213
Cell deformation
    measurement of, 158–161
    osmosis-induced increase of, 160
Cell detection/tracking and control
        algorithm, 134–138
Cell encapsulation, use of microfluidic-
        based technologies for, 127
Cell fusion, 127
Cell manipulation, 149
    experimental material preparation,
        155

force calibration, 155–156
optical stretching of human RBCs,
    157–158
optical tweezer system for, 153–155
results and discussion of optical
    stretching, 158–161
robotic manipulation of microbeads
    in RBCs, 156–157
Cell mechanical modeling, 150–153
Cell mechanics, human red blood cells,
    148–149
Cell membranes, deformation behavior
    of, 150
Cell size, stiffness measurements of
    single yeast cells and, 179–181
Cell stiffening, stretching-induced, 159
Cell stretching, optically induced, 149,
    157–158
Cell suction system, use of in automatic
    single-cell transfer design,
    130–131
Cell treatment, integration of
    microfluidic technology in,
    126–128
Cellular analyses, use of microfluidic
    technology for, 126–128
Cellular heterogeneity, 167
Central pattern generator. *See* CPG
Channel ratio, 228–230
Channel sequence recognition, 221
Cheetahs, Bio-Cycle inspired by
    movement of, 36–38
Chromaticity histogram, 211–212
Cloning, use of microfluidic-based
    technologies for, 127
Closed-loop CPG networks
    analysis of, 20–22
    control of snake-like robots using,
    17–20
    simulation of control of snake-like
    robots using, 22–26
Clutch/brake system
    design of in a multifunctional
    actuator, 241–242, 246–249
    pulse response in multifunctional
    actuator, 259
    torque generated from in
    multichannel actuators, 251
Cog, 298

Cogging force, 244
Colonoscopy, 206
Color, use of for computer-aided CE
    image recognition, 210–212
Color wavelet covariance (CWC)
    features, 214
Compound resistance system
    analysis of driving characteristics,
    44–46
    principle of, 46–47
Concordance correlation coefficient, 221,
    224–227, 233
Conical indenters, stiffness
    measurements using, 171–173
Contour-based shape recognition
    method, 212–213
Control
    case study of a golf swing robot,
    70–74
    design of system for snake-like
    robots, 28
    strategy for robotic neck, 116–117
CPG, 14
CPG networks
    analysis of, 20–22
    control of snake-like robots using,
    16–17
    with feedback connection, 17–20
CPG-based control systems,
    experiments, 26–29
Cross-correlation coefficient, 224
Cuneate neurons, response of to manual
    skin stimulation, 266–273
Cuneate nucleus, 265
Curvature, control of, 23–24
Cyclic inhibitory CPG model
    analysis of, 20–22
    controlling snake-like movement
    using, 18–20
Cylindrical indenters, stiffness
    measurements using, 171–173

D

Data glove system, 289–290, 292
DC motors
    design of BLPM, 243–244
    use of in robotic fish design, 89–90
Deformation processes of RBCs, 150

measurement of, 158–161
Designing mechanisms, 5
Desktop bioplant, 127
Detection/tracking and control
　　algorithm, 134–138
Diffraction limited modulation transfer
　　function, 133
Digestive tract, use of capsule
　　endoscopy for diagnosis of, 206
Digital images, relative size of pixels
　　in, 137
Distal interphalangeal joints,
　　rehabilitation of, 285
Donor cells, digital imaging of, 137
Double integration method, 170
Driving force, analysis of for Bio-Cycle,
　　45–46
Dynamic manipulation, 56
Dynamically coupled driving, 56–57, 82
　case study for, 65–67
　method to utilize, 67–74
　utilization of, 57–63
　utilization of actuators for, 62

E

E-SEM system, 168
　observations of biological samples
　　by, 177–179
EDDIE, artificial eyes in, 301–302
EEGs, 190–191
Elastic shear modulus, RBCs, 160
Electroencephalograms. *See* EEGs
Electron microscopes, nanorobotic
　　manipulations inside of,
　　176–177
Electrophysiological neuron modeling,
　　264
Eletrorheological (ER) fluids-based
　　actuators, 241
ELIAS, artificial eyes in, 300–301
Endoskeleton, hand rehabilitation
　　machines, 278–279
Environmental scanning electron
　　microscope nanorobotic
　　manipulation system. *See*
　　E-SEM system
Ergonomics, 39–40

EU SHOAL project, system
　　configuration of robotic fish
　　for, 95–97
Evans–Skalak material, 149
Excitatory synapses, 271
Exercise, necessity of, 240
Exercise motions, detection of, 47–50
Exoskeletons
　hand rehabilitation machines,
　　278–279
　lower extremity, 240
Extensor digiti minimi, 225
Extensor digitorum, 225
Extensor policis brevis, 225
Extensor policis longus, 225
Eye movements
　characterization of, 300
　handling of vergence with
　　teleoperations, 306
Eye tracker, use of in Wizard-of-Oz
　　scenario, 304–305, 308–309

F

Feedback control, 6
Fibroblasts
　suction of, 138–139
　use of in somatic cell cloning, 130
Finite element method, analysis and
　　modeling of multifunctional
　　actuators using, 249–250
Fish. *See also* Biological fish; Robotic fish
　fin configuration of, 87
　swimming behaviors of, 87–89
Fitness cycles, 34–36
　design of compound resistance
　　system for, 44–50
　ergonomic analysis and mechanism
　　design of, 39–44
　mechanism scheme-based multidrive
　　mode, 38–39
Flocking algorithm, 97–101
Fluorescent microscopy, 128
Force, identification of in hand
　　movements, 230–233
Force calibrations, 155–156
　use of to characterize properties of
　　RBCs, 153
Force–deformation relationship, 151–153

Foveated vision, 298
Functional magnetic resonance imaging (fMRI), 190
Functional near-infrared spectroscopy (fNIRS), 190–191

G

Gait cycle, 242–243
Gastrointestinal tract, cancers of, 206
Gastroscopy, 206
Gaze, different roles of, 297
Gaze-based communication, 299
Generation of rhythmic motion, CPG models for, 15–16
Genetic algorithms, 8–9
Goldman–Hodkin–Katz voltage equation, 264
Golf swing robot
    case study of, 70–74
    experimental results for, 77–82
    mechanism design of, 65–67
    simulation of, 74–77
Growth phases, stiffness measurement of single yeast cells and, 181–182

H

Hand fitness cycles, 34–35
Hand movements
    classification of, 223–230
    identification of force and speed of, 230–233
    muscles responsible for, 225
    neuronal system for, 264–265
    rehabilitation of with arm structure machine, 280–285
    use of sEMG for identification of, 220–221
    use of STFT method for determination of, 232
Hand rehabilitation
    arm structure design for machine-assisted, 280–285
    machine-assisted, 278
    work of arm structure machine design, 288–291
Hard nanoprobes, 174

fabrication of, 182–183
measurement of single-cell stiffness using, 175–176
Head movements, human-like, 296
Head tracker, use of in Wizard-of-Oz scenario, 304–305, 308–309
Head-worn communication devices, acoustic noises and, 106
Hertz–Sneddon continuum mechanics model, 175–176
Heterogeneity of cells, 167
HRP-2 serial neck, 106
HSI color space, use of for CE image recognition, 209–212
Hue, saturation, intensity color space. *See* HSI color space
Human eye movements, characterization of, 300
Human hand movements. *See also* Hand movements
    identification of, 220–221
Human red blood cells. *See* RBCs
Humanoid robots, 2
    vision systems of, 298
Hybrid Assistive Limb (HAL), 240
Hybrid nanorobotic manipulation system, 177
Hybrid sensor probe
    assistive device control experiment, 198–199
    assistive device control experiment results, 200–203
    device development, 194–195
    operation verification of, 196–197
    optical data collection experiment, 197–198
    optical data collection experiment results, 199–200
    signal processing and control board, 195–196
    verification of operation of, 199
Hyper dynamic manipulation, 82
    definition of, 56
    design of with smart structure, 57–63
    structure joint stop and, 63–65
Hypotonic solutions, effect of on RBCs, 159–161

I

iCub
    serial neck, 106
    vision system, 298
Image processing, use of to characterize
        properties of RBCs, 153
IMPC-based artificial muscle, 9
Indenter tips, stiffness measurements
        using different shapes, 171–173
Induced deformation, 149
Inhibition, 271
Integrated circuit (I2C) communication,
        use of in CPG-based control,
        27–28
Intestinal polyps, use of CE images for
        recognition of, 209–212
Inverse kinematics, robotic neck
        mechanism, 111–116
Ionic conducting polymer film (ICPF)
        actuators, 86
Ionic polymer–metal composites. *See*
        IMPC-based artificial muscle
Iterative learning control, 8

J

Joint stops, 56–57, 82
    case study for, 65–67
    experimental results for a golf swing
        robot, 78–82
    method to utilize in dynamically
        coupled driving, 67–74
    simulation results for golf swing
        robot, 75–77
    utilization of, 63–65
Joint structure hand rehabilitation
        machine, 279

K

Karakuri ningyo, 3
Kismet, 298

L

Lag phase, stiffness measurements of
        yeast cells in, 181–182

Lambert–Beer's law, use of to measure
        blood information of the brain,
        192–194
Lateral bending, robotic neck
        mechanism, 111–114
Layered control architecture, 90–92
    behavior layer, 92–93
    cognitive layer, 92
    swim pattern layer, 93–95
Legged robots, designing mechanisms
        of movement for, 5
Light absorbance, variation of with
        time, 193
Link mechanisms for exoskeleton-type
        machines, 279
    proposed design for, 280–285
Load-displacement relationship, shape
        of indenter tips and, 172–173
Locomotion
    control of curvature, 23–24
    control of speed of, 24
    control of the number of S-shapes,
        24–25
    movement with different curvatures,
        28
    S-shaped, 20–22
Log phase, stiffness measurements of
        yeast cells in, 181–182
Low-motion–noise robotic head/neck
        system. *See also* Robotic neck
    hardware development, 108–111
    programming head movements, 111
    system overview, 107–108
Lower extremity exoskeletons, 240

M

Macaulay's method, 170
Magnetic flux density, 249
Magnetoencephalography (MEG), 190
Magnetorheological fluid-based
        actuators. *See* Smart fluids-
        based actuators
Magnetorheological fluids. *See* MR
        fluids
Mammalian cloning, use of
        microfluidic-based
        technologies for, 127
Manipulators

control method for hyper dynamic manipulation, 70
controlling with dynamically coupled driving, 67–68
motion generation of, 68–70
revolute joint of, 56
use of dynamically coupled driving in design of, 59
Manual skin stimulation, responses of primary afferent and cuneate neuron to, 266–273
Median and/or paired fin propulsion. *See* MPF propulsion
Membrane theory, 150
Microbeads, robotic manipulation of in RBCs, 156–157
Microbial populations, heterogeneity of, 167–168
Microfluidic chips. *See also* PDMS chips
direction control in, 139–143
manufacture of, 131–132
Microfluidic technology, 126
materials and methods for on-chip closing using, 128–129
Microscopes, nanorobotic manipulations inside of, 176–179
MLP neural network, use of for computer-aided CE image recognition, 214
Modulation transfer function, 133
Motion classification, use of spectral method of square integral for, 226, 228
Motion control, 5–9
experimental setup for robotic neck, 117
robotic neck, 117
Motion generation, case study of a golf swing robot, 70–74
Motion noise test for robotic neck, 118–122
Motion planning, constraints on, 68–69
Motor, design of in a multifunctional actuator, 241, 243–246
Motor activity, necessity of, 240
Motor function
output power and power efficiency in multifunctional actuator, 257

torque *vs.* current and speed in multifunctional actuators, 256
Motors, use of in robotic fish design, 89–90
Movement, mechanisms of, 5
Movement control, function of the brain in, 264–265
Movement speeds, 221
identification of in hand movements, 230–233
MPF propulsion, 87–89
MR fluids, 241
influence of permanent magnets on, 249–250
use of in clutch/brake system in multifunctional actuators, 246–249
Multichannel sEMG sensor rings, 221
automatic relocation of sEMG electrodes in, 223–226
configuration of, 222
feature extraction from, 226–228
Multidrive system, mechanism scheme of, 38–39
Multifunctional actuators
analysis of, 249–251
configuration of, 248
control of, 254
design of, 241–243
design of clutch/brake system in, 246–249
modeling of, 251–254
motor design for, 243–246
prototype testing, 254–258
Multilayer perceptron neural network. *See* MLP neural network
Multistep acceleration, 61
Muscles, artificial, 9
Mutual inhibitory CPG model
analysis of, 20–22
controlling snake-like movement using, 18–20

N

Nanobiotechnology, evaluation of bio-samples using, 167

Nanoindentation, stiffness
measurement of single cells
using, 169–176
Nanomanipulation, 166–167
inside electron microscopes, 176–177
Nanoprobes
fabrication of, 182–183
stiffness measurement using, 173–174
Nanorobotic manipulation, background
of, 166–167
Nanosurgery system
elemental technologies of, 177
single-cell analysis and, 167–168
Nanotechnology, 166–167
Near-infrared spectroscopy (NIRS),
190–191
Neural oscillator, CPG models of, 16
Neuron modeling, 266
electrophysiological, 264
Nonverbal communication, 297–298
Nuclear transplantation, 127

O

Ocular torsion, 299
On-chip cloning technology
materials and methods for, 128–129
use of microfluidic technologies for,
127–128
On-chip microinjection, 127
Oocytes
cell cloning using, 129–130
digital imaging of, 137
suction of, 138–139
Open-loop CPG networks, control of
snake-like robots using, 16–17
Optical data
collection experiment results using
hybrid sensor probe, 199–200
collection experiment using hybrid
sensor probe, 197–198
measurement of blood information
of the brain using, 192–194
Optical force calibration, 155–156
Optical signals, measuring, 191–192
Optical stretching, 150–153, 158–161
human RBCs, 157–158
Optical tweezers
bead manipulation by, 156–157

cell manipulation with, 153–158
robotic manipulations technology
using, 149
Optically induced cell stretching, 149
Osmotic stress, 149, 160
Ostraciiform propulsion, 87–89
Overrunning clutches, 38–39

P

Parallel humanoid neck mechanisms,
106–107
PARO seal-mimetic robot, 4
Passive brain waves, 191–192
PDMS chips, 127–129
connecting cell suction system to,
130–131
direction control in, 139–143
manufacture of, 131–132
valve control principle for, 132–133
vision system for, 133–134
Pearson's product-moment coefficient,
224
Penicillin-streptomycin, use of in
automatic single-cell transfer
design, 130
Physical rehabilitation, machine-
assisted, 278
Pitch and roll motions, robotic neck
mechanism, 111–114
Planar manipulators, 59
Pneumatic actuators, 279
Pollutants
bio-inspired coverage of, 97–101
flock distribution of, 102
Pollution detection, use of robotic fish
for, 95–101
Polyacrylonitrile artificial muscle, 9
Polydimethylsiloxane chips. *See* PDMS
chips
Polyps
CE recognition of, 208
color and shape feature analysis of,
209–213
Position resistance, 46
Positron emission tomography (PET),
190
Primary afferents, 265

modeling of transformation of
information by cuneate
neurons to, 269–273
response of to manual skin
stimulation, 266–269
Propulsion energy, 86
types of, 87–89
Proximal interphalangeal joints,
rehabilitation of, 285

Q

QRIO humanoid robot, 3

R

Range of motion, determination of, 291
RBCs
cell deformation results, 158–161
cell mechanics of, 148–149
force calibration of, 155–156
manipulation of using optical
tweezer system, 153–155
mechanical properties of membranes
of, 150
optical stretching of, 157–158
robotic manipulation of microbeads
in, 156–157
Reactive control, 6–7
Recumbent fitness cycles, 34–35
Red blood cells. *See* RBCs
Region-based shape recognition
methods, 212–213
Rhythmic motion control, central
pattern generator in, 14–16
Rigidity maintenance, robotic neck,
116–117
RoboKnee, 240
Robot actuators, 9
Robotic eyes, human-like, 296
Robotic fish, 4, 86. *See also* Fish
bio-inspired coverage of pollutants
by, 97–101
biologically inspired, 89–90
layered control architecture for,
90–95
system configuration for pollution
detection using, 95–97

Robotic head/neck system, system
overview for, 107–108
Robotic neck
acoustic testing of, 121–122
control strategy for, 116–117
experimental setup and motion
control of, 117
hardware development for, 108–111
inverse kinematics and static
analysis of mechanism for,
111–114
motion control, 117
motion noise test, 118–122
programming head movements for,
111
system overview, 107–108
types of, 106–107
Robotic snakes, 3. *See also* Snake-like
robots
designing mechanisms of movement
for, 5
Robots, teleoperation of head and eye
movements in, 296–297
RoboTuna, 86
ROMAN serial neck, 106
Round motion, control of, 26
Rubbertuator, 9

S

S-shape locomotion, analysis of the use
of CPG networks for, 20–22
S-shapes
control of the number of, 24–25
movement with different numbers
of, 29
SARCOS robots, 298
Saturation phase, stiffness
measurements of yeast cells in,
181–182
Self-motion control, 289
sEMG electrodes
automatic relocation of, 223–226
placement of for identification of
hand movements, 220–221
sEMG signal processing, 223
experimental results of using STFT
method for, 232
use of STFT in, 230–231

sEMG-based sensing system,
configuration of, 222–223
Semi-active actuators, 241
Sensing, biologically inspired, 10–11
Sensing-perception-planning-control, 6
Sensors, use of in robotic fish design,
89–90
Serial humanoid neck mechanisms, 106
Service robots, gaze-based
communication of, 299
Servo motors, use of in robotic fish
design, 89–90
Shape, use of for computer-aided CE
image recognition, 212–213
Shape memory alloy (SMA), use of to
develop robotic lamprey, 86
Shell theory, 150
SHOAL robotic fish, 95, 98
control software architecture for, 96
hardware configuration for, 97
system configuration of, 95–97
Short-time Fourier transform. *See* STFT
method
Short-time Thompson transform. *See*
STTT
Sickle cell anemia, RBCs in, 160
Silicon nanoprobes
fabrication of, 182–183
stiffness measurement of single yeast
cells by, 184–185
Siliconizing, 130
Simulation of golf swing robot, 74–77
Single-cell analysis
nanosurgery system and, 167–168
principles of stiffness measurements,
169–171
stiffness measurements using
conventional AFM cantilevers,
179–182
stiffness measurements using
different indenter shapes,
171–173
stiffness measurements using hard
nanoprobes, 175–176
stiffness measurements using
nanoprobes, 182–185
stiffness measurements using soft
nanoprobes, 174–175
Single-cell loading and supply system

cell detection/tracking and control
algorithm for, 134–138
cell suction system, 130–131
cell types and preparation, 129–130
direction control in, 139–143
manufacture of microfluidic chips
for, 131–132
materials and methods for, 128–129
oocyte and fibroblast suction in,
138–139
valve control principle for, 132–133
vision system for, 133–134
Smart fluids, use of in assistive knee
braces, 241
Smart fluids-based actuators, 241
Snake-like robots, 3. *See also* Robotic
snakes
CPG network for control of, 16–22
designing mechanisms for, 5
experiments, 26–29
simulation of CPG-controlled, 22–26
Social robots, gaze-based
communication of, 299
Soft nanoprobes, 174
calibration of, 183–184
fabrication of, 182–183
measurement of single-cell stiffness
using, 174–175
Somatic cell cloning, 129
Sound absorption, 110–111
Sound insulation, use of in low-noise
robotic neck, 110–111
Spectral features of sEMG signals, 221,
233
Spectral flatness feature, 221, 232
based on STFT at different speeds,
236
Spectral method of square integrals,
226, 228
Spectral moment, features based on
STFT at different forces, 236
Speed
control of, 24
identification of in hand movements,
230–233
resistance, 46
Spherical indenters, stiffness
measurements using, 171–173
Spherical necks, 106–107

Spring-based necks, 106–107
Statics analysis, robotic neck mechanism, 111–116
Steady swimming behaviors, 88–89
Stewart-like necks, 106–107
STFT method
  experimental results of using for hand movement determination, 232
  features based on, 231–232
  results at different forces, 234
  results at different speeds, 235
  use of with sEMG signals, 221, 230–231
Stiffness measurements, principles of for a single cell, 169–176
Strain energy function, derivation of stretching deformation from, 151
Stretching deformation, derivation of from strain energy function, 151
Stretching force, 149
  relationship with axial deformation, 161
Structural joint stops, 56–57, 82
  case study for, 65–67
  experimental results for a golf swing robot, 78–82
  method to utilize in dynamically coupled driving, 67–74
  simulation results for golf swing robot, 75–77
  utilization of, 63–65
STTT, use of with sEMG signals, 221
Subcarangiform propulsion, 87–89
Support vector machines (SVM), use of for computer-aided CE image recognition, 214
Surface electromyography sensor electrodes. *See* sEMG electrodes
Swarm control, 8–9
Swing plane, 70

T

Telepresence setup

camera motion device used in, 302–304, 306–308
gaze-based, 299
teleoperation channel used in Wizard-of-Oz scenario, 305–306
use of eye and head tracker in, 304–305, 308–309
Temporal features of sEMG signals, 221
Tensionability, 116
Thunniform propulsion, 87–89
Torque control, assistive knee braces with, 241
Torque manipulators
  case study of golf swing robot, 70–74
  use of dynamically coupled driving in design of, 59
Torsional movements, 298
Transient swimming, 88–89
Trapping forces, 153
Tungsten hard nanoprobes, fabrication of, 182–183
Turning motion, control of, 25–26

U

Unilateral CPG networks, 17–20
Unsteady swimming motion, 88–89
Upright fitness cycles, 34–35

V

Valve activation, PDMS microfluidic chips and, 132–133
Velocity coupling torque, 60–61
Venous blood flow, measurement of, 193–194
Vergence movements, 298
  handling of with teleoperation, 306
Vision systems, state of the art, 298

W

WABIAN-RIV serial neck, 106
Walking Power Assist Leg (WPAL), 240
WE-4RII, 298
Wearable Walking Helper (WWH), 240
Wizard-of-Oz scenario

camera motion devices used in,
302–304, 306–308
evaluations of gaze-based human
-robot interaction, 296–297
handling of eye vergence in, 306
objectives of, 299–300
robotic platforms used in, 300–302
teleoperation channel used in,
305–306
use of eye and head tracker in,
304–305, 308–309

Y

Yaw motion
robotic head, 109–111
robotic neck mechanism, 111–114

Yeast cells
observation of by E-SEM system,
177–179
stiffness measurement of by
nanoprobes, 184–185
stiffness measurements and growth
phases of, 181–182
stiffness measurements and size of,
179–181
Young's modulus, estimation of for a
single cell, 175–176

Z

Zernike moments
experimental results of using for CE
image recognition, 214–215
use of for CE image recognition,
209–213